DIABETES

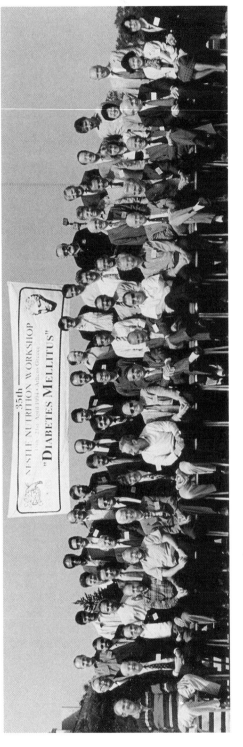

The 35th Nestlé Nutrition Workshop, Diabetes, was held in Athens, Greece, April 18–21st, 1994.

Workshop participants: (*left to right, first row*): A. Drash-USA; F. A. Van Assche-Belgium; R. Assan-France; F. W. Scott-Canada; R. N. Bergman-USA; O. Crofford-USA; P. M. Catalano-USA; G. F. Bottazzo-U.K.; R. M. Cowett-USA; R. Schwartz-USA; J. Girard-France; E. Marliss-Canada; J. J. Hoet-Belgium; G. Chiumello-Italy; K. Papadatos-Greece; C. Bartsokas-Greece; K. Unachak-Thailand; C. Dakou-Voutetaki-Greece; (*second row*) G. Jiang-China; P. Steenhout-Switzerland; J. Batubara-Indonesia; A. Carrascosa-Spain; E. Borrajo-Spain; M. Bueno-Sanchez-Spain; M. Nattrass-U.K.; C. Zoupas-Greece; K. Choo-Malaysia; M. Ratti-Malaysia; R. Jegasothy-Malaysia; S. Sampurno-Indonesia; G. Zoppi-Italy; V. Tripodi-Italy; A. Quinto-Italy; C. Panpitpat-Thailand; G. Biscatti-Italy; (*third row*) P. Swift-U.K.; F. Vargas Torcal-Spain; M. Oyarzabal-Spain; S. Batuna-Indonesia; F. J. Dorca-Spain; P. Beauvais-France; A. Otten-Germany; I. Barberi-Italy; L. Giuffre-Italy; A. Latronico-Italy; J. Rodriguez Pereira-Portugal; J. Sales Marquez-Portugal;' R. Carolino-Portugal; U. Vetter-Germany; A. Martins Mota-Portugal; H. Geiger-Germany; Lai-Italy, V. Tripodi-Italy; H. Grobe-Germany.

Nestlé Nutrition Workshop Series
Volume 35

DIABETES

Editor

Richard M. Cowett, M.D.

Professor
Department of Pediatrics
Brown University School of Medicine
Providence, Rhode Island, USA

NESTLÉ NUTRITION SERVICES

RAVEN PRESS ■ NEW YORK

Nestec Ltd., 55 Avenue Nestlé, CH-1800 Vevey, Switzerland
Raven Press, Ltd., 1185 Avenue of the Americas, New York,
New York 10036

Made in the United States of America

Library of Congress Cataloging-in-Publication Data

Diabetes / editor, Richard M. Cowett.
     p. cm.—(Nestlé Nutrition workshop series ; v. 35)
  "Nestlé Nutrition Services."
  "35th Nestlé Nutrition Workshop"—Pref.
  Includes bibliographical references and index.
  ISBN 0-7817-0324-7
  1. Diabetes—Congresses. I. Cowett, Richard M. II. Nestlé
Nutrition Services. III. Nestlé Nutrition Workshop (35th : April 21, 1994 :
Athens, Greece) IV. Series.
    [DNLM: 1. Diabetes Mellitus—congresses. W1 NE228 v.35 1994 / WK
810 D5369 1994]
  RC660.A1D47 1994
  616.4'62—dc20
  DNLM/DLC
  for Library of Congress   95-810

9 8 7 6 5 4 3 2 1

Preface

The 35th Nestlé Nutrition Workshop, *Diabetes Mellitus*, surveyed recent exciting discoveries in one of the major chronic diseases of our time. Diabetes mellitus has fascinated the curious since antiquity where, as discussed by one of the participants, it was first described in the Egyptian Papyrus Ebers in 1500 BC. The name of the disease is derived from the ancient Greek word for siphon as recorded by Aretaeus of Cappadocia (AD 81–138). The continuing importance of the disease is emphasized by its mention by medical giants through the ages including Galen, Avicenna, Claude Bernard, Langerhans, Minkowski, and von Mering. Of course, the modern era dates back to Banting and Best who, with MacLaod and Collip, are credited with the discovery of the pancreatic extract "insulin" in 1923. They named it after the Latin root for the islet cell of the pancreas.

Interest has focused on this disease for numerous reasons. Not only is it a major cause of morbidity and mortality, but it also affects the multiple stages of human existence from the fetus and neonate, the child and adolescent, the pregnant woman, to the middle aged and the elderly. Advances in medicine in general have paralled the successes in the understanding of diabetes mellitus by the various disciplines. These include studies of epidemiology, physiology, biochemistry, molecular biology, pathology, immunology, nutrition, genetics, and clinical evaluation at the various ages noted above. Many of these areas have been eloquently discussed in the chapters that comprise this volume.

This workshop conference brought together investigators who have contributed significantly to the advances of the recent past and are contributing to the potential for the immediate future.

We trust the interested reader will share the workshop's enthusiasm for the current successes in the understanding of this ancient malady.

RICHARD M. COWETT, M.D.
Professor
Department of Pediatrics
Brown University School of Medicine
Providence, Rhode Island, USA

Foreword

From the time of the first revolution of the 1920s when Banting and Best discovered insulin therapy, and that of the second revolution (at least for pediatric diabetologists) of the 1950s when the free diet was proposed and insulin treatment adapted to the level of blood glucose, urinary glucose, and ketones, no breakthrough occurred for the following 30 years in the field of diabetes mellitus. It has been only during the last 10 years that a tremendous number of discoveries and new concepts have reawakened interest in the subject.

The prevention of the complications of diabetes is now directed less toward acute hypoglycemia or hyperglycemia with acidosis; these should be avoided by strict monitoring and good education of the patient, even a young child. The current focus is more on the prevention of long-term complications such as blindness, renal insufficiency or, more generally, early atherosclerosis, and is based on the monitoring of glycosylated hemoglobin. The use of genetically engineered human insulin prevents some cases of immunologically induced insulin resistance. The use of a portable insulin pump may help to equilibrate the treatment in difficult circumstances, and pancreas transplant or transplant of islet cells may offer a better way of avoiding hyperglycemia and its long-term consequences.

But the most recent work consists of trying to identify the population of children and adolescents genetically at risk of developing insulin-dependent diabetes mellitus (IDDM), and to prevent autoimmune destruction of the β cells by different drug or diet therapy.

That bovine serum albumin (BSA) shares some epitopes with a protein of the β cell seems to be accepted, but the possibility of preventing insulin-dependent diabetes mellitus by a diet devoid of BSA in infancy is far from proved, and seems to be in contradiction with the observation that the two countries in the world where insulin-dependent diabetes mellitus is most frequent (Finland and Sweden) are also the two countries where use of cow's-milk-based infant formulas during the first months of life is the lowest among all the industrialized countries.

For prevention of non-insulin-dependent diabetes mellitus (NIDDM), diet is, in contrast, now well established through a weight reduction plan based on lowering the fat content of the diet rather than on a calorie count. This offers interesting possibilities for a food company to work in collaboration with the medical profession to reduce the incidence of this disease with its severe consequences and rapidly increasing incidence. This workshop and its publication is an important step forward.

PIERRE R. GUESRY, M.D.
Vice President of Research
Nestlé Research Center
Vers-Chez-Les-Blanc
Switzerland

Contents

Contributors

Speakers

Roger Assan
C.H.U. Bichat
Assistance Hôpitaux Publiques de Paris
46, rue H.-Huchard
75877 Paris, Cedex 18 France

Marian Benroubi
Polikliniki Anthinon
Pireos Str. 3
Athens, 10552 Greece

Richard N. Bergman
Department of Physiology and
Biophysics
Univeristy of Southern California
School of Medicine
1333 San Pablo St., MMR 626,
Los Agneles, California 90033, USA

Gian F. Bottazzo
Department of Immunology
The London Hospital Medical College
Turner Street
London, E1 2AD England

Patrick M. Catalano
Department of Reproductive Biology
Case Western Reserve University
MetroHealth Medical Center
2500 MetroHealth Medical Center
Cleveland, Ohio 44109-1998, USA

Richard M. Cowett
Department of Pediatrics
Brown University School of Medicine
101 Dudley Street
Providence, Rhode Island 02905-2401,
USA

Oscar B. Crofford
D-3100 Medical Center North
Vanderbilt University
Nashville, Tennessee 37232-2358, USA

Allan L. Drash
The Children's Hospital of Pittsburgh
Rangos Research Center
3705 Fifth Avenue
Pittsburgh, Pennsylvania 15213, USA

John H. Fuller
University College London Medical
School
Department of Epidemiology and Public
Health,
1-19, Torrington Place,
London, WC1E 6BT England

Edwin A. M. Gale
Department of Diabetes and
Metabolism
St-Bartholomew's Hospital
Centre for Clinical Research
59, Bartholomew Close
West Smithfield
London, EC1A 7BE England

Jean Girard
Centre de Recherche sur
l'Endocrinologie Moléculaire et le
Développement. CNRS
9, rue Jules Hetzel
92190 Meudon, France

Joseph J. Hoet
Cell Biology Laboratory
Catholic University of Louvain
5, Place Croix du Sud
1348 Louvain-la-Neuve, Belgium

xi

Nicholas Katsilambros
1st Department of Propedeutic Medicine
Athens University Medical School
Laiko General Hospital
17 Agiou Thomas street (Goudi)
Athens, 11527 Greece

Errol B. Marliss
McGill Nutrition and Food Science
* Centre*
Royal Victoria Hospital
687 Pine Avenue West
Montréal, Quebec H3A 1A1 Canada

Robert Schwartz
Department of Pediatrics
Rhode Island Hospital
593 Eddy Street
Providence, Rhode Island 02903 USA

Fraser W. Scott
Nutrition Research Division
Bureau of Nutritional Sciences Food
* Directorate*
Health Canada Sir Frederick Banting
* Research Centre*
Tunney's Pasture
Ottawa, Ontario K1A 0L2 Canada

David Sutherland
Department of Surgery
University of Minnesota
420 Delaware Street SE
Minneapolis, Minnesota 55455 USA

F. A. Van Assche
U.Z. Gasthuisberg
Department of Obstetrics and
* Gynecology*
Herestraat 49
3000 Leuven, Belgium

Session Chairmen

J. Alivisatos / *Athens, Greece*
Ch. Bartsocas / *Athens, Greece*
G. Chiumello / *Milan, Italy*
Richard Cowett / *Providence, RI, USA*

C. Dakou-Voutetaki / *Athens, Greece*
Robert Schwartz / *Providence, RI,*
* USA*
Ch. Zoupas / *Athens, Greece*

Invited Attendees

J. Alivisatos / *Athens, Greece*
Ignazio Barberi / *Messina, Italy*
Ch. Bartsokas / *Athens, Greece*
Jose Rizal Latief Batubara / *Jakarta,*
* Indonesia*
Sander Batuna / *Jakarta, Indonesia*
Paul Beauvais / *Mulhouse, France*
Giuliano Biscatti / *Cantù, Italy*
Emilio Borrajo / *Murcia, Spain*
Manuel Bueno Sanchez / *Zaragoza,*
* Spain*
Rui Carolino / *Ess, Portugal*
Antonio Carrascosa / *Barcelona,*
* Spain*
Giuseppe Chiumello / *Milan, Italy*

Keng Ee Choo / *Kota Bharu,*
* Kelantan, Malaysia*
P. Christakopoulos / *Athens, Greece*
C. Dakou-Voutetaki / *Athens, Greece*
Syahrir Dullah / *Surakarta, Indonesia*
H. Geiger / *Schwäbisch Hall,*
* Germany*
Liborio Giuffre / *Palermo, Italy*
H. Grobe / *Nürnberg, Germany*
Ravidran Jegasothy / *Seremban,*
* Malaysia*
Guoyan Jiang / *Beijing, China*
Ahmad Jufri / *Lhokseumawe,*
* Indonesia*
B. Karamanos / *Athens, Greece*
Amilcar Joaquim Martins Mota /
* Lisbon, Portugal*

Malcolm Nattrass / *Birmingham, England*
A. Otten / *Hamm, Germany*
Mirentxu Oyarzabel Irigoyen / *Pamplona, Spain*
Chanathip Panpitpat / *Udontani, Thailand*
C. Phenekos / *Athens, Greece*
Anna Quinto / *Napoli, Italy*
S. Raptis / *Athens, Greece*
Moti Lal Ratti / *Kuala Lumpur, Malaysia*
Jorge Rodriguez Pereira / *Aveiro, Portugal*
Giorgio Rondini / *Pavia, Italy*
Jorge Sales Marquez / *V.N. Gaia, Portugal*

Gian Paolo Salvioli / *Bologna, Italy*
Slamet Iman Sampurno / *Palembang, Indonesia*
Francesca Severi / *Pavia, Italy*
Ahmad Siadati / *Tehran, Iran*
Peter Swift / *Leicester, England*
N. Thalassinos / *Athens, Greece*
Ch. Theodorides / *Athens, Greece*
Mahmoud Touhami / *Oran, Algeria*
Vittorio Tripodi / *Napoli, Italy*
Kevalee Unachak / *Chiang Mai, Thailand*
Fernando Vargas Torcal / *Elche, Spain*
U. Vetter / *Berlin, Germany*
Giuseppe Zoppi / *Verona, Italy*
Ch. Zoupas / *Athens, Greece*

Nestlé Participants

Francisco Javier Dorca, *Barcelona, Spain*
Bianca-Maria Exl, *Münich, Germany*
Pierre R. Guesry, *Vers-chez-les-Blanc, Switzerland*

Alberto Latronico, *Milano, Italy*
George Makridimitris, *Athens, Greece*
Constantin Papadatos, *Athens, Greece*
Philippe Steenhout, / *Vevey, Switzerland*

Nestlé Nutrition Workshop Series

DIABETES

Diabetes, edited by Richard M. Cowett,
Nestlé Nutrition Workshop Series,
Vol. 35. Nestec Ltd.,
Vevey/Raven Press, Ltd., New York © 1995.

Hormonal Control of Glucose Metabolism

Jean Girard

*Centre de Recherche sur l'Endocrinologie Moléculaire et le Développement, CNRS,
9 rue Jules Hetzel, 92190 Meudon, France*

Plasma glucose concentration is normally maintained within a narrow range despite wide fluctuations in the supply (meal) and demand (exercise) for nutrients. In adult humans, plasma glucose concentrations throughout a 24-hour period average 90 mg/dl, with maximum values 60–90 minutes after meals, usually not exceeding 140 mg/dl, and values during a moderate fast or exercise usually remaining above 50 mg/dl. This relative stability contrasts with the situation for other fuels such as glycerol, lactate, free fatty acids (FFA), and ketone bodies (acetoacetate and β-hydroxybutyrate), the fluctuations of which vary more widely. The reason why plasma glucose concentration must be maintained in a narrow range of concentration is related to the deleterious effects of both hypoglycemia and hyperglycemia. Acute hypoglycemia is well known to have harmful effects on the brain. Glucose is usually the main fuel used by the brain; this is because plasma concentrations of one of the alternative fuels (ketone bodies) are low, while transport across the blood-brain barrier of the other alternative fuel (free fatty acids) is limited. As the brain has low energy stores, it is markedly dependent upon circulating glucose for its energy metabolism. When plasma glucose levels fall below 60 mg/dl, brain glucose uptake decreases and cerebral function is impaired. More severe and prolonged hypoglycemia can cause convulsions, permanent brain damage, and death. Chronic hyperglycemia also has deleterious effects. The functional and vascular changes in the eyes, nerves, aorta, and kidneys of diabetic patients seem to be related to increased metabolism of glucose via the polyol pathway. To maintain plasma glucose concentrations within a normal range, the changes in the dietary or endogenous glucose supply must be precisely matched by comparable changes in tissue uptake. Conversely, the changes in tissue glucose uptake (for example, during exercise) must be matched by appropriate changes in the exogenous or endogenous glucose supply.

The aim of this chapter is to review briefly the mechanisms by which the rate of glucose production and uptake is finely regulated during a 24-hour period in normal resting humans, and how they are coordinated by hormones and alternative substrates to maintain the plasma glucose level within a normal range. The cellular mechanisms by which hormones alter the rate of hepatic glucose production and peripheral tissue glucose utilization will also briefly be discussed.

OVERALL GLUCOSE HOMEOSTASIS IN HUMANS

In a normal human living in a Western society, the 24 hours of a normal day can be divided into three periods of approximately 4 hours, corresponding to the absorption and assimilation of the principal meals and to a postabsorptive period corresponding to the 12-hour overnight fast. During these periods, systemic glucose homeostasis is profoundly modified, as described in a recent review (1).

The Postabsorptive State

The postabsorptive period generally refers to the 12 hours following the last meal of the day during which transition from the fed to the fasting state occurs. At the end of this period, tissue glucose utilization in resting humans is approximatively 2 mg/kg/min. Approximatively 1 mg/kg/min is due to the obligatory uptake of glucose by the brain and other non-insulin-dependent tissues. Glucose uptake by insulin-dependent tissues (skeletal muscle, adipose tissue) accounts for less than 30–50% of glucose utilization. Tissue glucose uptake is precisely matched by the liver glucose output, and plasma glucose concentration remains constant.

The Postprandial State

Postprandial hyperglycemia is dependent upon the amount and form of carbohydrate ingested and on the amount of accompanying protein and fat [reviewed in (1)]. In general, complex carbohydrates are absorbed more slowly than simple sugars, and protein and fat delay absorption; both of these factors reduce postprandial glucose excursions. The time of the day when carbohydrates are ingested is also important since glucose tolerance is better in the morning than in the evening.

After a carbohydrate meal, plasma glucose levels increase after 15 minutes, glucose production is inhibited, and glucose utilization is enhanced. Plasma glucose, glucose production, and glucose utilization return to basal levels after 180 minutes. These changes are associated with a parallel increase in plasma insulin and a decrease in plasma glucagon. Plasma glucose concentrations after a meal are determined by the relative changes in the rates of glucose delivery and removal. The magnitude of these changes is largely determined by the secretion of insulin and glucagon.

The major tissues responsible for glucose removal after a carbohydrate meal are the liver, small intestine, brain, skeletal muscles, and adipose tissue [reviewed in (1)]. Skeletal muscles and splanchnic tissues (liver, small intestine) each probably account for 30%, brain for 20%, and adipose tissue for 10% of glucose taken up. The uptake of glucose by skeletal muscles and adipose tissue is influenced by both plasma glucose and insulin levels, whereas the uptake of glucose by the brain is only influenced by plasma glucose levels. Adipose tissue lipolysis and lipid oxidation are suppressed after carbohydrate ingestion. Of the glucose taken up by tissues, 60% is used for replenishment of liver and muscle glycogen stores, 30% is oxidized, and 10% is released as lactate into the circulation for further uptake by the liver for indirect glycogen formation.

CONTROL OF HEPATIC GLUCOSE PRODUCTION

The only tissues that contain significant amounts of glucose-6-phosphatase, the enzyme necessary for hydrolysis of glucose-6-phosphate to glucose and the subsequent release of glucose into the circulation, are liver and kidney. The liver is the main source of circulating glucose except in two situations: 1. after a prolonged fast, when kidney may provide up to 10% of circulating glucose; 2. after meals or administration of exogenous nutrients (for example, intravenous infusions, parenteral nutrition).

The liver provides glucose to the circulation through two metabolic pathways: 1. glycogenolysis, the breakdown of glycogen stores, and 2. gluconeogenesis, the formation of new glucose molecules from amino acids, glycerol, and lactate. The contribution of each of these pathways in humans has been estimated from different types of studies: the rate of decrease in glycogen from serial liver biopsies, balance of gluconeogenic precursors across the splanchnic bed, and incorporation of isotopically labeled gluconeogenic precursors into circulating glucose [reviewed in (1)]. It was initially estimated that glycogenolysis accounts for 70% of overall hepatic glucose output in the postabsorptive period. However, recent studies employing nuclear magnetic resonance to measure depletion of hepatic glycogen stores suggest that glycogenolysis may account for only 30% of overall hepatic glucose output (2). If fasting is prolonged to 48–60 hours, gluconeogenesis accounts for virtually all of the hepatic glucose output.

On a minute-to-minute basis, glucose, insulin, and glucagon are the major factors regulating hepatic glucose production. After ingestion of a meal, plasma insulin and glucose concentrations increase, plasma glucagon levels are suppressed, and hepatic glucose production is reduced. Conversely, as one proceeds from the fed into the fasted state, plasma insulin and glucose levels decrease, plasma glucagon levels increase, and hepatic glucose production is increased. Under stressful conditions, circulating epinephrine from the adrenal medulla and neurally released norepinephrine become involved and augment hepatic glucose production through β-adrenergic receptors in humans (3). Glucocorticoids have no direct effects on hepatic glucose production, but they markedly potentiate the effects of glucagon and adrenaline (permissive role).

By using the "pancreatic clamp" technique, it has been possible to delineate the respective role of glucose and different hormones in hepatic glucose production in dogs in the postabsorptive state [reviewed in (4–6)]. This technique involves the infusion of somatostatin into a peripheral vein to inhibit the secretion of insulin and glucagon and the infusion of the two pancreatic hormones into the portal vein to replace their endogenous secretion. It is thus possible to fix the levels of plasma glucose, insulin, glucagon, catecholamines, and cortisol to the desired values. The

TABLE 1. *Effect of hormones and substrates on glucose production and utilization*

Effect	Glucose	Insulin	Glucagon	Epinephrine	Norepinephrine
Glucose production					
Glycogenolysis	↓↓↓	↓↓↓	↑↑↑	↑↑	—
Gluconeogenesis	↓	↓	↑↑↑	↑	↑↑
Glucose utilization	↑↑	↑↑↑	—	↓	↓

rates of liver glucose production and net hepatic glucose uptake are assessed by radioactive tracer and arteriovenous difference techniques. The principal conclusions from these experiments [reviewed in (4–6)] will be summarized briefly below and in Table 1.

Role of Glucose in Hepatic Glucose Production

It has been clearly shown that changes in plasma glucose concentrations can regulate hepatic glycogenolysis independently of pancreatic hormones. Moderate (200 mg/dl) or marked (300 mg/dl) hyperglycemia induced a complete inhibition of hepatic glucose production in postabsorptive dogs. Since gluconeogenesis represents only 10–20% of overall glucose production in postabsorptive dogs, hyperglycemia acts mainly by inhibiting glycogenolysis. Gluconeogenesis is much less sensitive than glycogenolysis to inhibition by hyperglycemia.

Role of Glucagon in Hepatic Glucose Production

In postabsorptive dogs, selective glucagon deficiency induced a 70% decrease in hepatic glucose production, suggesting that two-thirds of the production is attributable to glucagon. A selective physiological increase in portal plasma glucagon brought about a rapid and marked increase in hepatic glucose production that, however, waned with time. The evanescent effect, despite raised plasma glucagon levels, was due to glycogenolysis since gluconeogenesis remained increased. The evanescent effect is probably due to the hyperglycemia that developed and counteracted the effect of glucagon on glycogenolysis. Dose-response studies have indicated that the levels of glucagon required for half maximum activation of glycogenolysis and gluconeogenesis *in vivo* are similar and coincide with the commonly occurring physiologic increases of glucagon.

Role of Catecholamines in Hepatic Glucose Production

A selective physiological increase in plasma epinephrine or norepinephrine increased hepatic glucose production moderately and transiently. The evanescent effect, despite increased plasma epinephrine or norepinephrine levels, was due to the ensuing hyperglycemia that counteracted the effect of epinephrine on glycogenolysis. The difference between epinephrine and norepinephrine was related to their effect on glycogenolysis. Norepinephrine did not increase glycogenolysis, whereas epinephrine stimulated it. In contrast, norepinephrine was more potent than epinephrine at stimulating gluconeogenesis.

Role of Insulin in Hepatic Glucose Production

A selective severe insulin deficiency brought about a rapid and marked increase in hepatic glucose production that, however, waned with time. Selective hypoinsulinemia also caused a progressive increase in gluconeogenesis. The evanescent effect, despite low plasma insulin levels, was due to the hyperglycemia that developed and counteracted the effect of insulin deficiency on glycogenolysis. A selective physiological increase in portal plasma insulin rapidly and efficiently inhibited hepatic glucose production. As hyperinsulinemia was ineffective in inhibiting gluconeogenesis, it has been suggested that gluconeogenesis is inhibited at low plasma insulin levels and that small decrement of plasma insulin markedly enhance this process. Dose-response studies have indicated that the levels of insulin required for half maximum inhibition of glycogenolysis *in vivo* are much lower than the levels of insulin required for half maximum inhibition of gluconeogenesis.

Mechanisms Involved in the Control of Hepatic Glucose Production

Control of Hepatic Glycogenolysis

The rate-limiting step in hepatic glycogenolysis is catalyzed by phosphorylase. This enzyme catalyzes the hydrolysis of 1,4 linkages of glycogen to yield glucose-1-phosphate. In liver, phosphorylase exists in both an active and an inactive form (Fig. 1). Active phosphorylase (phosphorylase a) is phosphorylated on a serine residue by phosphorylase kinase. Inactive phosphorylase (phosphorylase b) is dephosphorylated by a specific protein phosphatase-1. Phosphorylase kinase also exists in both an active and an inactive form. Active phosphorylase kinase (phosphorylase kinase a) is phosphorylated on a serine residue by the cyclic adenosine monophosphate (cAMP)-dependent protein kinase. Inactive phosphorylase kinase (phosphorylase kinase b) is dephosphorylated by a specific protein phosphatase-1.

The molecular mechanisms by which glucose is able to inhibit liver glycogenolysis involve the binding of glucose to phosphorylase a and its inactivation. In addition, when phosphorylase a has bound glucose, it is a much better substrate for protein phosphatase-1. The effect of high glucose concentration is, therefore, to cause the conversion of phosphorylase b to phosphorylase a and to arrest glycogenolysis. Furthermore, since phosphorylase a is a potent inhibitor of synthase phosphatase, its inhibition allows the latter enzyme to activate glycogen synthase and to initiate glycogen synthesis after a lag period of a few minutes.

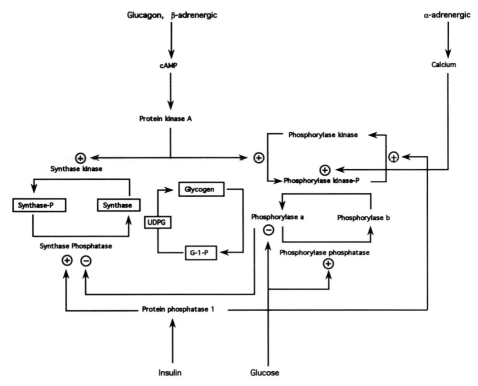

FIG. 1. Schematic representation of the control of glycogen metabolism in the liver. G-1-P, glucose-1-phosphate; UDPG, uridine diphosphate glucose; cAMP, cyclic AMP.

The molecular mechanisms by which glucagon stimulates glycogenolysis are relatively well known. After binding to plasma membrane receptors, glucagon induces an increase in intracellular cAMP levels. cAMP then binds to the regulatory subunit of cAMP-dependent protein kinase and releases its catalytic subunit. The catalytic subunit of cAMP-dependent protein kinase stimulates the phosphorylation of phosphorylase kinase and activates phosphorylase kinase. Active phosphorylase kinase then stimulates the phosphorylation of phosphorylase and increases glycogenolysis.

In humans, exogenous catecholamines act mainly via β-adrenergic receptors and thus activate phosphorylase and stimulate glycogen breakdown by mechanisms similar to those described above for glucagon. In rodents, it has been shown that catecholamines act mainly via α-adrenergic receptors and stimulate glycogen breakdown via a cAMP-independent mechanism. Catecholamines, via α-adrenergic receptors, activate plasma membrane phospholipase C, which hydrolyses phosphatidylinositol 4,5-diphosphate into inositol 1,4,5-triphosphate and 1,2-diacylglycerol. Inositol 1,4,5 triphosphate is a potent stimulator of calcium mobilization from intracellular calciosomes. The increase in intracellular calcium stimulates phosphorylase kinase, a calmodulin-sensitive protein kinase.

The mechanism by which insulin inhibits phosphorylase and glycogen breakdown has not been entirely clarified. After binding to its receptor, insulin activates the tyrosine kinase activity of the β subunit of the receptor, leading to the activation of a serine/threonine kinase by an unknown mechanism. An insulin-stimulated protein kinase has recently been identified in skeletal muscle (7). This enzyme is phosphorylated in response to insulin, leading to an activation of protein phosphatase-1 via phosphorylation on serine/threonine residues. Activated protein phosphatase-1 then stimulates the dephosphorylation of glycogen synthase and phosphorylase kinase, leading to an inhibition of glycogenolysis and an activation of glycogen synthesis. If this enzyme is present in liver and is activated by insulin, it could be involved in the inhibition of glycogenolysis.

Control of Hepatic Gluconeogenesis

Flux through the gluconeogenic pathway is regulated by different factors: 1. the provision of gluconeogenic substrates to the liver from peripheral tissues, 2. the activities of liver key enzymes that are influenced by substrates and hormones, and 3. by the provision of ATP and cofactors essential for these enzymes.

The major gluconeogenic precursors are lactate, amino acids, and glycerol. The supply of gluconeogenic precursor to the liver is regulated by various hormones (4,8). In the postabsorptive state and in most catabolic situations, amino acids (mainly glutamine and alanine) are released from skeletal muscle and glycerol is produced by adipose tissue. It has clearly been established that 1. insulin inhibits, whereas glucocorticoids stimulate, muscle proteolysis, and 2. insulin inhibits, whereas catecholamines (via β-adrenergic receptors) and growth hormone stimulate, adipose tissue lipolysis. In addition, glucocorticoids potentiate the lipolytic effect of catecholamines on adipose tissue. The regulation of lactate production by peripheral tissues is much less well known. The increased rate of free fatty acid delivery to peripheral tissues in the postabsorptive state and in most catabolic situations could play an important role, since fatty acids inhibit glucose oxidation and increase the release of lactate. Thus both hormones and free fatty acids play a crucial role in the regulation of the delivery of gluconeogenic substrate to the liver. Nevertheless, several different hormones have been shown to have a marked effect on the regulation of gluconeogenesis when the gluconeogenic supply is maintained at a constant level, such as in the perfused liver or in isolated hepatocytes (4,8). This indicates that crucial steps of liver gluconeogenesis and/or glycolysis are regulated. Gluconeogenesis cannot be viewed as a reversal of glycolysis since three steps of glycolysis, catalyzed by glucokinase, phosphofructokinase, and pyruvate kinase, are characterized by a large and negative free-energy charge and are essentially irreversible *in vivo*. These three steps are bypassed by a separate set of enzymes, catalyzing different reactions that function in gluconeogenesis (Fig. 2). The regulatory enzymatic steps controlling net flux along the gluconeogenic pathway are pyruvate carboxylase, phosphoenolpyruvate carboxykinase, fructose-1,6-diphosphatase, and glucose-6-phosphatase (9). Thus both glycolysis and gluconeogenesis are irreversible processes in

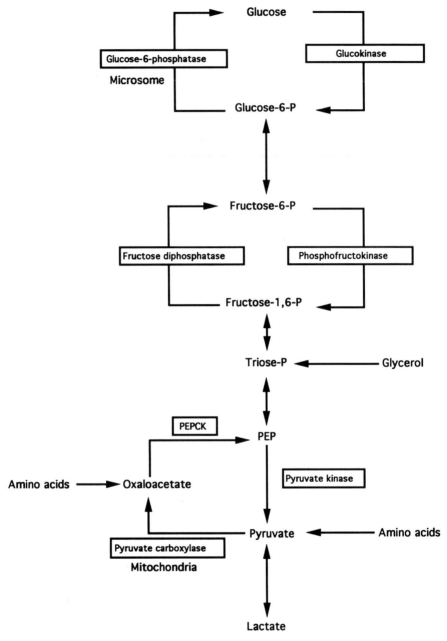

FIG. 2. Schematic representation of the pathway of glycolysis and gluconeogenesis in the liver. PEP, phosphoenolpyruvate; PEPCK, phosphoenolpyruvate carboxykinase.

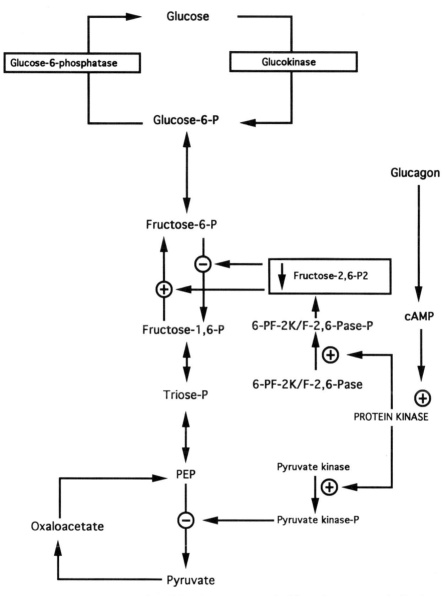

FIG. 3. Schematic representation of the short-term control of liver gluconeogenesis. Fructose-1,6-P, fructose-1,6-phosphate; fructose-2,6-P2, fructose-2,6-bisphosphate; cAMP, cyclic adenosine monophosphate; 6-PF-2-K/F-2,6-Pase, 6-phosphofructo-2 kinase/fructose 2,6-bisphosphatase; PEP, phosphoenolpyruvate.

cells that are independently regulated through controls exerted on specific enzymatic steps that are not common to the two pathways.

It has been clearly established that gluconeogenesis is subject to short-term regulation by hormones at the level of the fructose-6-phosphate—fructose 1,6-bisphosphate and phosphoenolpyruvate—pyruvate cycles (10,11). Glucagon and β-adrenergic agents increase liver cAMP and activate cAMP-dependent protein kinase. The catalytic subunit of cAMP-dependent protein kinase stimulates the phosphorylation of L-type pyruvate kinase and inactivates this enzyme. The inhibition of pyruvate kinase decreases the conversion of phosphoenolpyruvate (PEP) to pyruvate and allows more PEP to be directed through the gluconeogenic pathway (Fig. 3). In addition, the catalytic subunit of cAMP-dependent protein kinase stimulates the phosphorylation of a bifunctional enzyme (6-phosphofructo-2-kinase/fructose 2,6-bisphosphatase) and inactivates it (12–14). This produces a decrease in the level of fructose 2,6-bisphosphate, an activator of phosphofructokinase and an inhibitor of fructose-1,6-bisphosphatase. The resulting reduction in intrahepatic fructose-2,6-bisphosphate level inhibits glycolysis and promotes gluconeogenesis (Fig. 3). Insulin antagonizes the action of low concentrations of glucagon on pyruvate kinase and 6-phosphofructo-2-kinase/fructose-2,6-bisphosphatase, via a decrease in liver cAMP and fructose-2,6-bisphosphate.

Another important factor in the short-term regulation of liver gluconeogenesis is the alteration in fatty acid oxidation (11). A rise in fatty acid oxidation increases the acetyl-CoA/CoA and NADH/NAD$^+$ ratios and the ATP concentration. The increased mitochondrial acetyl-CoA leads to activation of pyruvate carboxylase, and the increased cytosolic NADH/NAD$^+$ ratio allows displacement of the equilibrium reaction catalyzed by the glyceraldehyde phosphate dehydrogenase in the direction of gluconeogenesis (Fig. 4).

Various recent studies have also shown that glucagon and β-adrenergic agents (via cAMP), glucocorticoids, insulin, and glucose modulate the expression of several

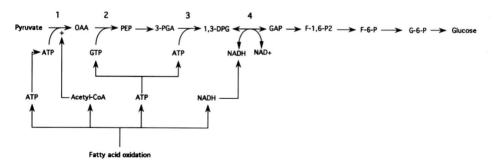

FIG. 4. Schematic representation of the role of free fatty acid oxidation in the regulation of liver gluconeogenesis. 1: pyruvate carboxylase; 2: phosphoenolpyruvate carboxykinase; 3: glyceraldehyde-3-phosphate dehydrogenase; 4: phosphoglyceraldehyde dehydrogenase. OAA, oxaloacetate; PEP, phosphoenolpyruvate; 3-PGA, 3-phosphoglycerate; 1,3-DPG, 1,3-diphosphoglycerate; F-1,6-P2, fructose-1,6-bisphosphate; F-6-P, fructose-6-phosphate; G-6-P, glucose-6-phosphate; NADH, reduced nicotinamide adenine dinucleotide; GTP, guanosine triphosphate.

TABLE 2. *Effect of hormones and substrates on expression of genes involved in hepatic carbohydrate metabolism*

Gene	Glucose	Insulin	Glucagon	Glucocorticoids	Thyroid hormones
Glycolysis					
Glucokinase	—	↑	↓	↑ P	↑
6-PF-2K/F-2,6-Pase	↓	↑	↓	↑	↑
Pyruvate kinase	↑	↑ P	↓	↑ P	↑
Gluconeogenesis					
PEPCK	—	↓	↑	↑ P	↑
Fructose 1,6-diphosphatase	?	↓	↑	↑ P	?
Glucose-6-phosphatase	?	?	?	?	?

6-PF-2K/F-2,6-Pase, 6-phosphofructo-2 kinase/Fructose 2,6 biphosphatase; PEPCK, phospho-enolpyruvate carboxykinase; P, permissive effect.

genes involved in the control of liver gluconeogenesis and glycolysis (15–17) (Table 2). It has been shown that cAMP increases the transcription of phosphoenolpyruvate carboxykinase (PEPCK) (15) and inhibits the transcription of glucokinase (18) and pyruvate kinase (17). Insulin inhibits the transcription of PEPCK (15) and increases the transcription of glucokinase (18). Glucose increases the transcription of pyruvate kinase, an effect that is potentiated by insulin (17).

Glucose-6-phosphatase is a microsomal enzyme that catalyzes the hydrolysis of glucose-6-phosphate to free glucose. The short-term regulation of this enzyme is not well known. It has been suggested that the enzyme is mainly controlled by the level of glucose-6-phosphate. The rise in glucose-6-phosphate in response to glucagon or catecholamines is sufficient to account for an increased flux through glucose-6-phosphatase with a concomitant increase in hepatic glucose production. In contrast, the fall in glucose-6-phosphate in response to an oral glucose load is sufficient to account for a diminished flux through glucose-6-phosphatase, with concomitant suppression of hepatic glucose production.

In summary, key factors affecting acute regulation of gluconeogenesis in humans include precursor supply, glucagon, insulin and lipid oxidation by the liver. Catecholamines released under stressful conditions can directly increase gluconeogenesis but probably exert their main action by providing additional precursors (for example glycerol and amino acids) and increasing intrahepatic lipid oxidation. Adrenocorticosteroids increase gluconeogenesis on a longer-term basis by increasing substrate supply and promoting increased synthesis of gluconeogenic enzyme. Their effects are synergistic with those of glucagon and catecholamines. The role of growth hormone remains to be defined.

CONTROL OF GLUCOSE UTILIZATION

The primary determinants of glucose utilization *in vivo* are plasma glucose concentration and, for certain tissues, plasma insulin concentration and the sensitivity of tissues to insulin. The sensitivity of tissues to insulin can be affected by hormones such as cortisol, growth hormone and catecholamines (Table 1) and also by changes in the availability of alternative substrates (for example, free fatty acids and ketone bodies). After an oral glucose load, skeletal muscles and liver probably account for 60% of glucose taken up. Thus the metabolism of glucose in these tissues will be discussed.

Control of Muscle Glucose Metabolism

Uptake of glucose by most tissues occurs by facilitated diffusion, a process that is not energy dependent and that follows Michaelis-Menten kinetics. Transport kinetics vary among tissues, depending to a large extent on the characteristics of glucose transporters expressed in these tissues and on whether the process is sensitive to insulin. Five glucose transporter isoforms have been identified, the distribution of which varies among tissues, as does their dependency on insulin (19). One of them, GLUT-4, is expressed in insulin-dependent tissue (muscle and adipose tissue) and has a specific role in the regulation of glucose utilization in response to insulin. Insulin controls the transport of glucose in muscle and adipose cells by two different mechanisms. It acutely accelerates glucose transport by promoting the translocation of GLUT-4 glucose transporters from an intracellular store to the cell membrane (translocation mechanism) (20). It also controls the concentration of GLUT-4 glucose transporters by promoting their synthesis (21,22).

Glucose taken up by muscle cells has two main fates: storage as glycogen or conversion to pyruvate (Fig. 5). Pyruvate can then be converted to lactate, which is released into the circulation, or it can be oxidized to CO_2 (Fig. 5). The relative proportion of glucose that is metabolized in these different pathways varies between tissues and is dependent upon the hormonal environment and the presence of alternative substrates, for example, free fatty acids or ketone bodies. Thus, in the postabsorptive state there is no net storage of glucose, and all glucose taken up is either completely oxidized or converted to lactate (or alanine) which can be recycled back to the liver to be used for gluconeogenesis. The glucose-lactate and glucose-alanine cycles account for 25–35% of glucose uptake in the postabsorptive state (23,24). In the brain, almost all of the glucose taken up is completely oxidized, whereas in skeletal muscle most of the glucose taken up undergoes glycolysis and is recycled back to the liver as either lactate or alanine. In contrast, after an oral glucose load, a significant part of glucose is stored as glycogen.

Mechanisms Involved in the Control of Glycolysis

Glycolysis involves the anaerobic breakdown of glucose to pyruvate and lactate. When oxygen is not available, the reduced NADH, which is formed during glycolysis but cannot readily be oxidized by the respiratory chain, is oxidized by the lactate

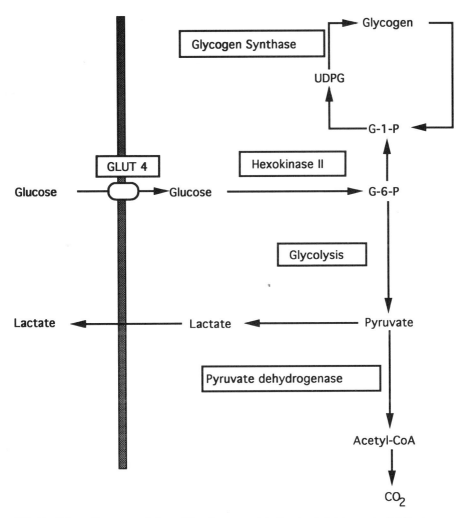

FIG. 5. Schematic representation of the glucose metabolism in skeletal muscle. G-1-P, glucose-1-phosphate; G-6-P, glucose-6-phosphate; UDPG, uridine diphosphate glucose.

dehydrogenase reaction, which catalyzes the conversion of pyruvate to lactate, thereby allowing glycolysis to proceed.

After the uptake of glucose into cells, there are numerous potential control points for glycolysis. The first is the phosphorylation of glucose to form glucose-6-phosphate. In non-hepatic tissues, this reaction is catalyzed by a hexokinase, which has a high affinity for glucose and is subjected to product inhibition by glucose-6-phosphate. Glucose taken up is immediately converted to glucose-6-phosphate. This allows a very low intracellular glucose concentration to be maintained that facilitates glucose transport in the direction of the glucose gradient. Until recently, hexokinase was not considered to be a major site of acute regulation of glycolysis, and transport of glucose was considered to be the rate limiting step for glucose metabolism in skeletal muscle. However, it has been shown that insulin-sensitive tissues express a specific hexokinase, hexokinase II, the synthesis of which is controlled by insulin (25). Thus hexokinase II could be involved, in association with GLUT-4, in the long-term regulation of muscle glucose uptake.

Glucose-6-phosphate formed within cells is either converted to glycogen (see above) or rapidly converted to fructose-6-phosphate by a reversible non-rate-limiting enzymatic step catalyzed by phosphohexose isomerase. The next potential control point of glycolysis is the conversion of fructose-6-phosphate to fructose-1,6-diphosphate. This is catalyzed by phosphofructokinase, the activity of which is markedly increased by fructose-2,6-bisphosphate. The concentration of fructose-2,6-bisphosphate increases following glucose or insulin administration or after a meal and decreases after fasting and in experimental models of diabetes (13,14). The next steps involve the conversion of fructose-1,6-disphosphate to PEP by reactions that are not highly regulated. The last step of glycolysis, the conversion of PEP to pyruvate, is catalyzed by pyruvate kinase, which is highly regulated. Once pyruvate is formed, the redox state of the tissue and the activities of pyruvate dehydrogenase and pyruvate carboxylase determine the extent to which the pyruvate undergoes oxidation in mitochondria in the Krebs cycle or is reduced to lactate by lactate dehydrogenase.

Mechanisms Involved in the Control of Glucose Oxidation

Pyruvate, which is formed in the cytoplasm, is transported into the mitochondria and, if adequate NAD^+ is available, is converted to acetyl-CoA and ultimately to CO_2 and H_2O. The key step determining pyruvate flux through the Krebs cycle is the pyruvate dehydrogenase complex.

Insulin activates pyruvate dehydrogenase by dephosphorylation. In most tissues, there is competition between glucose and free fatty acids as oxidative fuels, and free fatty acids are the preferred substrate. The preferential utilization of free fatty acids can have a profound effect on glucose metabolism by way of a complex series of steps collectively referred to as the glucose–fatty acid cycle (26), a concept that has now received widespread experimental support and is generally accepted as operating in humans. According to this concept, the steps of which are illustrated in Fig. 6, a rise in free fatty acid oxidation increases the mitochondrial acetyl-CoA/CoA ratio and cytosolic citrate levels. The increased acetyl-CoA/CoA ratio inhibits pyruvate dehydrogenase, reducing pyruvate formation and hence its oxidation. The increased cytosolic citrate levels inhibit phosphofructokinase, which results in an increase in glucose-6-phosphate, an inhibitor of hexokinase. Reduced activity of hexokinase via an increase in intracellular glucose will then reduce glucose transport (uptake) by tissues. This mechanism has been invoked to explain the reciprocal changes observed in glucose and lipid metabolism in a variety of physiological and pathological conditions (26). Thus, during starvation and diabetes, when rates of fat oxidation are

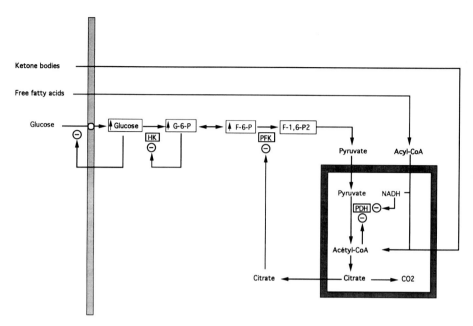

FIG. 6. Schematic representation of the glucose–fatty acid cycle. HK, hexokinase II; PFK, phosphofructokinase; PDH, pyruvate dehydrogenase. G-6-P, glucose-6-phosphate; F-6-P, fructose-6-phosphate; F-1,6-P2, fructose-1,6-bisphosphate.

increased, there is impaired tissue glucose uptake and oxidation. Reduced suppression of lipid oxidation after ingestion of a meal may impair glycogen formation in diabetes because of impaired glucose uptake. Furthermore, increases in lipid oxidation also promote increased gluconeogenesis. Thus, alterations in lipid metabolism can affect both the production and the utilization of glucose.

Control of Hepatic Glucose Metabolism

Under postabsorptive conditions it is not possible to elicit significant net glucose uptake by the liver or splanchnic bed with either hyperinsulinemia, hyperglycemia, or hypoglucagonemia, when imposed independently (27). Net glucose uptake by the liver is greater during enteral glucose administration or infusion of glucose into the portal vein than during peripheral venous glucose infusion. It has been postulated that there is a "portal signal" evoked during enteral or intraportal glucose delivery that enhances glucose uptake by the liver. The nature of the "portal signal" is not yet known. Both humoral and neural factors must be considered. Gastrointestinal peptides (glucagon-like peptide 1, gastrin, neurotensin) released during glucose ingestion could be involved. These peptides are all insulinotropic and contribute to the improved glucose tolerance following glucose ingestion by promoting peripheral glucose removal and inhibiting hepatic glucose production (incretin effect), but there are no data to suggest that they are directly involved in the enhanced hepatic glucose uptake. It appears that the enhanced glucose uptake by the liver in response to intraportal glucose delivery is not just the consequence of increased portal glucose levels but also involves the negative glucose gradient between arterial and portal venous blood. Because the ability of portal glucose delivery to enhance net hepatic glucose uptake is abolished by hepatic denervation (28), this suggests that the "portal signal" involves the autonomic nervous system. Whether this signal is generated locally or involves a comparison between portal venous glucose and the brain arterial glucose levels remains to be clarified. There is evidence for both afferent fibers in the hepatic branch of the vagus nerve and neurons in the lateral hypothalamus that can detect changes in glucose levels in the portal vein and efferent fibers that can alter net hepatic glucose uptake (29). Thus, a neural loop can serve to regulate hepatic glucose uptake.

Mechanisms Involved in the Control of Hepatic Glucose Uptake

The liver is considered to be "freely permeable to glucose" since GLUT-2, the principal glucose transporter expressed in this tissue, has a low apparent affinity for glucose ($K_m = 20$ mM). This allows equilibration between extracellular and intracellular glucose on a minute-to-minute basis. In this tissue, glucose phosphorylation by glucokinase, a specific hexokinase that has a low affinity for glucose ($K_m = 10$ mM) and is not inhibited by glucose-6-phosphate, is considered to be the rate-limiting step in overall glucose metabolism. Recently, the short-term regulation of hepatic glucokinase has been described (30). Glucokinase is inhibited by physiological levels of fructose-6-phosphate and this inhibition is released by fructose-1-phosphate. These effects are due to a modification of the affinity of glucokinase for glucose by means of a regulatory protein (31). The mechanism of action of this regulatory protein has recently been clarified (31). Fructose-6-phosphate binds to the regulatory protein and promotes the formation of a complex between glucokinase and the regulatory protein. Under these conditions, glucokinase is inactivated. Fructose-1-phosphate inhibits the formation of this complex and glucokinase is activated. The liver fructose-6-phosphate level is at least 10 μmol/liter in most physiological conditions. In the postabsorptive state, liver does not contain fructose-1-phosphate, and glucokinase is inhibited by the regulatory protein. After a meal that contains significant amounts of fructose, liver fructose-1-phosphate levels increase and the inhibition of glucokinase by the regulatory protein is released. Since fructose is present in most foods of vegetable origin, it can play a role as a signal to stimulate liver glucose utilization after a meal.

Mechanisms Involved in the Control of Hepatic Glycogen Synthesis

Following ingestion of a meal, hepatic glycogen stores are repleted via two metabolic pathways (32). In the first pathway, called the *direct pathway,* glucose is taken up, phosphorylated to glucose-6-phosphate, transformed to glucose-1-phosphate, converted to UDP-glucose, and then incorporated into glycogen (Fig. 1). The last reaction is catalyzed by glycogen synthesis and is considered to be the rate-limiting step in that process. The molecular mechanisms by which glucose is able to increase liver glycogen synthesis involve the binding of glucose to phosphorylase a and its inactivation (Fig. 1). Since phosphorylase a is a potent inhibitor of synthase phosphatase, its inhibition allows the latter enzyme to activate glycogen synthase and to initiate glycogen synthesis after a lag period of a few minutes. The molecular mechanisms by which insulin increases liver glycogen synthesis are much less established. Insulin could activate protein phosphatase-1 and stimulate the dephosphorylation of glycogen synthase, leading to an increase of glycogen synthesis (Fig. 1).

The other pathway, called the *indirect pathway,* initially involves the metabolism of glucose to gluconeogenic precursors (mainly lactate and alanine), which are subsequently converted to glucose-6-phosphate in the liver and then to glycogen by steps identical to those involved in the direct pathway. The exact proportion of glycogen formed via each pathway and the source of the gluconeogenic substrates used for the indirect pathway have not been precisely determined. The relative proportions depend on species, antecedent diet, and duration of fast. In humans fasted overnight, it has been estimated that the direct pathway may account for 40–60% (33,34).

The significance of the direct *versus* indirect pathways and the source of substrates used for the indirect pathway lies in the potential influence of peripheral (extrahepatic) glucose metabolism on the liver. It was originally proposed that production of these precursors occurred in skeletal muscle (32). However, balance studies in dogs have shown that neither skeletal muscle, (35) the brain (36), nor the gastrointestinal tract (37) are major sources of lactate and alanine after an oral glucose load. This leaves the liver itself as the possible site for generation of the gluconeogenic precursors. The liver is indeed capable of producing lactate, while also taking it up and converting it to glycogen (37). The liver may be a major source of the gluconeogenic precursors used for the indirect pathway of glycogen synthesis. This can be explained by the fact that periportal hepatocytes are mainly gluconeogenic, whereas perivenous hepatocytes are mainly glycolytic (38). After administration of an oral glucose load, the perivenous hepatocytes take up glucose, synthesize glycogen, and release lactate into the circulation. Lactate is then transported to the periportal hepatocytes and converted to glycogen via gluconeogenesis (38).

REFERENCES

1. Gerich J. Control of glycaemia. *Baillière's Clin Endocrinol Metab* 1993; 7: 551–86.
2. Rothman D, Magnusson I, Katz L, *et al*. Quantitation of hepatic glycogenolysis and gluconeogenesis in fasting humans with C-13 NMR. *Science* 1991; 254: 573–6.
3. Clutter W, Rizza R, Gerich J, Cryer P. Regulation of glucose metabolism by sympathochromaffin catecholamines. *Diabetes Metab Rev* 1988; 4: 1–15.
4. Cherrington AD. Gluconeogenesis: its regulation by insulin and glucagon. In: Brownlee M, ed. *Diabetes mellitus,* vol 3. New York: Garland STPM Press, 1981: 49–117.
5. Cherrington AD, Stevenson RW, Steiner KE, *et al.* Insulin, glucagon and glucose as regulators of hepatic glucose uptake and production in vivo. *Diabetes Metab Rev* 1987; 3: 307–32.

6. Cherrington A, Wada M, Stevenson R, *et al.* Hormonal regulation of hepatic glucose production. In: Diamond M, Naftolin F, eds. *Metabolism in the female life cycle.* Rome: Ares-Serono, 1993: 1–18.

7. Dent P, Lavoinne A, Nakielny S, *et al.* The molecular mechanism by which insulin stimulates glycogen synthesis in mammalian skeletal muscle. *Nature* 1990; 348: 302–8.

8. Exton JH. Hormonal control of gluconeogenesis. In: Klachko DM, Anderson RR, Heimberg M, eds. *Hormones and energy metabolism.* New York: Plenum Press, 1979: 125–67.

9. Scrutton MC, Utter MF. The regulation of glycolysis and gluconeogenesis in animal tissues. *Annu Rev Biochem* 1968; 37: 249–302.

10. Hers HG, Hue L. Gluconeogenesis and related aspects of glycolysis. *Annu Rev Biochem* 1983; 52: 617–53.

11. Hue L, Girard J. Gluconeogenesis and its regulation in isolated and cultured hepatocytes. In: Guillouzo A, Guillouzo C, eds. *Isolated and cultured hepatocytes.* London: J. Libbey, 1986: 63–86.

12. Hers HG, Van Schaftingen E. Fructose 2,6-bisphosphate 2 years after its discovery. *Biochem J* 1982; 206: 1–12.

13. Hue L, Rider MH. Role of fructose 2,6-bisphosphate in the control of glycolysis in mammalian tissues. *Biochem J* 1987; 245: 313–24.

14. Pilkis S, El Maghrabi M, Claus T. Fructose-2,6-bisphosphate in control of hepatic gluconeogenesis. *Diabetes* 1990; 13: 582–99.

15. Granner D, Pilkis S. The genes of hepatic glucose metabolism. *J Biol Chem* 1990; 265: 10173–6.

16. Pilkis S, Granner D. Molecular physiology of the regulation of hepatic gluconeogenesis and glycolysis. *Annu Rev Physiol* 1992; 54: 885–909.

17. Vaulont S, Kahn A. Transcriptional control of metabolic regulation genes by carbohydrates. *FASEB J* 1994; 8: 28–35.

18. Iynedjian PB. Mammalian glucokinase and its gene. *Biochem J* 1993; 293: 1–13.

19. Mueckler M. Family of glucose-transporter genes. Implications for glucose homeostasis and diabetes. *Diabetes* 1990; 39: 6–11.

20. Cushman S, Wardzala L. Potential mechanisms of insulin action on glucose transport in the isolated rat adipose cell. Apparent translocation of intracellular transport systems to the plasma membrane. *J Biol Chem* 1980; 255: 4758–62.

21. Kahn B. Facilitative glucose transporters: regulatory mechanisms and dysregulation in diabetes. *J Clin Invest* 1992; 89: 1367–74.

22. Klip A, Marette A. Acute and chronic signals controlling glucose transport in skeletal muscle. *J Cell Biochem* 1992; 48: 51–60.

23. Randle P, Kerbey A, Espinal J. Mechanisms decreasing glucose oxidation in diabetes and starvation: role of lipid fuels and hormones. *Diabetes Metab Rev* 1988; 4: 623–8.

24. Felig P. The glucose-alanine cycle. *Metabolism* 1973; 22: 179–207.

25. Printz RL, Koch S, Potter LR, *et al.* Hexokinase II mRNA and gene structure. Regulation by insulin and evolution. *J Biol Chem* 1993; 268: 5209–19.

26. Randle P, Garland P, Hales C, *et al.* The glucose-fatty acid cycle: its role in insulin sensitivity and the metabolic disturbances of diabetes mellitus. *Lancet* 1963; i: 785–9.

27. Pagliassotti M, Cherrington A. Regulation of net hepatic glucose uptake in vivo. *Annu Rev Physiol* 1992; 54: 847–60.

28. Adkins-Marshall BA, Pagliassotti MJ, Asher JR, *et al.* Role of hepatic nerves in response of liver to intraportal glucose delivery in dogs. *Am J Physiol* 1992; 262: E679–86.

29. Gardemann A, Puschel G, Jungermann K. Nervous control of liver metabolism and hemodynamics. *Eur J Biochem* 1992; 207: 399–411.

30. Van Schaftingen E, Vandercammen A. Stimulation of glucose phosphorylation by fructose in isolated rat hepatocytes. *Eur J Biochem* 1989; 179: 173–7.

31. Van Schaftingen E. A protein from rat liver confers to glucokinase the property of being antagonistically regulated by fructose 6-phosphate and fructose 1-phosphate. *Eur J Biochem* 1989; 179: 179–84.

32. McGarry J, Kuwajima M, Newgard C, *et al.* From dietary glucose to hepatic glycogen: the full cycle round. *Annu Rev Nutr* 1987; 7: 51–73.

33. Consoli A, Nurhjan N, Gerich J. Rates of appearance and disappearance of plasma lactate after oral glucose: implications for indirect pathway hepatic glycogen repletion in man. *Clin Physiol Biochem* 1989; 7: 70–8.

34. Shulman GI, Landau BR. Pathways of glycogen repletion. *Physiol Rev* 1992; 72: 1019–35.

35. Kelley D, Mitrakou A, Marsh H, *et al.* Skeletal muscle glycolysis, oxidation and storage after an oral glucose load. *J Clin Invest* 1988; 81: 1563–71.

36. Mitrakou A, Melde J, Michenfelder J, *et al*. Rates of lactate appearance and disappearance and brain lactate balance after oral glucose in the dog. *Horm Metab Res* 1989; 13: 343–6.
37. Mitrakou A, Jones R, Okuda Y, *et al*. Pathway and carbon sources for hepatic glycogen repletion in the dog. *Am J Physiol* 1991; 260: E194–202.
38. Jungermann K, Thurman RG. Hepatocyte heterogeneity in the metabolism of carbohydrates. *Enzyme* 1992; 46: 33–58.

DISCUSSION

Dr. Schwartz: The data you show really refer to the adult, whether canine or human, and I would like to point out that the young infant has a hepatic output that is two or three times that of the adult, so where you showed a value of 1 mg/kg/min, the young infant requires 2–4 and maybe even 4–6 mg/kg/min. I should also like to point out something we all recognize which is that the infant has a very large brain; the mass of the brain is most important in terms of glucose uptake. Could you comment on the role of other substrates? What about ketones and lactate for example?

Dr. Girard: Hepatic glucose production is indeed two- to threefold higher in newborn babies than in the adult. In neonates, gluconeogenesis is a very important pathway—much more important after an overnight fast than in the adult—so regulation by insulin is less efficient. It has been clearly shown that hyperglycemia in babies may be due to a lack of effect of insulin on gluconeogenesis.

The second question is the use of alternate substrates by the brain and other tissues. The food intake of breast-fed babies in the first week of life is high in fat. When you calculate the amount of carbohydrate provided by the milk, and compare it with the rate of glucose utilization by the brain, the amount of glucose provided is at most 40–50% of that needed by the peripheral tissues. So gluconeogenesis is a very important pathway of glucose homeostasis at that time. The other aspect is that immediately after birth the liver is capable of converting free fatty acids to ketones to provide additional substrate for the brain, not only for use as a fuel but also as substrate for lipogenesis, for brain myelin formation. So it is true that alternative fuels are very important and that babies who have a defect of both glucose production and fatty acid oxidation, for example, those with a deficiency of the enzyme that allows the entry of long-chain fatty acids into the mitochondria, carnitine palmitoyl transferase-1, are in a very difficult situation, since they have both very low blood glucose and ketone body concentrations.

Dr. Drash: I want to extend Dr. Schwartz's comments up the developmental scale a little to adolescence. Many things change during adolescence; in particular there is a state of insulin resistance. My colleague Dr. Silva Arslanian has been doing very elegant work, documenting major changes in energy flow as you go from pre-adolescence to adolescence (1,2). Adolescence is one of the few situations in which insulin resistance seems to be of positive value because it tends to push the system toward protein accretion. We think it is a major factor responsible for growth acceleration in adolescence. On the other hand, this is the time when we see the peak incidence of childhood diabetes. I think this may be at least partly related to this normal insulin resistance.

Dr. Girard: This is a very important point. I have no explanation for the appearance of insulin resistance at puberty. There is no evidence that the liver is involved in this process, but it is well known that there is a marked change in the mass of tissue, for example, both fat and protein accretion occur at this time. This is also the time when the sex hormones are secreted in increasing concentrations, and it is well known that some of these hormones have anti-insulin effects on skeletal muscle and peripheral tissues. So the state of insulin resistance could be due to sexual maturation and the secretion of hormones at this time, and I feel that the effect is largely taking place in peripheral tissues rather than in the liver.

Dr. Carrascosa: During puberty there is a progressive increase in insulin growth factor-1 levels, and this means that there is an increasing availability of this growth factor, which as you know has an insulin-like effect, at the level of peripheral tissues. Do you think this increasing insulin growth factor level during puberty may play any role in the insulin resistance of diabetics in this period?

Dr. Girard: I don't think so since insulin growth factor-1 has the same effect as insulin but at higher concentrations. If you infuse insulin growth factor-1 in humans, you can increase glucose utilization despite a state of insulin resistance. But if you are implying that insulin growth factor-1 is the result of oversecretion of growth hormone, then it should be pointed out that growth hormone has anti-insulin effects and these effects could be mediated through increased growth hormone secretion rather than through overproduction of insulin growth factor-1.

Dr. Cowett: What about the situation in very elderly people in whom there is a higher frequency of non-insulin-dependent diabetes? What is the possibility that there is altered enzyme sensitivity in the liver in elderly people?

Dr. Girard: In type 2 diabetes, hepatic glucose production after an overnight fast, is 50% higher than in normal people. In normal people, 50% of glucose production is derived from glycogen breakdown and 50% from gluconeogenesis. In type 2 diabetes, gluconeogenesis represents about 75% of hepatic glucose production. Perhaps what we describe as a state of liver insulin resistance could be due not only to a defect in transmission of the insulin message but also to the fact that the liver is using a different metabolic pathway for glucose production. I think it is very important to focus on this aspect. If you study patients with type 2 diabetes using the euglycemic clamp and you increase the insulin levels from 10 μunits/ml to 100 μunits/ml, what is clear is that you are capable of completely inhibiting hepatic glucose production whereas stimulation of glucose utilization is reduced only by 50%. This indicates that the liver is less sensitive to insulin but is not insulin resistant. My explanation is that the pathway used for producing glucose in type 2 diabetes is gluconeogenesis and that gluconeogenesis is less sensitive to insulin than glycogen breakdown.

Dr. Nattrass: Your illustrations tend to suggest that the endpoint of gluconeogenesis is glucose, although in one of your later figures it appears that glycogen may also be an endpoint. I wonder what effect this has upon the interpretation of, say, the effect of insulin on gluconeogenesis when you measure alanine and lactate uptake into glucose rather than into glycogen.

I should also like to emphasize the importance of the differential effects of insulin upon metabolism. I think this is very underappreciated by clinicians. For example, inhibition of lipolysis takes very little insulin, whereas stimulation of glucose uptake into cells takes a good deal.

Dr. Girard: Your question concerns what we call the *glucose paradox*. This is the situation where, between starvation and refeeding, part of the glycogen repletion in the liver is achieved not only by hepatic uptake of glucose but also by gluconeogenesis which, instead of providing glucose for the blood, provides glycogen for repletion. This was an active field of research about 5–6 years ago. It seems to me from reading the original publication (3) that if you consume a large amount of carbohydrate, the direct pathway (that is, the conversion of glucose to glycogen) should be the most important. But in a situation where you provide a mixed meal, where there is less glucose in the meal and also substrates for gluconeogenesis, then gluconeogenesis is partly used to replenish glycogen stores in the liver, up to a maximum of about 50%. These studies have mainly been done in rodents, and I am not sure the results can necessarily be extrapolated to humans.

Dr. Bergman: I agree with Dr. Girard. I think the issue that was being addressed is the question of whether it is necessary to suppress the gluconeogenic pathway in order to suppress glucose production from non-carbohydrate precursors. I believe there is evidence that hormonal control, rather than suppressing gluconeogenesis, actually suppresses the ultimate phase of carbohydrate metabolism as it goes up the pathway, whether it goes toward glycogen or toward glucose. It is the *direction* of the final glucose pathway, whether it goes toward glycogen or toward glucose in the blood, that may be under control rather than the pathway itself.

I should also like to add a comment following Dr. Nattrass's remarks (*above*) on the differential sensitivity of various tissues to insulin. One of the things that has impressed us recently is the fact that the concentration of insulin at the cells may be quite different from its concentration in the blood. In the liver, the hepatocytes are exposed to more or less the same concentration of insulin as in the portal blood because of good transfer characteristics across the capillary endothelium. On the other hand, in muscle, which has a very tight capillary endothelium and inefficient insulin transfer, the concentration of insulin at the muscle cell is much lower than it is in the blood. When we interpret the sensitivity of these tissues to insulin we need to think in terms not only of the blood insulin but of insulin in the lymph.

Dr. Marliss: My question relates to the stimulation of hepatic glycogenolysis in humans by catecholamines. Are you going to stand firmly by the premise that this is β receptor mediated or will you accept the possibility that this is not absolutely clear as yet?

Dr. Girard: From the work of Riza and De Fronzo (4,5) it is clear that, in the resting state, a large part of glycogenolysis is due to a β-adrenergic mechanism in the human. This conclusion is mainly based on the fact that if you use a β-adrenergic inhibitor you can completely suppress the effect of catecholamines. It is possible, however, that what occurs during the physiological release of catecholamines could be markedly different since it seems that norepinephrine and epinephrine are not acting in the same way or on the same metabolic pathways. From the work Cherrington (6), it seems that norepinephrine is a good stimulator of gluconeogenesis but not of glycogen breakdown. However, there is much controversy about this since the proportion of the catecholamine effect that is due to the activation of β-adrenergic or α-adrenergic receptors varies among the species. In the rodent, most of the effect of catecholamines acts through α-adrenergic receptors. In the human, it seems that much of the effect is mediated through β-adrenergic receptors, as in the dog.

Dr. Crofford: Another problem in interpreting these data is that most of the experiments performed in humans, and indeed most of the ones performed by Cherrington in dogs, were performed in the resting state; the effect of exercise, however, is dramatic in terms of the disposition of a particular meal or glucose load, and I think that should be taken into consideration when one interprets the fraction of the nutrient that is distributed and taken up by the various tissues.

Dr. Girard: It has been shown that, when exercise is stopped and glycogen stores are repleted, there is a predominance of skeletal muscle glycogen restoration over hepatic glycogen restoration. So I agree that we have to take into account that what I have described refers to the resting state.

REFERENCES

1. Arslanian S *et al.* Correlation of FFA and glucose metabolism: Possible explanation of the insulin resistance of adolescence. *Diabetes* 1994; 43: 908–14.

2. Arslanian S *et al*. Insulin resistance and protein metabolism in adolescence. *Pediatr Res* 1994; 35: 201A.
3. McGarry JD, Kuwajima M, Newgard CB, Foster DW. From dietary glucose to liver glycogen: The full circle round. *Ann Rev Nutr* 1987; 7: 51–73.
4. Rizza RA, Cryer PE, Haymond MW, Gerich JE. Adrenergic mechanisms of catecholamine action on glucose homeostasis in man. *Metabolism* 1980; 29: 1155–63.
5. Deiber DC, De Fronzo RA. Epinephrine-induced insulin resistance in man. *J Clin Invest* 1980; 65: 717–21.
6. Cherrington AD, Wada M, Stevenson RW, Steiner KE, Connolly CC. Hormonal regulation of hepatic glucose production. In: *Metabolism in the female life cycle*. Diamond MP, Natfolin F, eds. Rome: Ares-Serono Symposia Publications 1993: 1–18.

Diabetes, edited by Richard M. Cowett,
Nestlé Nutrition Workshop Series,
Vol. 35. Nestec Ltd.,
Vevey/Raven Press, Ltd., New York © 1995.

The Contributions of Epidemiology to the Understanding of the Etiology of Insulin-Dependent Diabetes Mellitus

Allan L. Drash

The Children's Hospital of Pittsburgh, 3705 Fifth Avenue, Rangos Research Center, Pittsburgh, PA 15213, USA

Why does insulin-dependent diabetes mellitus occur? What are the factors that account for the remarkable variability in the age and timing of onset of clinical disease? Are there adverse environmental factors that may stimulate early disease expression? Conversely, are there environmental influences that, if enhanced, may prevent or delay expression? Can insulin-dependent diabetes mellitus be prevented or cured?

The advances in knowledge of the multi-factorial nature of the etiology of insulin-dependent diabetes mellitus (IDDM) over the past two decades is one of the highlights of modern medicine. We now know that IDDM is not genetic in the usual Mendelian sense. Rather, several genetic alterations, most but probably not all of which are located on chromosome six within the major histocompatibility complex, result in an increased likelihood of β-cell damage (1–10).

The mechanism of β-cell damage and destruction is autoimmune. Substantial evidence suggests that antigens released from the β cell are seen as foreign proteins by the macrophage or antigen presenting cell (APC) that presents the altered antigen to a highly specialized HLA-linked receptor in a helper T cell. This process then initiates an active cellular and humoral response involving antibody production and lymphokine release. The final biochemical mediator of this toxic process is probably nitric oxide (11–16).

EPIDEMIOLOGIC VARIABLES THAT PROVIDE INSIGHT INTO IDDM ETIOLOGY

The original epidemiological inquiries set out to define the magnitude of the problem of diabetes in our society by determining incidence and prevalence rates. As these studies began to appear in various parts of the world, comparisons led to the surprising observation that this disease did not occur uniformly over time or space.

Attempts to define these curious observations further led to a variety of interlocking studies looking closely at geographic variation, secular trends, evidence of migrant drift, and epidemics. These studies have been extraordinarily important in defining new directions for research for clinical and basic scientists, geneticists and molecular biologists (17).

GEOGRAPHIC DISTRIBUTION OF IDDM

A conference on the epidemiology of IDDM held in 1983 identified clearly, and for the first time, the remarkable variation in expression of this disorder in various parts of the world (18). Many follow-up studies have confirmed this, with the finding of a high incidence of IDDM in the Scandinavian countries, intermediate levels in much of the West, and very low levels in the Far Eastern countries, including Japan, China, and Korea (19–25). This distribution is extraordinarily similar to that seen in the worldwide distribution of atherosclerosis and of morbidity and mortality from coronary artery disease. The latter is closely linked to the ingestion of saturated fat and cholesterol and to the dietary intake of dairy products. Conversely, atherosclerotic risk and IDDM incidence are inversely correlated with the content of naturally occurring antioxidants in the diet, traditionally high in the diet of the Orient and quite low in that of individuals living in Western countries (26–35).

Genetic studies carried out by our laboratories, in collaboration with many other investigators, have documented a remarkable parallel between the population distribution of the homozygous non-aspartic-acid status at codon 57 of the HLA-DQ β antigen and the national incidence of IDDM. That is, in many of the countries studied to date, the incidence of diabetes, either high or low, is directly correlated with this diabetes susceptibility gene distribution. The addition of the HLA-DQ α variation with arginine found at position 52 further defines diabetes susceptibility. However, it appears that somewhat less than one individual in 20 carrying gene alterations that increase susceptibility to diabetes will in fact develop overt diabetes, so environmental factors are still very important for actual disease induction (36–38).

SECULAR TRENDS IN IDDM INCIDENCE

If the incidence of IDDM were exclusively dependent upon the frequency of the diabetes susceptibility genes within the population, one would expect that the annual incidence would be remarkably similar year after year, reflecting the absence of or only very slow change in the distribution of diabetes-related genes in the population over time. That, in fact, is not the case. There is now substantial evidence, based on carefully constructed registry data extending in many countries over the last 20–40 years, that there have been substantial increases in IDDM incidence in many locations, particularly in the Scandinavian countries. The incidence of diabetes among Finnish children has almost doubled during the past 20 years. Similar observations have been made in Norway, Denmark, and Sweden. In our own experience in Allegheny County, Pennsylvania, we had observed an increase of approximately 1% per year in the incidence of IDDM until a more recent acute acceleration (39–44).

Probably the most dramatic evidence of a secular increase is given by the experience on the Italian island of Sardinia. The incidence of IDDM in Sardinia currently approaches 30/100,000 per year, just below that in Finland and approximately five times greater than the incidence of diabetes in Italian children living on the mainland of Italy. This high incidence is explained by the finding of a very high frequency of homozygous non-aspartic-acid genetic status in the population of Sardinia (36,37,45). However, a recent review of the earlier incidence of diabetes in Sardinia, not yet published or verified, suggests that the attack rate for this disease among Sardinian school children 20–30 years ago was in the neighborhood of 4–5/100,000 per year, the incidence rate now seen in the mainland of Italy. Obviously, there has been no significant increase in the genetic susceptibility to diabetes in Sardinia over the past quarter of a century. The increase in attack rate, if it is accurate, must reflect significant environmental changes that have occurred during that period, almost certainly associated with industrialization, changes in lifestyle patterns, and changes in dietary habits.

DIABETES EPIDEMICS

While secular changes in IDDM incidence over a period of several years stress the validity of a totally genetic-immunologic explanation for IDDM, acute increases in incidence, referred to by some as *diabetes epidemics,* truly defy genetic explanation and must be viewed as a consequence of acute environmental changes. There are now several well-documented examples of abrupt increases in IDDM incidence followed by a return to the baseline incidence in several countries, including Poland, Latvia, and England (46–50).

Our own recent experience in Pittsburgh is particularly important in this regard. Both in our Children's Hospital and in Allegheny County registry we have continued surveillance, both retrospectively and prospectively, covering approximately 40 years. While we have documented a slight and just statistically significant incidence increase of about 1% per year from 1965 through 1985, we have recently observed a major increase in incidence during the interval 1985–1989. This increase in incidence is seen predominantly in males, in younger children, and in African-Americans. It is statistically correlated with chicken pox epidemics, with a lag phase of between 2 and 3 years. Although we do not suggest that chicken pox is a primary etiologic factor in IDDM, we strongly believe that our recent observations of a highly significant increase in incidence among children in western Pennsylvania indicates changing environmental stressors. Our documentation of increasing frequency of IDDM in younger children is consistent with the clinical experience of many pediatric diabetologists in various parts of the world and again suggests environmental stressors appearing at earlier ages (51).

MIGRANT STUDIES

Although classical prospective migrant studies have not been carried out in IDDM, there are a number of important and valuable observations that strongly suggest that susceptibility to IDDM may be altered by changes in geography and life style. These conclusions result from the study of individuals of a particular geographic or nationality group living at a distance from their natural home, within a population that has an IDDM incidence significantly different from that of the study population. Such observations have documented that Japanese living in Hawaii have an IDDM incidence approximately five times greater than Japanese children living in their homeland. Similarly, there is an approximate doubling of the incidence of French and Italian children in Montreal when compared with the incidence in France and Italy (52,53). The incidence of IDDM in Indian children following migration from South Africa to England showed a dramatic increase from very low levels to that compatible with children in England (54).

These studies and others strongly support the thesis that environmental factors may either increase or decrease the expression in diabetes in susceptible individuals. The migrant study observations have been appropriately criticized by the absence of experiences documenting reduced risk in certain populations. However, the natural migrant drift in the past several decades is from east to west, from developing countries to Western countries, from poverty to affluence, and from tropical to temperate zones. All of these moves in general involve migration of individuals from countries at lesser risk for the development of diabetes to countries where the incidence rate is higher.

EVIDENCE FOR ENVIRONMENTAL FACTORS IN THE ETIOLOGY OF INSULIN-DEPENDENT DIABETES MELLITUS

Environmental factors may play one of several possible roles in processes involving β-cell destruction. At one extreme, there are undoubtedly cases of diabetes occurring as a direct result of ingestion of β-cytotropic agents, with no intervening genetic susceptibility or autoimmune mechanisms. At the other extreme, β-cell destruction results exclusively from genetically mediated autoimmune processes that are internally triggered without interaction with specific environmental stimulants. It seems likely, however, that most cases of IDDM fall in a middle ground where environmental factors, rather than being directly causative, act as stimulants or provocateurs of the immune system. Further it is my belief that, in the great majority of cases, IDDM does not result from a single environmental insult leading to a relentless autoimmune destructive process but rather that there are multiple hits from the environment, resulting in waxing and waning of the inflammatory process. What is the evidence? (55–57,10).

Four general environmental categories have been proposed as potential causative or provocative agents in the expression of IDDM. These include infectious agents, environmental toxins, nutrient factors, and physical and emotional stress. An additional interesting observation is that children who experience maternal-child blood group incompatibility are apparently at a fourfold increased risk for IDDM (57). Although it is likely that genetically susceptible individuals finally develop diabetes after multiple environmental insults, possibly involving adverse experiences from each of the four general environmental categories, these categories are discussed separately below.

ANIMAL STUDIES

In medicine, we have traditionally looked to animal models for insights and understanding of disease processes that cannot be elucidated fully in the human subject. Animal research has played a major role in the study of diabetes for well over 100 years. Strangely, those stringent advocates of an exclusively internally mediated autoimmune disease process accept the evidence of disease mechanisms from genetically susceptible models as important to the human condition. The animal experience can be summarized as follows.

1. Toxic agents, for example alloxan and streptozotocin, can regularly induce β-cell destruction and diabetes in both genetically susceptible and normal animals. Overt diabetes can be rapidly induced by a large dose of streptozotocin by direct toxic action of the drug, or probably by autoimmune mechanisms, using small doses of the toxin repeatedly. (This is reminiscent of the human situation with the drug Vacor^R in which the acute ingestion of a large dose results in rapid β-cell destruction, while chronic ingestion of small doses appears to induce autoimmune β-cell destruction) (58).

2. Various infectious agents can induce β-cell destruction in diabetes-susceptible and non-susceptible animal models. The identified agents include encephalomyocarditis (EMC) virus, Mengo virus, and coxsackie B virus variants. The β-cell destructive process may be either directly cytolytic or may cause the induction of β-cell damage leading to eventual autoimmune destruction (59).

3. Environmental manipulation will alter the expression of diabetes in genetically susceptible animal strains. The BB rat and the NOD mouse strains are immunologically defective animals that are at markedly increased risk for the development of β-cell destruction or overt diabetes, mimicking human IDDM in many respects. Environmental manipulation, particularly dietary alteration, can result in marked variation in the expression of disease in both of these animal models (60–62). This is particularly true in relation to cow's milk protein and/or beef in the animal chow. Adding bovine serum albumin or whole milk or beef protein to the chow increases the incidence of diabetes, while replacing the animal chow with synthetic proteins and amino acids reduces the expression of diabetes to near zero. This evidence strongly suggests that cow's milk protein or beef has a specific provocative effect on the immune system of these animals, resulting in progressive β-cell destruction.

4. Various immune suppressive or modulating strategies introduced well before

β-cell damage will reduce the expression of diabetes in genetically susceptible animal models. These observations provide cause for optimism that immunologic intervention before the onset of diabetes may prevent disease in the human situation (63–66).

INFECTIOUS DISEASES

Several viral infections have been associated with the development of IDDM, on the basis either of epidemiologic surveys or of individual case reports. The association between mumps infection and IDDM has been known for 100 years, and there have been periodic case reports of diabetes occurring in individual cases following mumps infection a few weeks previously. Coxsackie infections, particularly serotypes B3 and B4, have been associated with IDDM both in disease surveillance statistics and in a few isolated but highly important cases. Cytomegalovirus (CMV) has also been associated with carbohydrate intolerance and diabetes, and insulitis has been identified in the pancreas of infants dying with disseminated CMV infection. The best documented association between a specific viral infection and IDDM is found in the congenital rubella syndrome. Rubella infection, acquired by the fetus as a result of transplacental passage of the virus, results in a generalized rubella infection that may have devastating effects on the infant. In the great majority of cases, the infection burns out soon after delivery. However, it leaves behind an autoimmune destructive process that over a period of 5 to 20 years will result in β-cell destruction and overt diabetes. HLA studies indicate that diabetes eventually develops in those children with rubella syndrome who have a genetic predisposition to disease. The eventual development of diabetes may approach 100% in those individuals who are HLA DR3 and/or DR4. No DQ α or β studies have been reported on this group of patients but they should be done. The congenital rubella syndrome-diabetes association is strong evidence of a virus-induced autoimmune phenomenon leading to β-cell destruction. The recent studies of Yoon et al. documenting an increased frequency of CMV viral fragments in the genome of children with IDDM suggest that such patients either acquired CMV infections very early in life, which then initiated a β-cell destructive process, or that IDDM may be associated with persistence of the infection (67–74).

ENVIRONMENTAL TOXINS

It is well documented that several chemical agents have β-cell destructive properties. Streptozotocin, the agent used to induce diabetes in laboratory animals, has been used to destroy the pancreas in humans with severe hypoglycemia resulting from inoperable islet cell malignancy. The rodenticide Vacor[R] is highly toxic to the β cell, resulting in an acute induction of diabetic ketoacidosis following oral ingestion of a large dose (75,76). Inadvertent chronic small-dose ingestion, as apparently occurred in Korea when the rat poison was mixed with feed, is strongly reminiscent of low-dose streptozotocin-induced autoimmune destruction in laboratory animal models. Nitrosamines, produced when foods are cured by smoking techniques, have been implicated in cases of IDDM in Iceland (77,78). The possibility that the widely used technique of grilling or barbecuing beef may be a factor needs investigation. Furthermore, almost nothing is known about the health hazards of a large number of industrial environmental contaminants as they enter our food and water supply. The recent finding that the apparently benign inert silicone breast implant may be associated with autoimmune disease should raise increasing concern about the health hazards of so-called biochemical advances in our society.

NUTRIENTS

There is increasing evidence that nutrients may play either a protective or a provocative role in the development of IDDM. Of special interest is the accumulating evidence that the early introduction of cow's milk protein may be an important factor in the later expression of diabetes in genetically susceptible infants (79–81).

The recent studies of Karjalainen *et al.* (82) have focused attention on the possible relationship between early ingestion of bovine serum albumin and the later development of diabetes in genetically susceptible individuals. These investigators found that antibody to a specific fragment of bovine serum albumin, referred to as *Abbos,* is present in 100% of newly diagnosed diabetic Finnish children, while it is hardly ever present in non-diabetic children or normal adults. The Abbos epitope is immunologically cross reactive with a β-cell autoantigen, P69, which may, by virtue of molecular biological mimicry, explain why ingestion of this compound can induce β-cell inflammatory responses (82). Recent attempts in another laboratory to confirm the Abbos finding have been unsuccessful (83).

It is well documented that the antioxidant potential of the islet tissue of the pancreas is inherently deficient when compared with most of the other tissues and organs of the body. This means that the islet tissue is at increased risk of free radical damage. The balance between oxidant and antioxidant concentrations within the body fluids and tissues is a delicate one. Free radical excess or antioxidant deficiency will result in disease. Nutritional intake is an important factor in this balance, and antioxidant ingestion is achieving increasing prominence in the prevention of human disease. It is possible that the lower content of naturally occurring antioxidants that characterizes the Western diets may be inadequate to neutralize free radical accumulation, thus increasing the likelihood of β-cell damage and clinical diabetes. Conversely, the considerably lower incidence of diabetes in Oriental countries may be at least partially related to a high dietary intake of antioxidant compounds.

STRESS

The relationship between acute emotional stress and the induction of hyperthyroidism has been widely accepted among endocrinologists for many years. The anecdotal association between the two is convincing. Only recently has research begun to explore the complexities of the interrelationship between the endocrine and the immunologic systems. It is now quite clear that alterations in the hypothalamic-pituitary-adrenal axis, through the release of both ACTH and adrenal steroids, can result in major alterations in the effectiveness of the immunologic surveillance system. While the anecdotal association between emotional trauma and the onset of IDDM is not as strong in diabetes as it is in hyperthyroidism, there are, nonetheless, several studies suggesting such a cause-and-effect relationship (84–87).

THE FUTURE

The possibility of curing or preventing insulin-dependent diabetes mellitus rests solely on the continued accumulation of knowledge into causation. This includes a more complete understanding of the several genetic alterations that may be associated with either increasing risk for diabetes or protection against β-cell inflammation. Much more must be learned about the normal immunologic system and the alterations that occur in individuals who later develop IDDM. There is increasing focus on the development of new immunosuppressive or immunomodulatory interventions that may alter the immune reaction and thus prevent β-cell destruction. In addition, efforts must continually be directed toward further defining environmental risk factors and toward the development of epidemiologic methods for reducing these risks, with a major collaborative effort involving basic and clinical scientists. One can look to the future with optimism (88–90).

ACKNOWLEDGMENTS

This chapter is adapted from Drash AL, "Does beta cell death result exclusively from genetically-mediated autoimmune mechanisms? A polemic—the case for environmental factors in the etiology of insulin dependent diabetes mellitus." In: Dorman J, ed. The NATO ASI Series: *Standardization of epidemiologic studies of host susceptibility*. New York: Plenum 1994; 145–164.

REFERENCES

1. Todd JA, Bell JI, McDevitt HO. HLA-DQ beta gene contributes to susceptibility and resistance to insulin-dependent diabetes mellitus. *Nature* 1987; 329: 599–604.
2. Morel PA, Dorman JS, Todd JA, *et al*. Aspartic acid at position 57 of the DQ beta chain protects against Type I diabetes: a family study. *Proc Natl Acad Sci USA* 1988; 85: 8111–5.
3. Trucco M. To be or not to be ASP 57, that is the question. *Diabetes Care* 1992; 15: 705–15.
4. Segurado OG, Arnaizvillena A, Wank R, Schendel DJ. The multi-factorial nature of MHC-linked susceptibility to insulin dependent diabetes. *Autoimmunity* 1993; 15: 85–9.
5. Kumar D, Gemayel NS, Deapen D, *et al*. North American twins with IDDM—genetic, etiological and clinical significance of disease concordance according to age, zygosity and the interval before diagnosis in first twin. *Diabetes* 1993; 42: 1351–63.
6. Serjentson JW, Court J, MacKay IR, *et al*. HLA-DQ genotypes are associated with autoimmunity

to glutamic acid decarboxylase in insulin-dependent diabetes mellitus patients. *Hum Immunol* 1993; 38: 97–104.

7. Penny MA, Micovic CH, Cavan DA, *et al.* An investigation of the association between HLA-DQ heterodimers and type I (insulin-dependent) diabetes mellitus in five racial groups. *Hum Immunol* 1993; 38: 179–83.

8. Cruickshanks KJ, Jobim LF, Lawlerhevner J, *et al.* Ethnic differences in human leukocytes antigen markers of susceptibility to IDDM. *Diabetes Care* 1994; 17: 132–7.

9. Vanendert PM, Liblau RS, Patel SD, *et al.* Major histocompatability complex-encoded antigen processing gene polymorphism in IDDM. *Diabetes* 1994; 43: 110–7.

10. Trucco M. Immunogenetics of insulin-dependent diabetes mellitus: the second-event hypothesis. In: Belfiore F, Bergman RN, Molinatti GM, eds. *Current topics in diabetes research,* vol 12. Basel: Karger, 1993: 124–46.

11. Gepts W. Pathologic anatomy of the pancreas in juvenile diabetes mellitus. *Diabetes* 1965; 14: 619–33.

12. Drell DW, Notkins AL. Multiple immunologic abnormalities in patients with type I (insulin dependent) diabetes mellitus. *Diabetologia* 1987; 30: 132–43.

13. Bottazzo GF. Death of a beta cell: homicide or suicide? *Diabetic Med* 1986; 3: 119–30.

14. Eisenbarth GS. Type I diabetes mellitus. An autoimmune disease? *N Engl J Med* 1986; 314: 1360–8.

15. Kolb H, Kolb-Bachofen V. Nitric oxide: a pathogenic factor in autoimmunity. *Immunol Today* 1992; 13: 157–60.

16. Laron Z, Karp M, eds. *Genetic and environmental risk factors for type I diabetes (IDDM),* including a discussion on the autoimmune basis. London: Freund Publishing House, 1992.

17. Dorman J, ed. *Standardization of epidemiologic studies of host susceptibility.* The NATO ASI Series. New York: Plenum 1994; 145–164.

18. LaPorte RE, Tajima N, Akerbloom HR, *et al.* Geographic differences in the risk of insulin dependent diabetes mellitus. The importance of registries. *Diabetes Care* 1985; 89: 101–7.

19. Diabetes Epidemiology Research International. Geographic patterns of childhood insulin dependent diabetes mellitus. *Diabetes* 1988; 37: 1113–9.

20. WHO DIAMOND Project Group. WHO multinational project for childhood diabetes. *Diabetes Care* 1990; 13: 1062–8.

21. Tuomilehto J, Dabee J, Karvonen M, *et al.* Incidence of IDDM in Mauritian children and adolescents from 1986 to 1990. *Diabetes Care* 1993; 16: 1588–91.

22. Pociot F, Norgaard K, Hobolth N, Andersen O, Nerup J. A nationwide population-based study of the familial aggregation of type I (insulin-dependent) diabetes mellitus in Denmark. *Diabetologia* 1993; 36: 1870–5.

23. Kocova M, Trucco M, Konstantinova M, Dorman JS. A cold spot of IDDM incidence in Europe-Macedonia. *Diabetes Care* 1993; 16: 1236–40.

24. Staines A, Bodansky HJ, Lelley H, Stephenson C, McNally R, Cartright R. The epidemiology of diabetes mellitus in the United Kingdom: the Yorkshire regional childhood diabetes registry. *Diabetologia* 1993; 36: 1282–7.

25. Karvonen M, Tuomilehto J, Libman I, LaPorte R. A review of the recent epidemiological data on the worldwide incidence of type I (insulin-dependent) diabetes mellitus. *Diabetologia* 1993; 36: 883–92.

26. Gey F, Puska P, Paul J, *et al.* Inverse correlation between plasma vitamin E and mortality from ischemic heart disease in cross-cultural epidemiology. *Am J Clin Nutr* 1991; 53: 326S.

27. Gey F, Moser UK, Jordan P, *et al.* Increased risk of cardiovascular disease at suboptimal plasma levels of essential antioxidants: an epidemiological update with special attention to carotene and vitamin C. *Am J Clin Nutr* 1993; 57:(suppl 5) 787S–797S.

28. Steinberg D, Parthasarathy S, Carew T, *et al.* Beyond cholesterol: modification of low-density lipoprotein that increases its atherogenicity. *N Engl J Med* 1989; 320: 915–24.

29. Riemersma R, Wood D, Macintyre CCA, *et al.* Risk of angina pectoris and plasma concentrations of vitamins A, C and E and carotene. *Lancet* 1991; 337: 1–5.

30. Grei B. Ascorbic acid protects lipids in human plasma and low-density lipoprotein against oxidative damage. *Am J Clin Med* 1992; 54: 113S.

31. Keizo S, Nikim E, Shimasaki H. Free radical-mediated chain oxidation of low-density lipoprotein and synergistic inhibition by vitamin E and vitamin C. *Arch Biochem Biophys* 1990; 279: 402–5.

32. Halliwell B, Gutteridge J, Cross CE. Free radicals, antioxidants, and human disease: where are we now? *J Lab Clin Med* 1992; 119: 598–620.

33. Olson JA, Kobayashe S. Antioxidants in health and disease: overview. *Proc Soc Exp Biol Med* 1992; 200: 245–7.
34. Asayama K, Uchida N, Makane T, *et al.* Antioxidants in the serum of children with insulin dependent diabetes mellitus. *Free Radic Biol Med* 1993; 15: 597–602.
35. Wolff SP. Diabetes-mellitus and free radicals. *Br Med Bull* 1993; 49: 642–52.
36. Dorman J, LaPorte R, Stone R, *et al.* Worldwide differences in the incidence of type I diabetes are associated with amino acid variation at position 57 of the HLA-DQ Beta chain. *Proc Natl Acad Sci USA* 1990; 87: 7370–4.
37. Contu L, Carcassi C, Trucco M. Diabetes susceptibility in Sardinia. *Lancet* 1991; 338: 65–6.
38. Lipton R, Kocova M, LaPorte R, *et al.* Autoimmunity and genetics contribute to the risk of insulin-dependent diabetes mellitus in families: islet cell antibodies and HLA-DQ heterodimers. *Am J Epidemiol* 1992; 146: 503–12.
39. Diabetes Epidemiology Research Internation Group. Secular trends in incidence of childhood IDDM in 20 countries. *Diabetes* 1990; 39: 858–64.
40. Metcalfe M, Baum J. Incidence of insulin dependent diabetes in children aged under 15 years in the British Isles during 1988. *BMJ* 1991; 302: 443–7.
41. Joner G, Sovik O. Increasing incidence of diabetes mellitus in Norwegian children 0–14 years of age (1973–1982). *Diabetologia* 1989; 32: 79–83.
42. Nystrom L, Dahlquist G, Rewers M, *et al.* The Swedish childhood diabetes study. An analysis of the temporal variation in diabetes incidence 1978-1987. *Int J Epidemiol* 1990; 19: 141–6.
43. Tuomilehto J, Rewers M, Reunanen A, *et al.* Increasing trend in type I (insulin-dependent) diabetes mellitus in childhood in Finland. Analysis of age, calendar time and birth cohort effects during 1965–1984. *Diabetologia* 1991; 34: 282–7.
44. Green A, Gale EA, Patteson CC. Incidence of childhood-onset insulin-dependent diabetes mellitus. The EURODIAB ACE study. *Lancet* 1992; 339: 905–9.
45. Mutoni S, Songini LM. High incidence rate of IDDM in Sardinia. *Diabetes Care* 1992; 15: 1317–22.
46. Rewers M, LaPorte R, Walczakj M, *et al.* Apparent epidemic of insulin-dependent diabetes mellitus in midwestern Poland. *Diabetes* 1987; 36: 106–13.
47. Rewers M, Stone R, LaPorte R, *et al.* Poisson regression modeling in temporal variation in incidence of childhood insulin-dependent diabetes mellitus in Allegheny County, Pennsylvania, and Wielkopolska, Poland. *Am J Epidemiol* 1989; 129: 569–81.
48. Wagenknecht L, Rosemann J, Herman W. Increased incidence of insulin-dependent diabetes mellitus following an epidemic of coxsackie virus B5. *Am J Epidemiol* 1991; 133: 1024–31.
49. Laron Z, Karp M, Modan M. The incidence of insulin dependent diabetes mellitus in Israeli children and adolescents 0–20 years of age: a retrospective study 1975–1980. *Diabetes Care* 1985; 8: 24–8.
50. LaPorte RE, Tan M, Podar T, *et al.* Childhood diabetes, epidemics, and epidemiology—an approach for controlling diabetes. *Am J Epidemiol* 1992; 135: 803–16.
51. Dokheel T, and the Pittsburgh Diabetes Epidemiology Research Group. An epidemic of childhood diabetes in the United States? Evidence from Allegheny County, Pennsylvania. *Diabetes Care* 1993; 16: 1606–11.
52. Mimura G. Present status and future view of the genetic study of diabetes mellitus. In: Mimura G, Baba S, Goto Y, Kobberling J, eds. *Clinico-genetic genesis of diabetes mellitus.* Amsterdam: Excepta Medica, 1982.
53. Colle E, Siemiatyeti J, West JR, *et al.* Incidence of juvenile onset diabetes in Montreal: demonstration of ethnic differences and socio-economic class differences. *J Chron Dis* 1981; 34: 611–6.
54. Burden AC, Burden ML, Willimas ER, *et al.* Evidence of frequent epidemics of childhood diabetes. *Diabetes* 1991; 40: 373A.
55. Orchard T, Dorman J, LaPorte R, *et al.* Host and environmental interactions in diabetes mellitus. *J Chron Dis* 1986; 36: 979–1000.
56. Drash A. Reflection on the beta cell and its demise, diabetes in the young. *Bull ISGD* 1988; 19: 233–59.
57. Dahlquist G. Etiological aspects of insulin dependent diabetes mellitus: an epidemiological prospective. *Autoimmunity* 1993; 15: 61–5.
58. Kolb H. Mouse models of insulin dependent diabetes: low dose streptozotocin-induced diabetes in nonobese diabetic (NOB) mice. *Diabetes Metab Rev* 1987; 8: 751–78.
59. Yoon J. Role of viruses in the pathogenesis of IDDM. *Ann Med* 1991; 23: 437–45.

60. Elliott R, Martin J. Dietary protein: a trigger of insulin dependent diabetes in the BB rat? *Diabetologia* 1984; 26: 297–9.
61. Daneman D, Fishman L, Clarson C, *et al*. Dietary triggers of insulin-dependent diabetes in the BB rat. *Diabetes* 1987; 5: 93–7.
62. Coleman D, Kuzava J, Leiter E. Effect of diet on incidence of diabetes in nonobese diabetic mice. *Diabetes* 1990; 39: 432–6.
63. Sumoski W, Baquerizo H, Rabinovitch A. Oxygen free radical scavengers protect rat islet cell from damage by cytokines. *Diabetologia* 1989; 32: 792–6.
64. Drash AL, Rudert WA, Borquaye S, *et al*. Effect of probucol on development of diabetes mellitus in BB rats. *Am J Cardiol* 1988; 62: 27B–30B.
65. Like AA, Anthony M, Buberski DL, *et al*. Spontaneous diabetes mellitus in the BB/W rat: effect of glucocorticoids, cyclosporin A and antiserum to rat lymphocytes. *Diabetes* 1983; 32: 326–30.
66. Murase N, Lieberman I, Nalesnk M, *et al*. Prevention of spontaneous diabetes in the BB rat with FK-506. *Lancet* 1990; 336: 373–4.
67. Harris HF. A case of diabetes mellitus following mumps. *Boston Med Surg J* 1987; 140: 645–9.
68. Gamble DR, Taylor KW, Cumming H. Coxsackie viruses in diabetes mellitus. *BMJ* 1984; iv: 260–2.
69. Yoon JW, Austin M, Ondera T, *et al*. Virus induced diabetes mellitus: isolation of a virus from the pancreas of a child with diabetic ketoacidosis. *N Engl J Med* 1979; 300: 1173–9.
70. Forrest JM, Menser MA, Burgess JA. High frequency of diabetes mellitus of young adults with congenital rubella. *Lancet* 1971; ii: 332–4.
71. Drash AL. Evidence for viral infections in the etiology of insulin-dependent diabetes mellitus. In: Czernichow P, Dorchy H, eds. *Diabetologie pédiatrique*. Paris: Doin, 1990.
72. Roberts SS. New clues to IDDM origins: IDDM may arise from a case of mistaken identity in which the immune system mistakes a normal beta cell antigen for a virus. *Diabetes Care* 1992; 15: 137–9.
73. Fohlman J, Friman G. Is juvenile diabetes a viral disease? *Ann Med* 1993; 25: 569–74.
74. Hyoty H, Hiltunen M, Reunanen A, *et al*. Decline of mumps antibodies in type I (insulin-dependent) diabetic children and a plateau in the rising incidence of type I diabetes after introduction of the mumps-measles-rubella vaccine in Finland. *Diabetologia* 1993; 36: 1303–8.
75. Karam J, Prosser P, Lewitt P. Islet cell surface antibodies in a patient with diabetes mellitus after rodenticide ingestion. *N Engl J Med* 1978; 299: 1191 (letter).
76. Karam J, Lewitt P, Young C, *et al*. Insulinopenic diabetes after rodenticide (Vacor) ingestion: a unique model of acquired diabetes in man. *Diabetes* 1980; 29: 971–8.
77. Helgason T, Jonnasson MR. Evidence for a food additive as a cause of ketosis-prone diabetes. *Lancet* 1981; ii: 716–20.
78. Helgason T, Ewen SWB, Ross IS, Stowers JM. Diabetes produced in mice by smoked/cured mutton. *Lancet* 1982; ii: 1017–22.
79. Gerstein HC. Does cow's milk cause type I diabetes mellitus? A critical overview of the clinical literature. *Diabetes Care* 1994; 17: 13–9.
80. Kostraba JN. What can epidemiolgy tell us about the role of infant diet in the etiology of diabetes? *Diabetes Care* 1994; 17: 87–91.
81. Drash AL, Kramer MS, Swanson J, Udall J. Infant feeding practices and their possible relationship to the etiology of diabetes mellitus. *Pediatrics* (in press).
82. Karjalainen J, Marin J, Knip M, *et al*. Evidence for a bovine albumin peptide as candidate trigger of type I diabetes. *N Engl J Med* 1992; 327: 302–7.
83. Atkinson MA, Bowman MA, Kao KJ, *et al*. Lack of immune responsiveness to bovine serum albumin in insulin dependent diabetes. *N Engl J Med* 1993; 329: 1853–8.
84. Bateman A, Singh A, Kral T, Solomon S. The immune-hypothalamic-pituitary-adrenal axis. *Endocr Rev* 1989; 10: 92–112.
85. Gupta D. Pathophysiology of immune-neuroendocrine network. *Network Lett* 1992; 14: 1–19.
86. Lager J, Attvall S, Eriksson BM, *et al*. Studies on the insulin antagonistic effect of catecholamines in normal man. *Diabetologia* 1986; 29: 409–16.
87. Surwit RS, Schneider MS. Role of stress in the etiology and treatment of diabetes-mellitus. *Psychosom Med* 1993; 55: 380–93.
88. Skyler JS, Marks JB. Immune intervention in type I diabetes mellitus. *Diabetes Rev* 1993; 1: 15–42.
89. LaPorte RE, Baba S. Magic bullets, reportable disease, and the prevention of childhood diabetes. *Diabetes Care* 1992; 15: 128–31.
90. Alberti KG. Preventing insulin dependent diabetes mellitus. *BMJ* 1993; 307: 1435–6.

DISCUSSION

Dr. Cowett: Would you discuss the antioxidants?

Dr. Drash: I am very interested in antioxidants, as are several other people in the field. We need to look more toward the use of antioxidants as preventives. We also need to examine the distribution of antioxidants in the diet, since in the Western world the frequency distribution of diabetes is negatively correlated with the natural occurrence of dietary antioxidants. So I would raise the question with you as to whether the level of naturally occurring dietary antioxidants may be a factor in the initiation of β-cell damage in a genetically predisposed individual. We should consider the pediatric experience; the first two years of life is the only time when nearly everyone is given vitamins, and diabetes is very uncommon in this period. Could this be a factor in the low incidence of diabetes in early life? Should we consider vitamin supplementation on a routine basis later in life?

Dr. Bergman: All sorts of factors may challenge the β cell. For example, insulin sensitivity diminishes if you take an Indian population and move them to Leicester, so past history cannot be ruled out. Insulin resistance develops during puberty and adolescence. Infectious diseases also cause insulin resistance.

Dr. Drash: I agree that there are multiple mechanisms for β-cell damage, and I personally feel that this is a "multiple-hit" disease. I think it is very rare for an individual to be exposed to something that sets off the whole process which then progresses inevitably to disease. I think there is a waxing and waning of the process leading eventually to damage, but if the precipitating factors don't occur often enough the disease does not develop. I think milk is very important. We have just come to some firm conclusions about the danger of early introduction of cow's milk protein. I believe that in some individuals this is a significant factor. However, I don't think we have any idea what proportion of the childhood population gets β-cell damage following early exposure to cow's milk protein.

Dr. Assan: If you adjust for the DR3 antigen from the Finnish data and the data from all the European countries, can you assess the part that is due to the DR3 gradients from the north to the south of Europe and can you then delineate better the possible part played by nitrosamines or cow's milk, for instance? In a particular community, do DR3 individuals who drink cow's milk become diabetic more frequently than the others?

Dr. Drash: The study that will answer this is, we hope, about to get under way in the coming months, led by a group in Canada. This will examine newborns in families in which there are diabetics, and in which the parents have been definitively HLA typed. The newborns will also be typed, so one will be able to say which are at very high risk. They will then be randomized to an exclusively breast-fed group or, if the mother does not want to breast feed, to a standard formula preparation group or to a Nutramigen group. The study is still on the drawing board but it really needs to move forward to define the relative roles of milk factors and high genetic sensitivity.

Dr. Dakou: Overall, Greece has among the lowest incidences of diabetes in the world, but the incidence is quite high in Athens and the Piraeus, almost double that in towns of less than 10,000 inhabitants. This supports an environmental cause because we don't think there is a different genetic population in Athens from that in the cities of less than 10,000 inhabitants. In certain other areas of Greece, we also see a localized high incidence of the disease. We do not find a seasonal variation. What I would like to ask is whether you have broken down your data on "bad genes" according to age of onset. In the old fashioned HLA-ABC studies we have done in our population we found that children with onset of diabetes below the age of 4 years had almost double the risk if they had bad genes.

Dr. Drash: Yes, we are currently working on that precise question. Early analysis suggests that individuals with early onset do have more "bad genes." An important paper has appeared in *Diabetes Care* from Switzerland. This is a study by Schoenle EJ *et al.* from Zürich based on military records. In Switzerland, all males have to do military service. Schoenle has been able to go back about 15 or 20 years in this population and determine the development of diabetes, and he has obtained data that may be similar to the Greek data. The first analysis shows that individuals growing up in urban communities in larger cities had a much higher incidence of diabetes than those growing up in rural communities (about twice as high). This supports the view that stress and the hurly burly of lifestyle in the city are factors in the pathogenesis, which might be consistent with your data. Because Schoenle had the military dataset, which stays in the system until the person dies, he was able to examine the continued expression of diabetes over time. He has found that by 40 or 45 years of age there is essentially an equal distribution of the incidence of type 1 diabetes in urban and rural areas. What the data seem to be saying is that if you are genetically susceptible the disease will catch up with you eventually, but if you live in a stressful environment the expression of the disease may occur earlier. This is very important information that I think will soon be verified by other groups (1).

Dr. Zoupas: How can you measure stress?

Dr. Drash: This is obviously a difficult area for quantitative data. However, we have accepted for many years that stress can provoke the expression of hyperthyroidism, for example, and we know a great deal more now in terms of the hypothalamic-pituitary-adrenal relationship and its interaction with the immunologic system. So certainly there is good evidence of an effect of the endocrine system on the immunologic system. How to quantitate this is a different matter. I think Fuller reported several years ago on the development of diabetes after parental death or divorce, both stressful life events, and there are several papers on this subject in the literature. But I agree with you, it is very difficult to quantitate.

Dr. Bartsocas: Athens has a particularly high incidence of diabetes compared with the rest of Greece. For example, in Macedonia the incidence is only 4.5 per 100,000, while in Athens it is almost 9.5 per 100,000. My second point is that DR2 does not protect Greek people from developing IDDM since the same incidence of HLA-DR2 exists in the IDDM population.

Dr. Bottazzo: I wish everything were as clear cut as the Swiss data, but it isn't. For example, a recent paper from Yorkshire, UK, which appeared in *Diabetologia,* showed exactly the opposite (2). Apparently in that area, there are more cases of IDDM in rural than in urban areas. We have also looked at this aspect in Sardinia (Songini, personal communication) and we found there is no difference between rural and urban areas. Although stress may be important, it should not be assumed that city dwelling is necessarily a risk factor for IDDM.

Dr. Scott: It is very difficult to determine what people eat, and I don't think we should be too ready to correlate certain dietary habits with the risk of type 1 diabetes.

Dr. Drash: I agree that it is a very difficult task. I think the reason it has not been done before is that it is so difficult to characterize eating habits in a way that is precise enough to obtain scientific data.

Dr. Alivisatos: Would you like to comment on the risk of developing diabetes in small-for-dates babies (babies with intrauterine growth retardation)?

Dr. Drash: I am not sure that this has been adequately looked at. We know that the very small-for-dates baby is at risk of transient diabetes in the newborn period. This is really a reflection of intrauterine starvation. I don't know whether true diabetes is seen with greater frequency in that population.

REFERENCES

1. Schoenle EJ *et al*. Epidemiology of IDDM in Switzerland: increasing incidence rate and rural-urban differences in Swiss men born 1948–1972. *Diabetes Care* 1994; 17: 955–60.
2. Staines A, Bodansky HJ, Lilley HE, Stephenson C, McNally RJ, Cartwright RA. The epidemiology of diabetes mellitus in the United Kingdom: the Yorkshire Regional Childhood Diabetes Register. *Diabetologia* 1993, 36: 1282–7.

Diabetes, edited by Richard M. Cowett,
Nestlé Nutrition Workshop Series,
Vol. 35. Nestec Ltd.,
Vevey/Raven Press, Ltd., New York © 1995.

The Etiology of Type 1 Diabetes:

Nature and Nurture

Fraser W. Scott

*Nutrition Research Division, Bureau of Nutritional Sciences, Food Directorate,
Health Canada, Sir Frederick Banting Research Centre, Tunney's Pasture,
Ottawa, Ontario, K1A 0L2, Canada*

The development of type 1 (insulin-dependent) diabetes mellitus requires genetic susceptibility (1). This disease is thought to be the result of an organ-specific autoimmune process in which the immune system reacts abnormally against the body's own insulin secreting β cells in the pancreatic islets. Several elements have been studied in the search for causes of type 1 diabetes, such as diabetes-related genes, immune factors, and environmental factors [mainly diet, viruses, and diabetogenic chemicals; for reviews see (1–5)]. The exact identity of the factors involved in the etiology of type 1 diabetes in humans is difficult to ascertain because the prodromal period is measured in years (6), and it is not yet possible to predict who in the general population will become insulin dependent. Only 10% of all patients with type 1 diabetes have a first-degree relative with the disease. If there is no family history of diabetes, the risk of developing type 1 diabetes is about 1% by the age of 50 years (7).

As a result, most studies have been carried out in first-degree relatives of patients with type 1 diabetes. In this group, the risk of developing the disease is increased and depends on which relative had the disease (7). It ranges from ~1–2% for mother and ~6% for father to 10% by 50 years if a sibling had the disease. The highest risk is reported in identical twins, 34–50%. The lack of concordance in identical twins has been taken as evidence that environmental factors play a role in the etiology of the disease.

Not all genetically susceptible people develop diabetes and, despite much greater genetic homogeneity, neither do all diabetes-prone BioBreeding (BBdp) rats or non-obese diabetic (NOD) mice. However, in all three species it is genes in the major histocompatibility complex (MHC) region that impart the main risk of developing diabetes. Moreover, there is marked geographic variation in diabetes incidence in countries around the world, and this is also evident in colonies of BBdp rats and NOD mice. The highest incidence of human type 1 diabetes occurs in Finland, the Scandinavian countries, and certain "hot spots" such as Sardinia and Prince Edward

Island, Canada, while the lowest incidence is seen in China, Japan, Korea, and Macedonia (8). There are also indications that migrant populations, such as the Japanese who moved to Hawaii and the French Canadians in Montreal, have an increased diabetes incidence compared with their country of origin (9). There have been reports that the incidence of diabetes is increasing in several areas, and there may even be "epidemics" (10). All these data are generally taken as further indication that environmental factors are involved.

The purpose of this review is to discuss briefly the evidence of a role for both genetics and the environment, with a particular emphasis on dietary factors, in the etiology of type 1 diabetes in humans and in the two spontaneous animal models of this disease, the BBdp rat and the NOD mouse.

NATURE

Susceptibility Genes for Type 1 Diabetes

Type 1 diabetes is not inherited in a Mendelian fashion, rather, it is the susceptibility to develop type 1 diabetes that is inherited (11). It is a polygenic disease and, as with many autoimmune diseases, susceptibility or resistance is closely associated with polymorphism in the class II genes of the major histocompatibility complex (MHC) (12).

In Caucasians, type 1 diabetes was originally found to be associated with MHC class I HLA-B8 and HLA-B15. The focus then shifted to the MHC class II HLA-DR locus, which showed a strong association of DR3 or DR4 with the disease; of those who become diabetic, approximately 90% have DR3 or DR4 genes. The presence of DR2 was shown to be protective. In 1987, an important discovery was reported by Todd *et al.* showing that HLA-DQ alleles with aspartic acid at position 57 of the β chain were associated with decreased susceptibility, protection, or neutral effects. Susceptibility was associated with the presence of an uncharged amino acid at this position; hence HLA-DQβ (non-Asp57) was identified as a significant risk factor. Studies of various racial groups support the concept that one of the strongest gene associations with diabetes is the DQA1*0301-DQB1*0201 combination and having both DR2 and DQB1*0602 confers strong protection (13,14).

The picture is, in fact, even more complex (15). Having an arginine at position 52 of the HLA-DQα molecule (DQα, Arg52) as well as DQβ, non-Asp57 is a combination that results in high genetic risk for type 1 diabetes. Still further data will be required to explain why 10–20% of type 1 diabetic patients do not have the common DQA1-DQB1 high-risk combinations.

Nonetheless, certain gene combinations, particularly of the *cis*- and *trans*-encoded DQ molecules, are associated with susceptibility or protection from diabetes and DQ-determined resistance is dominant over susceptibility. These associations could permit the identification of approximately 2% of the general population who are HLA-DR3 and DR4 (DQw2 and DQw8) heterozygous, with risk as high as 8%, a figure similar to siblings of diabetic patients (3). Strong linkage disequilibrium, which Thors-by & Rønningen (15) define as specific allelic variants often present together on the same chromosomal complex, means that, even if these MHC associations are not *the* actual susceptibility genes, the risk genes are likely to be located in or close to this area (16).

It is only recently that yeast artificial chromosome (YAC) and cosmid clones for the whole of the MHC have been isolated. In this region, there are at least 70–100 other expressed sequences, some of which affect the immune response, including certain complement proteins, cytokines such as tumor necrosis factor (TNF) α and β, and the peptide transporters TAP1 and TAP2 (17). Recent studies of gene polymorphism in this region indicate that two proteins believed to be involved in antigen processing and presentation by class I molecules, large multifunctional protease (LMP) and the transporter associated with antigen processing (TAP), are unlikely to be associated with development of type 1 diabetes, but some controversy exists (16). Genes outside the MHC region may also be important, but less is known about this connection. Non-MHC-region genes such as insulin and insulin-like growth factor 2 may modify susceptibility in DR4 individuals (18).

In the NOD mouse and BBdp rat, the genetics are no less complex than in humans, and several genes predispose these animals to diabetes. The NOD mouse was discovered serendipitously in 1974 in Japan during an inbreeding program established to try to isolate a strain with high cataract development (19). Approximately 80–100% of females and about 20–30% of males become diabetic by 16–20 weeks. Macrophages and mononuclear cells surround and infiltrate the islets (insulitis) beginning at around weaning several weeks before diabetes onset. The MHC haplotype of the NOD mouse, designated H-2g^7, has a unique H-2 (MHC class II) I-A complex, I-A NOD, and I-E expression is lacking. NOD mice have an I-Aβ chain with a serine at position 57 and are therefore "non-Asp57" similar to human type 1 patients who are HLA-DQβ, non-Asp57. However, it should be noted that the diabetogenic I-Aβ of NOD is also present in the Swiss (ICR) mice from which NOD was derived, yet these mice are diabetes resistant.

Including the previously mentioned genes, there are at least eight other genes, designated idd-2 to idd-9, involved in NOD diabetes (2,20). Most of these influence immune reactivity [for example, genes are linked to the IL-1 receptor (idd-5), the Thy1/Alp-1 genes (idd-2), impaired IgG Fc receptor (idd-3), and infection response genes (Lsh/Ity/Bcg)] or they are thought somehow to control the progression of insulitis and diabetes. Another gene that is linked to the Bcl-2 locus outside the MHC region has a role in apoptosis and is involved in insulitis and sialitis (2).

The BBdp rat was discovered in an outbred colony of Wistar rats at the BioBreeding Laboratories near Ottawa, Canada, in 1974 (21). In most colonies, 70% or more of BBdp rats develop insulin-dependent diabetes at between 60 and 120 days of age and mononuclear cells can be seen at the periphery and inside the islets 2–3 weeks prior to overt diabetes. The genetics of the BBdp rat have been extensively studied (22–24), and it appears that the diabetes trait is an autosomal recessive with incomplete penetrance, related to both MHC and non-MHC genes. There are at least three genes required: a class II MHC (DR equivalent), RT1^u, a lymphopenia gene, Lyp, and an as yet uncharacterized gene. The BBdp rat has a serine at position 57 of both class II β chains, RT1.Bβ and RT1.Dβ, in keeping with the "non-Asp" model, but the diabetes resistant BB rat (BBdr), the Lewis rat (RTI^l) and the BUF rat (RT1^b) also have either serine or tryptophan (*i.e.*, non-Asp) at this position. Therefore, the non-Asp residue at position 57 of the class II β chain is probably not a diabetes susceptibility marker in the rat.

Thus in humans, BBdp rats, and NOD mice, there is a requirement for certain diabetes susceptibility MHC haplotypes that are insufficient alone to produce diabetes (Table 1). As suggested by Leiter (37), it is likely that diabetes is the result of several common alleles in the presence of unfavorable conditions. This emphasizes again the fact that not all genetically susceptible individuals will develop diabetes, and there are possibly other diabetes susceptibility genes and non-genetic factors involved.

Prediction

Much progress has been made in the ability to predict who among the first-degree relatives of patients with type 1 diabetes will develop diabetes and when the disease will appear (3,38). There is general agreement that type 1 diabetes is a cell-mediated disease, but the pre-diabetic period is also associated with the appearance of several autoantibodies. In the years since islet cell antibodies were first reported by Bottazzo *et al.* (39), it has become clear that type 1 diabetic patients have autoantibodies to numerous antigens such as glutamic acid decarboxylase (GAD, formerly 64 kDa), a 38 kDa protein, insulin (IAA), proinsulin, carboxypeptidase H, amylin, heat shock proteins, glucose transporter, thymic hormones, thyroid, adrenal cortex, and others (1,2,38). These antibodies can be measured several years before overt diabetes, and they are probably a secondary phenomenon resulting from the progressive destruction of β cells (2). They are nonetheless useful in predicting the course of β-cell destruction and may well provide clues to the nature of the autoantigens that trigger or sustain the autoimmune process.

Attempts to predict who among high-risk subjects will develop diabetes have focused on the presence of certain islet cell antibodies, insulin autoantibody (IAA), anti-GAD (64 kDa), and metabolic signs of β-cell destruction (3,38). Eisenbarth and colleagues have developed a linear regression model in which measurements of competitive insulin autoantibodies and first-phase insulin response to intravenous glucose can predict with a high degree of success when islet cell antibody positive first-degree relatives of patients with type 1 diabetes will themselves become diabetic. At the present time, the tests available to predict diabetes susceptibility are useful in those at high risk, namely first-degree relatives. However, these tests lack the predictive power (4) to use in screening for the 85–90% of patients who do not have a family history of type 1 diabetes. More recent data suggest that measurement of antibodies

TABLE 1. *Characteristics of human, BB rat and NOD mouse diabetes*[a]

	Human	BBdp rat	NOD mouse
Insulin-dependent	Yes	Yes	Yes
Insulitis	Yes	Yes	Yes
Lymphopenia	No	Yes	No
Gender distribution	Equal	Equal	Usually ♀ predominance
Non-MHC genes	Possible[b]	Yes	Yes
MHC susceptibility genes	Yes	Yes	Yes
HLA-DQβ, non-Asp57 or equivalent	Yes	Yes, but also in BBdr	Yes
HLA-DQα, Arg52 or equivalent	Yes	No	No
Viruses ↑ incidence	Some evidence[c] for rubella virus, coxsackie, cytomegalovirus mumps (?)	No evidence of virus involvement in BBdp but Kilham rat virus can cause diabetes in BBdr rats.[d]	Endogenous β cell retrovirus present but role in pathogenesis not known
Viruses ↓ incidence	Not known	LCMV injection protects; gnotobiotic BBdp still get diabetes	LCMV injection protects; immunization with retroviral proteins protects (?)[e]
Other microbial agents	Not known, but role for bacteria proposed[f]	OK 432 (lyophilized streptococcus prep) protects; complete Freund's protects	Injection of complete Freunds's adjuvant protects. BCG injected I.V. protects, as does OK 432.
Diet	Possible connection with early diet[g]; meta-analysis shows significant but weak OR ($<\sim$1.5); cow milk protein (BSA) link proposed[h] but remains controversial.[i]	Major determinant of BBdp diabetes[j]: casein and hydr. casein protect; no effect of high starch, sugars or energy restriction or fat source (except EFA deficiency); wheat, soy, occasionally milk and possibly alfalfa diets are diabetogenic[k,j]	Major determinant of NOD diabetes: casein,[l] hydr. casein[l–n] and high vitamin E[o] diets protect; wheat flour[m] diabetogenic

Hydr, hydrolyzed; LCMV, lymphocytic choriomeningitis virus; BSA, bovine serum albumin; BCG, bacille Calmette-Guérin, attenuated *mycobacterium tuberculosis*; EFA, essential fatty acids

[a] From Rossini et al. (1); Yoon J-W et al. (2); Thai A-C et al. (3); Skyler et al. (4); Scott FW et al. (5).
[b] From Juller C et al. (18)
[c] From Yoon J-W et al. (2); Yoon J-W et al. (25).
[d] From Crisa L et al. (23).
[e] From Yoon J-W et al. (25).
[f] From Morris JA (26).
[g] From Gerstein H (27).
[h] From Karjalainen J et al. (28).
[i] From Atkinson MA et al. (29).
[j] From Scott et al. (30); Hoorfar J et al. (31); Scott FW et al. (32).
[k] From Rossini AA et al. (1).
[l] From Coleman DL et al. (35).
[m] From Hoorfar J et al. (33).
[n] Elliott RB et al. (34).
[o] From Hayward AR et al. (36).

against the β-cell autoantigen, GAD, has greater predictive value in the general population than islet cell antibodies or competitive insulin autoantibodies. Thus, with more relevant autoantibodies [GAD, 38 kDa (?)], better genetic data, and measurements of remaining β-cell function, it may be possible in the near future to predict who in the general population will become diabetic.

This brings up the question of what preventive measures can then be offered to these individuals. Skyler and Marks have reviewed the numerous immunotherapies that have been or are being tried (4). Several of these approaches are relatively nonspecific, of unknown efficacy, and not without risk. They reflect the incompleteness of our current understanding of how the immune system functions as well as the lack of knowledge of gene-environment interaction, particularly the timing of initiation, dose, duration, and frequency of exposure to diabetogenic agents in the environment. It is likely that immune interventions in newly diagnosed type 1 diabetic patients occur too late in the process to spare sufficient β-cell function to provide a lasting cure. For this reason, prevention strategies that avoid initiation or that dampen the early phases of the destructive immune process are most likely to provide long-term success.

NURTURE IDENTIFYING AND CHARACTERIZING ENVIRONMENTAL FACTORS

Indirect Evidence from Human Studies

In human populations, it has been difficult to identify and characterize the environmental factors involved in type 1 diabetes. The well-known studies of identical twins have provided data suggesting that the environment influences expression of type 1 diabetes. For example, Olmos *et al.* (40) reported that about 34% of unaffected identical twins in twin pairs with one type 1 diabetic patient become concordant for the disease. Also, the rate of disease appearance decreased rapidly in co-twins after diagnosis in the index twin, suggesting a process that occurred over a defined period of time. The incidence of the disease peaks at about 15 years in the general population and then declines sharply. Olmos *et al.* suggested that this pattern, combined with a lack of clustering or outbreaks, is consistent with a period of susceptibility to an environmental agent rather than exposure to the agent(s). It has been proposed that the generation of diversity whereby T cell receptor genes and immunoglobulin genes undergo random recombination, making each individual unique with respect to the immune system, could account for the results seen in the twin studies. Indeed, this might be part of the explanation. This same argument might be invoked to justify the involvement of environmental factors (infections, toxins, dietary chemicals) early in life when twins would be likely to be exposed to similar environmental influences. Alternatively, the discordance may reflect different environmental exposures later in life.

Evidence from the twin studies was the seed for epidemiologists to examine the question further. The Diabetes Epidemiology Research International (*DERI*) group adopted a strategy used in cancer research and found several indications that environmental factors are involved in the etiology of type 1 diabetes (9). The gist of the approach was to look at the following five questions. (i) Cancer can be produced in animals by external agents. Type 1 diabetes can also be induced chemically in animals using direct β-cell cytotoxic agents (alloxan, a single high dose of streptozotocin or other toxin) or multiple low doses of streptozotocin. Oral ingestion of the rodenticide, Vacor®, in humans also produced type 1 diabetes. (ii) There are geographic differences in cancer incidence. There is also marked geographic variation in type 1 diabetes incidence ranging from 0.5/100,000 in China to >35/100,000 in Finland. (iii) Rapid changes in cancer incidence have occurred that are not due to genetic change. For type 1 diabetes, the incidence has also increased in several countries, epidemics have been reported, and hot (Sardinia) and cold (Macedonia) spots have been identified. (iv) Migrants adopt the cancer risk of their new home. There is some limited evidence to suggest that this also occurs in the development of type 1 diabetes in Japanese moving to Hawaii as well as in Canadians of Jewish and French descent living in Montreal. (v) Environmental agents such as smoking, alcohol consumption, and asbestos cause cancers. Reliable epidemiologic data are difficult to obtain because, if available at all, they are mostly retrospective, and long-term prospective data on individuals who become diabetic are simply not available. Ideally, a sufficiently large prospective study would be carried out in individuals from birth to about 20 years of age in various populations with different risk levels to begin to ascertain the true interaction of genetic and environmental factors.

It is likely that the next few years will see even greater advances in characterizing the diabetes genes and the natural history of the disease. However, prevention is always preferable to cure, and the area with greatest potential for safe and cost-effective prevention is the modification of exposure to environmental factors.

Trying to identify nongenetic factors that might trigger or promote the process that leads to diabetes is exceedingly difficult in humans. Therefore information on environmental agents is very often indirect or comes from studies in susceptible animals. The main environmental factors considered in the etiology of type 1 diabetes have been chemical toxins, stress, diet, and infectious agents, mostly viruses.

Chemical Toxins and Stress

There are many chemical agents that can cause cytotoxic effects in β cells, and some also have effects on the immune system: alloxan, streptozotocin, Vacor® (N-3-pyridylmethyl-N'-P-nitrophenyl urea), chlorozotocin, cyproheptadine, pentamidine, cyclosporin, and others. These have been reviewed in detail elsewhere (41,42) and will not be considered further here. There is at least one study in BBdp rats that showed that diabetes-prone animals submitted to "multiple, concurrent and unpredictable" environmental stresses such as restraint, rotation, crowding, and random cage reassignment developed diabetes sooner than animals kept under normal conditions; the final diabetes incidence was not significantly different from the control group (43). The link between the neurochemical, endocrine and immune networks is only just beginning to be understood and may yet prove to be important in the development of type 1 diabetes.

Viruses

Viruses have been implicated in diabetes pathogenesis since the report by Harris nearly 100 years ago of a case in which mumps preceded the onset of type 1 diabetes [cited in (44)]. Since that time there have been many anecdotal reports of viral infection preceding the onset of diabetes. Mumps has often been implicated, as have rubella, cytomegalovirus, polio, measles, influenza, and tick-borne encephalitis (44). The viruses most often implicated are rubella and coxsackie B4. Congenital rubella syndrome is a unique and important example of an association between a viral infection followed by development of autoimmune diabetes in humans (25,45). Approximately 20% of these patients developed diabetes, with a latency period of between 5 and 20 years. The patients who became diabetic were more likely to be HLA-DR3, and DR2 was less frequent in this group. The mechanism of this interaction is not known.

Epidemiological studies have implicated coxsackie B4 virus in some cases of type 1 diabetes. It has been shown that this virus can infect and destroy β cells in Patas monkeys. A variant of coxsackie virus isolated from a young diabetic patient who died produced diabetes when inoculated into SJL/J mice but not in CBA/J, C57BL/6J or BALB/c mice (25).

More recently, Yoon has categorized the diabetogenic potential of viruses as follows: (i) *triggering agents for β cell autoimmunity:* retrovirus, rubella, cytomegalovirus, reovirus, mumps virus, and parvovirus (Kilham's rat virus, KRV); (ii) *cytolytic infection of β cells:* encephalomyocarditis (EMC) virus, mengovirus, and coxsackie B viruses; and (iii) *viruses protective against development of type 1 diabetes:* both NOD mice and BBdp rats can be protected from developing autoimmune diabetes by inoculation early in life with lymphocytic choriomeningitis virus (LCMV). Also, the diabetes that follows injection of diabetogenic EMC virus in susceptible mice can be prevented by live attenuated vaccine or immunization with a nondiabetogenic EMC virus.

It was pointed out that it is exceedingly difficult to show *in vivo* that viruses infect and destroy β cells, producing diabetes in humans. Nonetheless, there is indirect evidence in humans (congenital rubella syndrome) and direct evidence in animals (coxsackie B4 inoculation into susceptible SJL/J mice and Patas monkeys) that viruses can in some circumstances result in diabetes. Viruses such as the Kilham rat virus can cause diabetes in BBdr rats, but there is no evidence that viruses play a role in autoimmune-mediated diabetes in the BBdp rat (23). By contrast, the NOD mouse may contain an endogenous retrovirus, and there is speculation that this could lead to expression of viral antigen on the β-cell surface or alter expression of cellular genes (25). The role of viruses in the etiology of type 1 diabetes and the proposed mechanisms of action have been reviewed in detail recently (1,2,25).

Dietary Factors

The concept that diet might affect development of diabetes can be traced at least as far back as the 1930s to the studies of Himsworth and colleagues (46). Unfortunately, the problem with studies up until about 1981 was that individuals under 16 years in the case of Himsworth's study and those under 30 years of age in West's study (47) were excluded and adequate differentiation between type 1 and type 2 diabetes was lacking. These caveats meant that the early work was of little value in looking at diet and the development of type 1 diabetes.

Willett has pointed out that nutritional epidemiology is anything but simple because diet is not a single variable and very few dietary components can be described as simply present or absent (48). Obtaining representative food intake values for individual children is difficult, and several studies have shown that information provided by children is often less reliable than that from adults. Most often data are collected retrospectively and are not representative of the individual's usual intake. The quality of data obtained retrospectively is always open to question. An example was recently given by Kostraba (49) to illustrate the pitfalls of relying solely on retrospective case-control studies. In the long debate over the role of cow's milk in atopic allergy, case-control studies were able to detect the protective effect of exclusive breastfeeding, but it was not recognized until prospectively collected data were analyzed that the benefits of breastfeeding were attributable to avoidance of food antigens rather than benefits due to breast milk *per se*. This example highlights only a few of the difficulties in linking dietary intake to disease development (48).

For these reasons, much of the work linking diet and type 1 diabetes has been carried out in the BBdp rat and NOD mouse. In fact it was not until the availability of these spontaneous models that the first experimental evidence of an effect of diet on autoimmune type 1 diabetes was shown (50). Interest in dietary modification of autoimmunity dates from the work in the early 1970s on energy restriction in the systemic lupus erythematosus (SLE)-prone, (NZB $\times$ NZW)F_1 mouse. Most of the diet manipulations tried in this model of multisystem autoimmune disease have involved single nutrient and energy modification. By contrast, the work in the models of organ-specific autoimmunity, the BBdp rat and NOD mouse, has focused mainly on foods and food components (5).

The initial findings in the BBdp rat showed that semipurified AIN-76A diets based on cow's milk casein as the protein source, starch or starch/sucrose as the carbohydrate, corn oil as the fat source, plus cellulose as a source of "fiber," and supplemented with micronutrients, completely inhibited the expression of diabetes. The phenomenon is quite marked. Laboratory rodent diets such as Purina 5001 or NIH-07 contain a kaleidoscope of chemicals derived mainly from plant protein sources, and feeding these mixtures routinely results in a diabetes frequency of about 68% (n = 7 experiments) in BBdp rats by 130–150 days of age. However, several protein sources are not diabetogenic. Feeding diets containing casein, hydrolyzed casein, fish meal, canola flour, corn (or others) as the protein sources markedly inhibits the development of diabetes. We use two negative control, diabetes retardant, diets based on casein or hydrolyzed casein as the amino acid source. The diabetes frequency in BBdp rats fed casein-based diets is about 9% (n = 7 experiments) and hydrolyzed casein diets produced approximately 12% diabetes frequency (n = 7 experiments). The marked effect of various diets on insulitis and diabetes frequency is shown in Fig. 1.

The protective effect of semipurified diets containing diabetes-retardant protein sources is equally apparent if the test animals are fed from weaning at about 23 days or if the dams are also fed the diets when the pups are suckling. In fact, the diabetogenic effect of NIH-07 is still apparent if feeding this diet is delayed to 50 days and a non-diabetogenic diet is fed from weaning to 50 days. The only effect is to delay age at onset by 3–4 weeks; the rate of disease appearance and the final diabetes incidence remain unchanged. This suggests that the timing of the diet-diabetes interaction extends over a long period, reaching into what would be early puberty for the rat.

Other studies showed that semipurified (casein-based) diets high in sucrose or starch (β-cell stimulation as opposed to β-cell rest) were diabetes retardant, and changing the fat source from 5–20% corn oil or 20% lard did not increase diabetes frequency above background. Qualitative and quantitative studies of numerous protein sources confirmed that the protein source determined the diabetes outcome (31,51). When all the major components of the diabetogenic NIH-07 diet were tested individually, it was clear that wheat gluten and soybean meal were diabetogenic. Tests of cow's milk protein diets containing various amounts of casein and whey proteins showed that whey protein diets had a variable diabetes-inducing potential and were, with two or three exceptions, diabetes retardant or only mildly diabetogenic. A diet with large amounts of alfalfa seeds was moderately diabetogenic.

Others have also shown that casein (35) and hydrolyzed casein-based diets (33–35) inhibit diabetes development in NOD mice, but skim-milk-based diets were not diabetogenic (35). A recent study confirmed the observation that hydrolyzed casein inhibits the development of diabetes in NOD mice and also showed that a wheat flour diet produced a diabetes frequency of 60%, while soybean meal diets resulted in a 45% diabetes frequency (33). These results support our findings in the BBdp rat and suggest that characterizing plant food diabetogens may provide a way of modifying some of the key environmental factors in the etiology of type 1 diabetes. We believe that it should be feasible to identify and characterize foods that contain autoimmunogens (agents that trigger a process resulting in inappropriate immune response against one's own tissues) with the aim of expanding food-oriented interventions along with studies of individual diet components. The identification and characterization of food

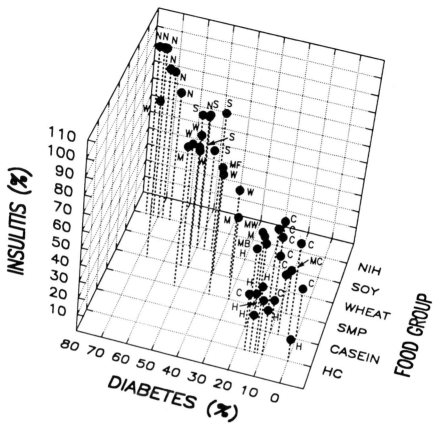

FIG. 1. Modification of insulitis and diabetes frequency by different foods and food components. BBdp rats were fed a standard laboratory rodent diet, NIH-07, or modified AIN-76A diets as described previously (31) from weaning usually to ~150 days of age and sometimes up to 240 days. Animals were considered diabetic if urine glucose was >2+ using Testape, fasting blood glucose was >200 mg/dl (11.1 mmol/liter), or if weight loss or failure to gain weight was observed. These rats were killed within 24 hours of diagnosis by exsanguination while under light anesthesia (3–5% halothane or isoflurane in O_2); degree of islet inflammation and damage was assessed as previously described. [From Hoorfar J *et al.* (31)] Each symbol represents a separate group of rats (n = 10–60/group). Various diets were assigned to Food Groups as follows: NIH = NIH-07 [N], an open formula diet (known % composition) that is highly diabetogenic and served as positive control; SOY, soybean meal, flakes, or flour [S]-based diets in which all amino acids were supplied from these materials; WHEAT, wheat gluten [W], the protein concentrate from wheat flour following water extraction, 80% protein, supplied all protein and was supplemented with certain amino acids; SMP, skim milk powder or other cow milk protein containing diet [M, SMP-based, MW, milk whey (10%) + casein (10%), MB, casein + 0.1% BSA (equivalent to amounts found in normal laboratory diets), MC, cow colostrum (8%) + hydrolysed casein, MF, cow's milk-based infant formula]; CASEIN, 20% casein based AIN-76A diet [C] which was consistently diabetes retardant; HC, hydrolyzed casein based [HC] diabetes-retardant diet.

autoimmunogens or immunomodulatory foods, as distinct from single nutrient modifications, is a relatively recent phenomenon and may prove useful in the prevention of diabetes and other autoimmune diseases.

If the food diabetogens can be characterized, it might even be possible to provide advice about diabetogenic or protective foods without the necessity of screening the general population. Conceivably, it should be possible to engineer diabetogen-free plant foods.

Diet is a major factor in the etiology of autoimmune diabetes in the BBdp rat and NOD mouse. The nature of the protein source is important: laboratory rodent diets, which are commonly plant based (for example, NIH-07 has 83% plant material), usually result in a diabetes incidence of about 68% in BBdp rats and 70–100% in female NOD mice. We see a dose response to NIH-07 diet, suggesting that there are food diabetogens in this diet mixture.

In our BBdp rats, nutritionally adequate diets, in which wheat gluten (80% protein) or soybean meal (52% protein) are the sole dietary protein sources, result in a diabetes frequency of around 50%. This level of diabetes is significantly higher than either of our negative control diets that are casein or hydrolyzed casein based and produce a diabetes incidence of 9–12%.

The low rates of diabetes observed in animals fed the control diets may be the true baseline or natural rates of the disease in these animals. Recall that when the BBdp rat was first discovered in 1974, the rate of diabetes was 10% (21). The difference between these rates and the diabetes frequency of 68% seen in BBdp rats fed NIH-07 (or other plant-based laboratory diets such as Purina 5001) represents diet-inducible diabetes in the BBdp rat, that is, about 86% of their diabetes is due to dietary factors.

The Cow Milk Protein Hypothesis

Much excitement has been generated concerning the possibility that a 17 amino acid peptide called ABBOS (a peptide sequence from bovine albumin that differed from the corresponding region of human, rat, and mouse albumin) might trigger the autoimmune process that causes type 1 diabetes (28). The basic hypothesis suggests that there could be an immune response against the ABBOS peptide resulting in cross reaction to a 69 kDa protein (ICA69, purported to contain a peptide fragment homologous to part of ABBOS) on the β-cell surface. Karjalainen et al. (28) reported that 100% of newly diagnosed children with diabetes had raised levels of IgG bovine serum albumin (BSA) antibodies. A polyclonal rat anti-ABBOS serum reacted against the ICA69 islet protein and other smaller proteins in liver, muscle, and heart. The authors concluded that their finding of the ubiquitous presence of anti-BSA antibodies in newly diagnosed type 1 diabetic children and the cross reactivity with ICA69 might somehow, in concert with recurring infections in the prediabetic period, be part of the process that destroys β cells.

This intriguing study caused much heightened interest and concern that there might be a link between dietary bovine serum albumin and type 1 diabetes. Atkinson *et al.* (29), using some of the same techniques as the previous group, measured BSA antibodies and the response of peripheral blood mononuclear cells from newly diagnosed type 1 diabetic patients, people at varying degrees of risk for diabetes (islet cell antibody positive or negative first-degree relatives), and people with other autoimmune diseases such as thyroiditis, rheumatoid arthritis, or systemic lupus erythematosus. They found only 10% of newly diagnosed diabetic patients were BSA antibody positive and this was not significantly different from control subjects. Hardly any of their subjects showed increased incorporation of labeled thymidine in the presence of ABBOS or BSA. Findings were similar in islet cell antibody positive or negative first-degree relatives, showing no association between islet cell antibody positivity and cellular response to BSA or BSA antibodies. However, they did find that BSA antibodies were more common in relatives of type 1 diabetic patients (nine out of 42 were BSA antibody positive) and in patients with thyroiditis. They concluded that BSA antibodies may reflect a defect in immunological tolerance associated with susceptibility to autoimmune disease. That only 10% of their newly diagnosed type 1 diabetic patients were BSA antibody positive compared with the 100% found by Karjalainen *et al.* and the absence of a cellular immune response to BSA or ABBOS, does not support a role for BSA in the development of type 1 diabetes.

Another group proposed a similar hypothesis in rheumatoid arthritis, invoking reactivity against an overlapping but nonidentical BSA peptide close to ABBOS (52). This peptide showed high homology with vitamin D binding protein, human collagen type I, and complement component C1q. They reported that some rheumatoid arthritis patients have high titers of BSA antibodies. This is in keeping with the finding of Atkinson *et al.* suggesting that oral tolerance may be abnormal in people prone to autoimmune diseases. It also suggests, perhaps not surprisingly, that protein homologies are either more common than previously thought or that there is greater access to protein databases.

In NOD mice, Coleman *et al.* found that an AIN-76A diet with an additional 10% skim milk powder was not diabetogenic (35). Leiter reported that anti-BSA antibodies were not present in NOD mice fed a highly diabetogenic diet based largely on wheat, and there was no correlation between an immune response to BSA and diabetogenesis (53). Our data in the BBdp rat suggest that BSA antibodies are not predictive of diabetes and the antibodies do not occur in all rats. Similarly, feeding studies with semipurified diets indicate that various BSA-containing diets are only occasionally diabetogenic and there is no correlation between daily dose of dietary BSA and diabetes frequency. It is not clear why milk protein diets should produce this variability.

These data suggest that a role for BSA in the pathogenesis of diabetes is at the very least controversial. Considering these concerns and the complete absence of data in humans on the required time of introduction, duration, and chemical identity of food diabetogens, it is premature to consider using the cow's milk hypothesis as the basis of an intervention trial. It is clear, however, that diet has major effects in the development of diabetes in the BBdp rat and NOD mouse. Identifying and characterizing food diabetogens could lead to safe and effective means of primary prevention of this disease in susceptible humans.

REFERENCES

1. Rossini AA, Greiner DL, Friedman HP, Mordes JP. Immunopathogenesis of diabetes mellitus. *Diabetes Rev* 1993; 1: 43–75.
2. Yoon J-W, Park YH, Santamaria P. Autoimmunity of Type 1 diabetes. In: Flatt PR, Ionnides C, eds. *Drugs, diet and disease*, vol 2. *Mechanistic approaches to diabetes*. London: Ellis Horwood, 1994 (in press).
3. Thai A-C, Eisenbarth GS. Natural history of Type I diabetes. *Diabetes Rev* 1993; 1: 1–14.
4. Skyler JS, Marks JB. Immune intervention in type I diabetes mellitus. *Diabetes Rev* 1993; 1: 15–42.
5. Scott FW, Cui J, Rowsell P. The role of food in autoimmunity. *Trends Food Sci Technol* 1994; 5: 111–6.
6. Gorsuch AN, Spencer KM, Lister J, McNally JM, Dean BM, Bottazzo GF. Evidence for a long prediabetic period in type I (insulin-dependent) diabetes mellitus. *Lancet* 1981; ii: 1363–4.
7. Moy CS. *Diabetes 1993. Vital statistics*. Alexandria, VA: American Diabetes Association, 1994.
8. Kocova M, Trucco M, Konstantinova M, Dorman JS. A cold spot of Type I diabetes in Europe. *Diabetes Care* 1993; 16: 1236–40.
9. LaPorte RE, Dorman JS, Orchard TJ *et al.* and the Diabetes Epidemiology Research International Group. Preventing insulin-dependent diabetes mellitus: the environmental challenge. *BMJ* 1987; 295: 479–81.
10. Dokheel TM, for the DERI Group. An epidemic of childhood diabetes in the United States? *Diabetes Care* 1993; 16: 1606–11.
11. Cahill GF, McDevitt HO. Insulin-dependent diabetes: the initial lesion. *N Engl J Med* 1981; 304: 1454–65.
12. Sinha AA, Lopez MT, McDevitt HO. Autoimmune diseases: the failure of tolerance. *Science* 1990; 248: 1380–8.
13. Todd JA, Bell JI, McDevitt HO. HLA-DQβ gene contributes to susceptibility and resistance to insulin-dependent diabetes mellitus. *Nature* 1987; 329: 599–604.
14. Todd JA. The emperor's new genes. The 1993 R D Lawrence lecture. *Diabetic Med* 1994; 11: 6–16.
15. Thorsby E, Rønningen KS. Particular HLA-DQ molecules play a dominant role in determining susceptibility or resistance to Type 1 (insulin-dependent) diabetes mellitus. *Diabetologia* 1993; 36: 371–7.
16. Van Endert PM, Liblau RS, Patel SD, *et al.* Major histocompatibility complex-encoded antigen processing gene polymorphism in Type I diabetes. *Diabetes* 1994; 43: 110–7.
17. Campbell RD, Milner CM. MHC genes in autoimmunity. *Curr Opin Immunol* 1993; 5: 887–93.
18. Julier C, Hyer RN, Davies J, *et al.* Insulin-IGF2 region on chromosome 11P encodes a gene implicated in HLA-DR4-dependent diabetes susceptibility. *Nature* 1991; 354: 155–9.
19. Leiter EH, Serreze DV, Prochazka M. The genetics and epidemiology of diabetes in NOD mice. *Immunol Today* 1990; 11: 147–9.
20. Todd JA, Aitman TJ, Cornall RJ, *et al.* Genetic analysis of autoimmune Type 1 diabetes mellitus in mice. *Nature* 1991; 351: 542–7.
21. Marliss EB, ed. The Juvenile Diabetes Foundation Workshop on the Spontaneously Diabetic BB rat: its potential for insight into human juvenile diabetes. *Metab Clin Exp* 1983; 32 (suppl. 1): 1–166.
22. Colle E. Genetic susceptibility to the development of spontaneous insulin-dependent diabetes mellitus in the rat. *Clin Immunol Immunopathol* 1990; 57: 1–9.
23. Crisa L, Mordes JP, Rossini AA. Autoimmune diabetes mellitus in the BB rat. *Diabetes Metab Rev* 1992; 8: 9–37.
24. Jacob HJ, Pettersson A, Wilson D, Mao Y, Lernmark Å, Lander ES. Genetic dissection of autoimmune type I diabetes in the BB rat. *Nature Genet* 1992; 2: 56–60.
25. Yoon J-W, Park YH. Viruses as triggering agents of insulin-dependent diabetes mellitus. In: Leslie RDG, ed. *Causes of diabetes*. London: John Wiley, 1993: 83–103.
26. Morris JA. A possible role for bacteria in the pathogenesis of insulin dependent diabetes mellitus. *Med Hypoth* 1989; 29: 231–5.
27. Gerstein H. Cow's milk exposure and type I diabetes mellitus. *Diabetes Care* 1994; 17: 13–9.

28. Karjalainen J, Martin JM, Knip M, *et al.* A bovine albumin peptide as a possible trigger of insulin-dependent diabetes mellitus. *N Engl J Med* 1992; 327: 302–7.
29. Atkinson MA, Bowman MA, Kao K-J, *et al.* Lack of immune responsiveness to bovine serum albumin in insulin-dependent diabetes. *N Engl J Med* 1993; 329: 1853–8.
30. Scott FW, Marliss EB. Conference summary: Diet as an environmental factor in development of Type I diabetes mellitus. *Can J Physiol Pharmacol* 1991; 69: 311–9.
31. Hoorfar J, Scott FW, Cloutier HE. Dietary plant materials and development of diabetes in the BB rat. *J Nutr* 1991; 121: 908–16.
32. Scott FW, Elliott RB, Kolb H. Diet and autoimmunity: prospects of prevention of type 1 diabetes. *Diabetes Nutr Metab* 1989; 2: 61–73.
33. Hoorfar J, Buschard K, Dagnaes-Hansen F. Prophylactic nutritional modification of the incidence of diabetes in autoimmune non-obese diabetic (NOD) mice. *Br J Nutr* 1993; 69: 597–607.
34. Elliott RB, Reddy SN, Bibby NJ, Kida K. Dietary prevention of diabetes in the non-obese diabetic mouse. *Diabetologia* 1988; 31: 62–4.
35. Coleman DL, Kuzawa JE, Leiter EH. Effect of diet on incidence of diabetes in non-obese diabetic mice. *Diabetes* 1990; 39: 432–6.
36. Hayward AR, Shriber M, Sokol R. Vitamin E supplementation reduces the incidence of diabetes but not insulitis in NOD mice. *J Lab Clin Med* 1992; 119: 503–7.
37. Leiter EH. The NOD mouse meets the "Nerup hypothesis": is diabetogenesis the result of a collection of common alleles present in unfavorable combinations? In: *Frontiers in diabetes research. Lessons from animal diabetes III.* London: Smith-Gordon, 1990: 54–8.
38. Palmer JP. Predicting type I diabetes mellitus: use of humoral immune markers. *Diabetes Rev* 1993; 1: 104–15.
39. Bottazzo GF, Florin-Christensen A, Doniach A. Islet cell antibodies in diabetes mellitus with autoimmune polyendocrine deficiencies. *Lancet* 1974; ii: 1279–83.
40. Olmos P, A'Hern R, Heaton DA, *et al.* The significance of the concordance rate for Type I (insulin-dependent) diabetes in identical twins. *Diabetologia* 1988; 31: 747–50.
41. Wilson GL, LeDoux SP. The role of chemicals in the etiology of diabetes mellitus. *Toxicol Pathol* 1989; 17: 357–63.
42. Yoon J-W, Kim CJ, Pak CY, McArthur RG. Effects of environmental factors on the development of insulin-dependent diabetes mellitus. *Clin Invest Med* 1987; 10: 457–69.
43. Carter WR, Herrman J, Stokes K, Cox DJ. Promotion of diabetes onset by stress in the BB rat. *Diabetologia* 1987; 30: 674–5.
44. Notkins AL. Virus-induced diabetes mellitus, brief review. In: Podolsky S, Viswanathan M, eds. *Secondary diabetes: the spectrum of the diabetic syndromes.* New York: Raven Press, 1980: 471–86.
45. Menser MA, Forrest JM, Bransby RD. Rubella infection and diabetes mellitus. *Lancet* 1978; i: 57–60.
46. Himsworth HP, Marshall EM. The diet of diabetics prior to the onset of the disease. *Clin Sci* 1935; 2: 95–115.
47. West KM, Kalbfleisch JM. Influence of nutritional factors on prevalence of diabetes. *Diabetes* 1971; 20: 99–108.
48. Willett W. Nutritional epidemiology: issues and challenges. *Int J Epidemiol* 1987; 16: 312–7.
49. Kostraba JN. What can epidemiology tell us about the role of infant diet in the etiology of IDDM? *Diabetes Care* 1994; 17: 87–91.
50. Scott FW, Trick KD. Dietary modification of spontaneous diabetes in the BB Wistar rat. *Proc Can Fed Biol Soc* 1987; 26: 222.
51. Scott FW, Sarwar G, Cloutier HE. Diabetogenicity of various protein sources in the diet of the BB rat. In: Camerini-Davalos RA, Cole HS, eds. *Prediabetes.* New York: Plenum Press, 1988: 277–85.
52. Pérez-Maceda B, López-Bote JP, Langa C, Bernabeu C. Antibodies to dietary antigens in rheumatoid arthritis—possible molecular mimicry mechanism. *Clin Chim Acta* 1991; 203: 153–65.
53. Leiter EH. The role of environmental factors in modulating insulin-dependent diabetes. In: DeVries RRP, Cohen IR, Van Rood JJ, eds. *The role of micro-organisms in non-infectious diseases.* London: Springer Verlag, 1990: 39–55.

DISCUSSION

Dr. Dakou: The child who is breastfed has a different environment in an early and very critical period. Do you think this may be important?

Dr. Scott: Of the 16 or so published case-controlled studies, about half find a link between breastfeeding and type 1 diabetes. Some find no link. In two of the studies in which there are what we might call prospective data, nurses went into the home and wrote down how the infant was being fed. From those studies there was no relationship between early exposure to cow's milk or breastfeeding and the development of diabetes. I think one of the difficulties here is that we are trying to simplify what is really a very complex relationship. The infant is also weaned onto different foods in different cultures and at different ages and these weaning foods could also be important.

Dr. Otten: I am one of those who found a protective effect of breastfeeding. Could you tell us what you fed your rats before you did your nutritional studies.

Dr. Scott: We fed the animals protective casein or hydrolyzed casein-based diets or the diabetogenic, cereal-based laboratory diets (1). The nature of the pre-weaning diet did not change diabetes outcome. We can expose animals as late as 50 days and they still get diabetes. This is a key point. If we find the effect this late in animals, it suggests that the exposure need not occur only in early infancy; later sustained exposure may also be important.

Dr. Guesry: I completely agree with Dr. Scott when he says that the issue about the importance of breastfeeding is very complex. If we draw a parallel between the development of IDDM and the development of cow's milk allergy in infants at risk of developing allergy, we know that breastfeeding can partially suppress sensitization to cow's milk in the infant. There is a reduction of about 50%, but not a total suppression. We also know that lactating mothers secrete heterologous proteins in their milk, I mean protein from other origins, either animal or vegetal. For example in Finland, I am sure that mothers secrete reindeer milk protein in their milk, and in Sardinia they probably secrete goat's milk protein. Since we also know that goat's milk and cow's milk share about half the same antigens, I am very surprised when I hear that there is a direct correlation between switching from goat's milk to cow's milk and the likelihood of developing IDDM.

Dr. Assan: How early after birth did you give the bovine protein? Many things are currently said about induction of oral immune tolerance, but I understand the earlier the better.

Dr. Scott: In the experiment that I showed you, the animals were tolerized at around 40–45 days. The point you raise is important. In an attempt at earlier exposure to dietary constituents, we orally dosed control and diabetes-prone animals between days 4 and 7 with Pregestimil[R], which is based on hydrolyzed casein as a protein source (in other words it is not diabetogenic), and with the complex diabetogenic mixture (NIH-07), and then, at weaning, the animals were weaned to either the hydrolyzed casein diet or the NIH-07 diet—that is, the nondiabetogenic or the diabetogenic diet. When we first exposed the animals to a nondiabetogenic hydrolyzed protein material for 4–7 days in infancy and then weaned them to a nondiabetogenic diet, none of the seven animals became diabetic up to 140 days. In the positive control, the animals were dosed with hydrolyzed casein and then weaned to NIH-07; in this case 60% of them became diabetic. However, when we exposed the animals early to NIH-07 orally and then weaned them to the same material, 12.5% of them became diabetic. This experiment indicates that there could be a possibility of tolerizing animals early on to this dietary mixture and preventing disease, but it needs to be repeated.

Dr. Beauvais: So far as breastfeeding is concerned, we have many people in our population who come from Algeria and Morocco—they represent 15% of our population, and 50% of our cases of diabetes. However, all these patients have been breastfed until the age of 9 months.

Dr. Drash: Is it the absence of human breast milk or the negative effect of the cow's milk protein that is harmful? As pediatricians, we praise the mother for all the wonderful things she gives her baby through breastfeeding, but my reading of the literature suggests that it is not the positive effect of human breast milk but the presence of a negative factor in cow's milk protein that may be diabetogenic.

Dr. Scott: I have some difficulty with the human literature. I think the studies are very difficult to interpret. As I said, the only two where there are prospective data do not really support the hypothesis well. One of the key things that has not been addressed is the timing of the interaction between diet and genetic susceptibility. We also do not know whether it is only the first 6 or 9 months of life that are important or whether it could be the first 10 years.

Dr. Drash: But isn't it truly amazing that those studies suggest that cow's milk protein is a factor when we are dealing with a population in which only a small number of children are genetically susceptible? The only way to get the answer, it seems to me, is to focus a careful study on individuals who are identified as being at genetic risk.

Dr. Scott: As I said, the difficulty I have is that most of the data are retrospective and contradictory. The milk hypothesis based on BSA is controversial. If the evidence were more convincing, one would be more encouraged to follow it up. It is also a problem that we know so little about the timing.

Dr. Carrascosa: Overproduction of free radicals has been implicated in the damage to the β cells. What do you think about this possibility? Do you think that overproduction of free radicals could be a common type of nutritional and environmental influence in the progressive destruction of the β cell?

Dr. Scott: We get back to the comment I have been making about nutritional epidemiology. I have some experience with this because colleagues have been doing dietary surveys in Canada. The available information is not extensive. It gives no real indication of free radical content and indeed it would be virtually impossible to obtain this. Not only that, but if you are looking at antioxidants in the diet you are only looking at one side of the story because we are dealing with a very complex system of protective and damaging components.

Dr. Crofford: Most of us here understand the difference between epidemiologic studies in humans that can point out the associations between variables (and are so important in the formulation of hypothesis) and the randomized intervention trials that are necessary in order to establish the validity of these hypotheses. Unfortunately this distinction is not well understood by the general population and, even worse, it is not well understood by the people who write for the general population by interpreting scientific literature. Often this leads to overinterpretation of these epidemiologic experiments, and the public believes that causality has been established. This can result in panic or in people making unwise health decisions. So I think it is always worth pointing out that we, as scientists, have a very profound responsibility to emphasize over and over again the fact that the associative studies do not necessarily establish causality, and to try to minimize the overinterpretation of such studies, as happens so often in the press and on television.

Dr. Bergman: I am curious to know what one can do to protect against the possible effect of changes in diet that may lead to changes in the need for insulin secretion, thus possibly contributing to diabetes as an end point. If you change the composition of the diet, how do you control for the possibility that the animal is more or less sensitive to insulin, and therefore that there is more or less stress on the pancreas, leading to earlier or later onset of diabetes?

Dr. Scott: This is a difficult problem to approach. What I can say is that we have tested dozens of diets and have categorized them as to their diabetogenic potential; in many cases what we have done is to substitute what we consider to be very similar protein sources, and when we measure the insulin levels we find they are similar. I think what you are talking about relates also to the concept of β-cell rest or stressing the β cell, which then produces more antigens on the surface.

Dr. Marliss: Several people have tried more or less successfully to bridge the metabolism-immunology gap. Buschard *et al.* very successfully demonstrated a decrease in diabetes incidence with exogenous insulin treatment (2), and this has been confirmed by others (3). This has led to current trials that may run into problems because of the difficulty in predicting who is actually going to get type 1 diabetes among humans. However, from the results of various other experiments, it is entirely predictable that if, for one reason or another, individuals susceptible to type 1 diabetes have a need to secrete more insulin to achieve their metabolic goals, these individuals will ultimately be more susceptible to the development of diabetes; this is likely to be one of those extremely difficult variables to control in any dietary type of study. There are several ways of approaching the problem, but if one uses either C-peptide secretion or excretion of C-peptide in urine it would appear that as much as 80% of the total amount of insulin that will be secreted in a day is secreted in relation to meals; thus one would anticipate that anything that is ingested in a meal that is capable of being an insulin secretogogue may well play a role in the etiology of diabetes, and it may play this role over a very prolonged period of time.

REFERENCES

1. Scott F. Food, diabetes and immunology. In: Forse RA *et al.* eds. *Diet, nutrition and immunity.* Boca Raton, FL: CRC Press, 1994: 73–95.
2. Gotfredsen CF, Buschard K, Frandsen EK. Reduction of diabetes incidence of BB Wister rats by early prophylactic insulin treatment of diabetes-prone animals. *Diabetologia* 1985; 28: 933–5.
3. Vlahos WD, Seemayor TA, and Yale JF. Diabetes prevention in BB rats by inhibition of endogenous insulin secretion. *Metabolism* 1991; 40: 825–9.

Diabetes, edited by Richard M. Cowett,
Nestlé Nutrition Workshop Series,
Vol. 35. Nestec Ltd.,
Vevey/Raven Press, Ltd., New York © 1995.

On the Pathogenesis of Insulin-Dependent Diabetes Mellitus (IDDM): Advances in Defining Immune Markers for Accurate Prediction of the Disease

Gian Franco Bottazzo, Vincenzo Sepe, Manuelita Lai,
*Stefano Genovese, *Ezio Bonifacio and *Emanuele Bosi

*The Department of Immunology, The London Hospital Medical College, Turner Street,
London E1 2AD, UK; and *Department of Internal Medicine, Instituto Scientifico San
Raffaele, Via Olgettina, 60, 20132 Milan, Italy*

EVIDENCE IN FAVOR OF AN AUTOIMMUNE PATHOGENESIS OF INSULIN-DEPENDENT DIABETES MELLITUS

There is general agreement that insulin-dependent diabetes mellitus (IDDM) is an autoimmune disease (reviewed in 1–7). Evidence supporting this concept includes selective lymphocytic infiltration in and around affected islets (that is, insulitis) at the time of diagnosis (8); detection of islet-specific autoantibodies (9), and of sensitized (10) and activated (11) lymphocytes; variation in the numbers of these cells present in the circulation of affected individuals (reviewed in 6); association with certain human leucocyte antigen (HLA) alleles (reviewed in 12); and frequently the concomitant presence of other organ-specific autoimmune manifestations, either in the patients or in their family members (13). Further support for the concept comes when one compares similarities between the human disease and the known spontaneous animal models of autoimmune diabetes (reviewed in 14,15), when one observes prolongation of β-cell survival after immunosuppression (16,17), or when one detects recurrence of lymphocytic insulitis in pancreases transplanted among identical twins or HLA-matched siblings, where the proband suffered from IDDM but the donor did not (18,19; reviewed in 20).

The factors that induce and sustain this autoimmune process are unknown, but most likely include an interaction between environmental agents and genetic susceptibility. Regardless of the mechanisms leading to the autoimmune process, considerable advances have been achieved in identifying the antigen targets of the autoimmune attack. Identification and characterization of the autoantigens in IDDM is of fundamental importance for accurate prediction of the disease and for potentially specific (that is, antigen-driven) immunotherapeutic intervention.

ISLET-RELATED ANTIBODIES AND OTHER AUTOANTIBODIES

Cytoplasmic Islet Cell Antibodies

Cytoplasmic islet cell antibodies (ICA) were first described in 1974 in IDDM patients who had other coexistent autoimmune disorders (9) and, subsequently, in up to 90% of newly diagnosed IDDM patients, with or without associated autoimmunities (21–23). They are usually detected in fewer than 3% of individuals in control populations (23). Islet cell antibodies are measured by indirect immunofluorescence on cryosections of human blood group O pancreas, and standardization programs have defined their quantitative measurement in reference Juvenile Diabetes Foundation units (JDF-u) (24). Islet cell antibodies are exclusively of the IgG class (25), with restriction of certain IgG subclasses (26,27), and are able to fix complement (28). Classically, but not invariably, islet cell antibody positive sera react with the cytoplasm of all the cell types of the islet, that is, α, β, δ, and PP cells (29), suggesting that at least one of the target antigens of the islet cell antibody is common to all the islet endocrine cells.

Despite the fact that the first description of islet cell antibodies dates back almost 20 years, the nature of the islet autoantigen(s) with which they react remains undefined. This is perhaps due to a multiplicity of target antigens with different biochemical properties. The initial biochemical characterization suggested that a major target of islet cell antibodies was a glycolipid (reviewed in 30). This suggestion was based on the observation that sera containing the antibodies reacted with neuraminidase-treated sections of pancreas (31) and that the antibodies could be inhibited by a lipid extract from islets (32). Direct binding of islet cell antibodies to a β-cell-specific sialoganglioside is, however, still lacking, but a monosialoganglioside, chromatographically migrating between GM1 and GM2, has been proposed as a candidate (32). Other glycolipids suggested as islet cell antibody autoantigens include the rat ganglioside GT3. Indeed, direct binding of antibodies to GT3 has been demonstrated (33), but its relevance to IDDM is questionable because of the apparent absence of this ganglioside in human islets (34). However, the possible role of gangliosides as islet autoantigens in IDDM is attractive, especially considering their functional importance in a number of cell physiological activities, including signal transduction, differentiation, etc., and not simply as membrane structural entities (35). It has also been proposed that sulfatides are glycolipids with islet cell antibody autoantigen characteristics (36), but although antibodies to these molecules have been reported in newly diagnosed IDDM patients no correlation was found between the presence of islet cell antibodies and anti-sulfatide antibodies in the same sera (37). Independently of these uncertainties in the IDDM field, it is interesting to recall that antibodies to both gangliosides and sulfatides have been described in several immune-mediated neurological (38) and other disorders, which is not surprising because the islets and the nervous system have a common embryogenesis. However, these latter considerations decrease the IDDM-disease specificity of the autoantibodies of these molecules.

Early evidence for heterogeneity within islet cell antibodies was their temporal behavior. In most patients, the antibodies disappear soon after the clinical onset of IDDM, possibly reflecting the progressive decline of the residual β-cell mass (22), whereas in others they persist almost indefinitely at significant titers long after β-cell destruction has been completed (39). Further evidence of islet cell antibody heterogeneity came at the detection level. In addition to the putative glycolipid autoantigens, it is now well established that the immunofluorescent staining by islet cell antibodies can also be contributed to by antibodies to protein components. Distinct islet cell antibody staining patterns have been demonstrated. Using four layer immunofluorescence, we showed (40) that some islet cell antibodies stain predominantly β cells (β-selective), whereas a second pattern confirmed the staining of all the cells within the islets (whole-islet ICA). Others demonstrated that those islet cell antibodies corresponding to the β-selective pattern, defined as restricted, could be further distinguished by their reactivity to mouse islets (41); and using blocking studies, a third group reported a dichotomy in the ability to block islet cell antibody immunofluorescence patterns (42). We further demonstrated that the β-selective islet cell antibodies were completely inhibited by preincubation with sera containing rat brain homogenate, but not when the same homogenate had been pre-cleared with anti-GAD (glutamic acid decarboxylase) antiserum (40). In contrast, the titers of whole islet ICA were unaffected by the preincubation with brain homogenate containing GAD. This indicates that GAD is not only the antigen corresponding to the immunoprecipitable 64 kDa islet protein but it is also the predominant autoantigen of the β-selective islet cell antibody. Another report also confirmed the contribution of GAD to islet cell antibody reactivity when it was shown that preabsorption of ICA-positive sera with recombinant GAD65 and GAD67 reduced or blocked islet cell antibody reactivity in sera from patients with IDDM and from unaffected ICA-positive individuals (43). All of these findings suggest a multiplicity of islet cell antibody specificities, which might occur alone or in combination.

64 kDa and GAD Antibodies

Autoantibodies that immunoprecipitate a protein of 64 kDa from detergent lysates of 35S-methionine-labeled human and rodent islets in IDDM sera were first described in 1982 (44). 64 kDa antibodies have later been reported to be at least as frequent as cytoplasmic islet cell antibodies (45). In contrast to islet cell antibodies, 64 kDa antibodies tend to persist longer in the circulation after diagnosis (46). The 64 kDa autoantigen was reported to be membrane-bound (47) and β-cell specific in an analysis of many tissues, which, however, did not include the brain (48). Despite their clinical relevance, the detection of 64 kDa antibodies involves cumbersome and expensive assays that have not allowed large population screening programs.

Antibodies to GAD, the biosynthesizing enzyme of the inhibitory neurotransmitter gamma-aminobutyric acid (GABA) were first reported in a single patient with "stiff man syndrome," a rare disorder of the nervous system (49). This patient was a female and also had IDDM with associated autoimmune polyendocrinopathy and a high titer of islet cell antibodies (50). Subsequently, antibodies to GAD were detected in 60% of a larger series of patients with stiff man syndrome (51). These observations provided the direct proof of the existence of an autoimmune variant of stiff man syndrome, in addition to paraneoplastic and (still) idiopathic types (52). In those original cases (51), GAD antibodies were associated with islet cell antibodies, expression of GAD staining in islets, and other organ-specific autoimmunities, including IDDM in a third of the cases.

In 1990, the identity of the 64 kDa autoantigen was determined to be GAD (53). This enzyme is selectively expressed in GABAergic neurons (54) and, outside brain, primarily in pancreatic β cells (55). Other extraneuronal tissues expressing GAD at lower levels are kidney, liver, adrenal, ovary, and testis (56–58). Two forms of GAD with molecular weights of 65,000 (GAD65) and 67,000 (GAD67), encoded for by separate genes located on chromosomes 10 and 2, respectively, have been cloned and sequenced from different species (59–66). Amino acid sequence homology between the two isoforms is 70% and both are present in brain and islets, with no qualitative differences (67,68). In brain, GAD65 and GAD67 interact differently with their cofactor pyridoxal phosphate and have a different intraneuronal distribution, GAD65 being widely distributed throughout the neurons and GAD67 being more concentrated in axon terminals (69). In β cells, GAD65 is more abundant and concentrated at the cytoplasmic surface of synaptic-like microvesicles (70). These are closely related to neuronal small synaptic vesicles (71) and are thought to be involved in storage and release of GABA by β cells (70). Although the function of GABA in β cells is unclear, it seems that this neurotransmitter plays a paracrine role in the islets (72). In β cells, GAD67 is hydrophilic and soluble, whereas GAD65, synthesized in a hydrophilic form, is posttranslationally modified into an amphiphilic form that can be either soluble or membrane anchored (73). GAD65 in β cells is present in two immunogenic isoforms, α and β, which differ in molecular mass by ~1 kDa (47,73).

Identification of islet 64 kDa as the enzyme GAD was based on various experimental data, including complete immunological cross-reactivity, identical size, and isoelectric focusing on two-dimensional gel electrophoresis, generation of identical products after trypsin digestion of the two proteins, and GAD enzymatic activity of the 64 kDa immunoprecipitates (53). Further characterization revealed that both GAD65 and GAD67 from islets or brain are immunogenic in IDDM and in stiff man syndrome (53), whereas GAD forms derived from other tissues are not (74). In IDDM, autoantibodies are predominantly directed against GAD65 (75). The epitopes recognized by these antibodies are localized in the middle and C-terminal domains of GAD65 (76).

Using a variety of methods for their determination, the prevalence of GAD antibodies has been reported to be between 25% and 70% at the time of diagnosis of IDDM (77–81). This large variability most probably depends on intrinsic differences in the assays used. A serum exchange program aimed at standardizing the measurement of GAD antibodies has been undertaken by the Immunology and Diabetes Workshops (IDW) and has, at least in part, clarified the differences in the reported prevalence (82). As in stiff man syndrome, there seems to be an association between GAD antibodies and other autoimmune polyendocrine manifestations affecting the same patients (77). In fact, they are detected more frequently in patients with high levels of islet cell antibodies and in female patients with thyrogastric antibodies.

Antibodies to the Tryptic Fragments of the Main 64 kDa Islet Autoantigen

Analysis of antibody reactivity by immunoprecipitation of trypsin-digested islet homogenates results in three major fragments of 50 kDa, 40 kDa, and 37 kDa (83). IDDM sera can precipitate all three fragments, the 50 kDa fragment alone, or the 37/40 kDa doublet. Antibodies that recognize the 50 kDa fragment also bind the intact 64 kDa antigen and correlate with its ability to cause immunoprecipitation of GAD. In contrast, antibodies to the 37/40 kDa fragments, also defined as the "37k antigen," do not correlate with GAD antibodies, and they appear to recognize tryptic determinants on the 64 kDa antigen complex that are exposed to proteolitic cleavage. On the basis of recent data, it is thought that the 50 kDa fragment and the 37k antigen are derived from distinct 64 kDa proteins with different antigenic and biochemical properties (84). The 50 kDa fragment derives from GAD, whereas the 37k antigen apparently does not. This is based on the demonstration that recombinant GAD65 is able to block the binding of antibodies to the 50 kDa tryptic fragment, but not to the 37k antigen; second, GAD antibodies recognize the 50 kDa fragment but not the 37k antigen; third, the 37k antigen is detectable after trypsin treatment of immunoprecipitates from insulinoma cells that lack expression of the major GAD isoforms.

Approximately 70% of IDDM patients possess antibodies to all three tryptic fragments of the 64 kDa islet autoantigen. At the time of diagnosis, more than 90% of IDDM patients have antibodies to at least one of the fragments (83).

Antibodies to Secretory-Granule-Associated Islet Autoantigens

Secretory granules that fuse with the plasma membrane, releasing their contents and exposing the internal membrane to the extracellular milieu, appear suitable candidates as autoantigen-containing structures in IDDM.

Insulin Autoantibodies

Spontaneous insulin autoantibodies, the major secretory granule component, were first identified in untreated newly diagnosed IDDM patients in 1983 (85, reviewed in 86). Two methodologies were set up to measure these specificities, the fluid phase radiobinding assay (RIA) (87) and the solid phase enzymatic assay (ELISA) (88), but there has long been debate as to which of the two should be chosen to assess insulin autoantibodies. The IDW program for insulin autoantibody standardization has demonstrated substantial discordance between the two most widely used techniques (89). The lack of concordance remains when the assays are performed while incorporating displacement with excess antigen to correct for nonspecific binding, clearly showing that these differences are not artifacts but reflect the detection of separate populations of insulin autoantibodies (90). It is known that RIA preferentially detects high-affinity antibodies, whereas ELISA, in which there is an excess of available antigen, also detects low-affinity antibodies (91). RIA produces significantly higher specific signals for insulin autoantibodies in newly diagnosed IDDM than ELISA (92), possibly reflecting a high-affinity response generated as part of the β-cell immunopathogenic process. Moreover, measurements from different RIA assays were more comparable to each other than those from ELISA. On that basis, the IDW Committee for insulin autoantibody standardization now recommends fluid phase radioassays for assessing IDDM-related insulin autoantibodies (92).

By the presently available sensitive and specific RIA, insulin autoantibodies are detected in around 50% of newly diagnosed IDDM patients (93), and there is a peculiar inverse correlation with age, that is, they are detected more frequently in young individuals (94).

Autoantibodies to Proinsulin

Autoantibodies to proinsulin have also been demonstrated in untreated IDDM patients but at a lower frequency than insulin autoantibodies and are not invariably associated with them (95). They have been detected by both ELISA and RIA, but it remains to be established which of the two techniques detects the most disease-specific proinsulin autoantibodies.

Antibodies to Carboxypeptidase H

Another autoantigen within the secretory granule includes carboxypeptidase H, the enzyme involved in the conversion of proinsulin to insulin, which has a molecular weight of 52–57 kDa. It was found that 25% of diabetic sera contain antibodies to a recombinant protein that corresponds to this enzyme (96). Antibodies binding to a 52 kDa rat insulinoma cell protein have also been found in the sera of a high proportion of NOD mice and in 30% of humans with IDDM (97). Apparently, these antibodies are different from those to carboxypeptidase H, despite the fact that they recognize a protein of similar molecular weight to the secretory granule associated enzyme (Karounos, *personal communication*).

Antibodies to Heat Shock Protein (HSP)-65

Humoral and T lymphocyte responses to HSP-65 of *Mycobacterium tuberculosis* have been shown in the NOD mouse model of IDDM (98). In humans, it was suggested that this HSP-65 antigen may also be the equivalent of the 64 kDa islet antigen (99), but others have not confirmed these initial findings (100). HSP-65 is a ubiquitous protein and therefore unlikely to contribute to the restricted tissue specificity of the

64 kDa reactivity, but the possibility cannot be disregarded that HSP-65 and GAD share sequence homology in their molecules (101).

Antibodies to Glucose Transporter

Immunoglobulin from IDDM patients inhibited the uptake of 3-O-methyl-β-D-glucose by dispersed rat islet cells. This inhibitory effect was abolished by preincubation of islet cells with membranes from hepatocytes, which contain the same glucose transporter, but not from erythrocytes, which lack it, suggesting that IDDM sera might contain antibodies to the glucose transporter (102). Such antibodies could act to impair glucose-stimulated insulin secretion *in vivo*. However, confirmation of the existence of these antibody specificities in IDDM is still lacking.

Autoantibodies to Surface Islet Autoantigens

In the past, much emphasis has been placed on the surface location of putative autoantigens, caused by the assumed availability of such antigens to destructive immune effector mechanisms. Current knowledge of the mechanisms of antigen presentation, whereby internal peptides can be presented on the cell surface by the HLA molecules, has obviated, in principle, the necessity for a constitutive external location of putative autoantigens to explain the autoimmune recognition and destruction of the target-affected cells.

In IDDM, islet cell surface antibodies (ICSA) were initially detected using viable cultured rodent (103) or human fetal islet cells (104), and it was suggested that there were separate specificities for α-, β- and PP-cells (105). Despite the potential relevance of these initial findings, their existence was questioned when highly purified adult human islets were used instead (106). In fact, no evidence for ICSA binding could be demonstrated on the surface of their corresponding endocrine cells. These data suggest that the ICSA autoantigen is not expressed on the surface membrane of human islet cells and therefore raise doubts about their relevance to the pathogenesis of IDDM. Nevertheless, early *in vitro* studies showed that serum from IDDM patients was cytotoxic to cultured islet cells and could interfere with glucose-stimulated insulin release (107), and as mentioned IDDM sera might contain antibodies to the glucose transporter, thus acting by impairing glucose-stimulated insulin secretion *in vivo* (102).

Other Autoantibodies and Antibodies in IDDM

Not only do IDDM patients elicit a specific autoantibody response against islet cell components, including separate autoantibodies to α and δ cells (108), but their sera often contain a variety of other organ-specific and non-organ specific autoantibodies (reviewed in 2,109). Cytoplasmic pituitary antibodies have been demonstrated in IDDM probands and in their first-degree relatives (110), and surface antibodies to rat pituitary cells have been reported in the sera of the same patients (111). Antilymphocytic antibodies have also been found in IDDM patients (112). The presence of these additional autoantibodies indicates that in IDDM there is a general tendency to autoimmunity, but it remains unclear whether these other humoral specificities have any direct role in the pathogenic process that destroys β cells.

Antibodies to exogenous antigens have also been reported in association with IDDM. Recently, major emphasis has been placed on antibodies to a number of cow's milk proteins, such as β-lactoglobulin (113,114) and bovine serum albumin (BSA) (115). It has been hypothesized that antibodies to BSA may crossreact with ICA-69, another recently identified islet autoantigen (116) that shows homologies with BSA—and in particular with "ABBOS," an apparently immunodominant peptide present on the BSA molecule—thus reflecting a link between environmental triggers and autoimmunity. Although some of these findings have recently been questioned (117), it cannot be excluded that, if not these, then other antibodies to exogenous antigens may act in IDDM as autoantibodies in molecular mimicry (reviewed in 118), as suggested for other autoimmune diseases (119).

CELL-MEDIATED IMMUNE ABNORMALITIES

Extensive research has been carried out on the cell-mediated immune process involved in the autoimmune destruction of the β cells. The first demonstration of the involvement of cell-mediated immunity was the leukocyte migration inhibition test (LMIT), which showed that newly diagnosed IDDM patients were sensitized to pancreatic antigens (10, reviewed in 120). Quantitative abnormalities of T cell phenotypes are also detected, but most commonly found are increased levels of the activated CD4$^+$ T cell subpopulation (11). In addition, lymphocytes of IDDM patients produce cytotoxicity to various islet cell targets *in vitro* (121, reviewed in 122). More recently, T cell reactivity to a 38 kDa antigen specific to fetal pig proislets has been shown (123), as has reactivity against the 38 kDa nuclear transcription factor jun-B (124), but it is not clear whether these antigens are identical. In addition to these antigens, T cells of IDDM patients respond, in conventional proliferation assays, to both GAD isoforms (125,126). It has to be emphasized that the T cell stimulation index is apparently not very high when GAD is used as an antigen. In addition, contrasting reports have appeared as to which peptide in the GAD molecule is recognized by the T cells, one group favoring the C-terminal portion of the molecule (127), as for autoantibodies to GAD (76), and others (128,129) favoring the amino acid sequence shared by GAD and a nucleocapsid protein of the coxsackie virus (78). It is vital to reach an agreement on these particular data, because there are important pathogenic implications. In fact, coxsackie viruses have often been indicated as potential causative agents of human IDDM (reviewed in 130), even though their precise role in the initial damage of the β cells has been questioned (reviewed in 4).

Although several abnormalities of cell-mediated immunity have been identified in

IDDM, they are not always consistent, suggesting low precursor frequencies in the circulation. Only by cloning can the islet-specific T lymphocytes be identified. Autoreactive CD4$^+$ T cell clones have been produced from peripheral blood lymphocytes of IDDM patients (131,132). The reactivity against islets was HLA-DR restricted, with unexpected cytotoxic properties when exposed to autologous islets (131), and some of these recognized a 38 kDa protein derived from insulin secretory granules but also present in other tissues of neuroendocrine origin (133). Peripheral blood lymphocytes from IDDM patients also have reactivity to this fraction (134). We still await the generation of an autoreactive CD8 cytotoxic T cell line from IDDM patients. The cytotoxic T cells are those most abundant in the insulitis observed at diagnosis (135) and in the recurrence of diabetes seen in identical twins with IDDM or in patients transplanted with part of the pancreas of unaffected co-twins or identical siblings, respectively (reviewed in 20).

PREDICTING INSULIN-DEPENDENT DIABETES MELLITUS

Despite the fact that IDDM is characterized by an acute clinical onset in the majority of cases, a long prodromal period precedes the appearance of clinical symptoms, during which a variety of autoimmune phenomena are present in susceptible individuals predisposed to the disease (reviewed in 136). This latency is totally asymptomatic, but it can be revealed by the detection of circulating autoantibodies. Indeed, although β-cell destruction is thought to be mediated by autoreactive T lymphocytes rather than by immunoglobulins (reviewed in 7), the investigation of IDDM-associated autoantibodies is of great relevance, because of the potential value of these serological specificities as disease predictors. Although the ultimate perspective of preventing IDDM is strictly dependent on achievements in the fields of epidemiology, genetics, and immunology of the disease, accurate prediction is necessary before therapeutic strategies aimed at preventing IDDM or, more realistically, its insulin-dependent stage can be practically applied. The postulated multifactorial etiopathogenesis of IDDM offers, at least in theory, a multiplicity of markers, each representative of single determinants and therefore a potential predictor of the disease. Nonetheless, the predictive value of any given marker needs to be carefully validated and quantified.

In order to use any marker for the prediction of a given disease, an understanding of Baycs' theorem is important (reviewed in 137). From this theorem, the usefulness of a marker depends upon its specificity (negative in health) and sensitivity (positive in disease) and the prevalence of the disease in the population tested. Both specificity and sensitivity are dependent upon the test used to measure the marker, in particular the threshold of positivity used. The specificity of the test will usually increase when higher positive thresholds are used.

Immunological Markers in the Prediction of IDDM

As previously reviewed, several islet-specific autoantibodies have been identified in the last two decades. However, those that have been shown to confer the highest risk for future development of IDDM, at least in first-degree relatives of affected individuals, are the following: the classical cytoplasmic islet cell antibodies (9), auto-antibodies to insulin (85), to the 64 kDa islet protein (44) of which part is GAD (53), and to the "37k antigen" of the 64 kDa main islet protein (83). Other autoantibodies reported to be associated with IDDM but yet to be validated as possible predictors of the disease include those against: carboxypeptidase-H (96), glucose transporter 2 (GLUT 2) (102), islet glycolipids (31), sulfatides (36,37), ICA-69 (117), and another immunoprecipitable 38 kDa islet protein (44) that is distinct from the 37k antigen. Apart from the islet-related autoantibodies, HLA alleles and insulin response to intra-venous glucose are also considered important markers of pre-IDDM. Although more time consuming and less easy to standardize than autoantibody tests (reviewed in 138), cell-mediated immunity assays are also gradually entering into clinical practice for prediction of IDDM.

Islet Cell Antibodies in the Prediction of IDDM

Cytoplasmic islet cell antibodies are still the most widely used serological markers in IDDM and pre-IDDM, especially now that their measurement has been quantified (139). Despite uncertainty about their autoantigen specificities [as previously men-tioned, islet gangliosides have been suggested (32)], and despite the difficulties still encountered in certain laboratories engaged in their measurement (140), islet cell antibodies represent the baseline screening for any program designed to predict the disease.

Family Studies

It was the prospective measurement of islet cell antibodies in first-degree relatives of IDDM patients that initially established that the clinical onset of IDDM is delayed by up to several years (141). This concept was subsequently amply confirmed (142, and reviewed in 143), including studies in identical twins (144). The predictive value of islet cell antibodies for future IDDM in unaffected first-degree relatives of diabetic children has been calculated. Overall, 22% of relatives with detectable islet cell anti-bodies are projected to develop diabetes within 5 years, compared to fewer than 0.1% of those with undetectable antibodies. The risk appears proportional to the antibody titer, being around 5% in relatives with titers of 4–19 JDF-u, but reaching 35% at 5 years and 60–70% at 10 years in those with titers of >20 JDF-u (reviewed in 145). However, in cases with titers of >80 JDF-u, first-degree relatives have a risk for IDDM that approaches 100% (reviewed in 130). In applying these data to the Bayes' theorem, one can extrapolate that, by using the high threshold of positivity, although almost all those identified will develop IDDM, the majority of first-degree relatives who will develop IDDM have islet cell antibody titers of <80 JDF-u and therefore would not be identified (false negatives). In contrast, at a threshold of 4 JDF-u, almost all of those developing IDDM will be positive for islet cell antibodies, but the predictive value of the test is substantially reduced, because a significant number of those who do not develop IDDM will also be positive (false positives).

Studies in the Population at Large

The majority of individuals who develop IDDM do not have a family history of the disease—the so-called "sporadic" cases. Thus, for effective prediction, any tests used should be applicable to the general population. In contrast with the data obtained in families, the predictive value of islet cell antibodies is relatively low when detected in nondiabetic individuals without a family history of the disease (146), even though the prevalence of these antibodies is increased in countries where there is a high incidence of IDDM (147), such as Finland (148) and Sardinia (149). This may not be surprising, since IDDM in the general population is at least 10 times less frequent than in first-degree relatives of affected children. On the other hand, the prevalence of islet cell antibodies in the general population is just slightly lower than that in relatives of IDDM families (approximately 2–4% *vs* 4–7%, respectively), thus indicating that the risk of developing IDDM in an individual found to have an islet cell antibody titer of >20 JDF-u but without a family history of the disease is expected to be less than 10% at 5 years. This is best exemplified in the United Kingdom, where, with a risk of IDDM of approximately 0.3% (150), around 3% of school children have detectable islet cell antibodies (146). Therefore at best the estimated predictive value of islet cell antibodies at a threshold of 4 JDF-u in the general population would be 10%. At a threshold of 80 JDF-u, the predictive value would increase to around 50%. Because of the very low incidence of IDDM in the general population, islet cell antibodies on their own cannot provide 100% predictive value. From these data, it appears that islet cell antibodies, while having significant power to predict IDDM in relatives of already affected individuals, have limited value when detected in the general population. However, since the large majority of cases of IDDM occur in the absence of a family history of the disease, new marker tools are greatly needed in order to circumvent the limited predictive value of islet cell antibodies in such cases (reviewed in 151). Thus the predictive value will be enhanced if islet cell antibodies are used in combination with other markers (reviewed in 45). In recent years, increasing numbers of new immunoserological specificities have been used to enhance prediction.

Insulin Autoantibodies in the Prediction of IDDM

In contrast to islet cell antibodies, the frequency of insulin autoantibodies is inversely correlated with age, reaching nearly 100% in children developing the disease before the age of 5 years, with a progressive decline with increasing age (152). However, when they are present on their own they are of poor predictive value for the disease, although their detection at any age in association with islet cell antibodies increase the risk. Insulin autoantibodies are more frequently associated with the presence of the HLA-DR4 allele (153). Furthermore, in a prospective study of off-spring of diabetic mothers, insulin autoantibodies were detected before islet cell anti-bodies in the small number of antibody-positive cases studied (154).

Autoantibodies to the 64 kDa Mr Islet Protein and to GAD in the Prediction of IDDM

Both these serological markers are found in most individuals before the onset of IDDM (155–157). On the basis of the reported frequency of 64 kDa antibodies, it is expected that GAD antibodies have a sensitivity of around 80% (156), very similar to islet cell antibodies. GAD antibodies, however, are not absolutely specific for IDDM, being also detected (as previously mentioned) in the autoimmune variant of stiff man syndrome (reviewed in 158). The value of GAD antibodies, either alone or in combination with islet cell antibodies and other markers, for predicting IDDM is under extensive evaluation, and the availability of more refined and sensitive assays, where RIA with the recombinant molecule seems the most promising (159,160), will certainly help in this direction. In some initial studies, GAD antibodies were shown to be of value (161,162), but this was not always the case (163).

It is important to note that when GAD antibodies are detected alone, in the absence of any other IDDM-related autoantibodies such as islet autoantibodies, they are poor predictors of IDDM. This conclusion has been borne out by prospective studies of patients with overt endocrine- or organ-specific autoimmune manifestations (164). It was first shown that, within the two islet cell antibody fluorescent patterns, β-selec-tive (40) or restricted (41) islet cell antibodies conferred a relatively low risk for IDDM, while whole islet or unrestricted islet cell antibodies conferred a higher risk. In contrast to the classical whole islet ICA, the β-selective islet cell antibodies were found in those patients with autoimmune polyendocrine involvement who progressed very slowly, or did not progress at all, to clinical IDDM (40). The same applied to first-degree relatives of diabetic patients, where again the β-selective islet cell anti-bodies were associated with infrequent progression to IDDM (41). Another feature of the detection of β-selective islet cell antibodies in patients with autoimmune poly-endocrinopathy was that it was not associated with IDDM-susceptible HLA class II alleles (165). Again, the proportion of islet cell antibodies blocked by rat brain homogenate was high in ICA-positive individuals who did not progress to IDDM, whereas it was low in those who subsequently developed the disease.

After this initial evidence was presented, it was soon found that the majority of patients with autoimmune polyendocrinopathy who were found to have the β-selec-tive islet cell antibody had indeed only GAD antibodies. It was confirmed that, despite the high titers of these specificities, but in absence of other IDDM-related autoanti-bodies, the majority of them continued to remain IDDM free, and the few who did not had a slow onset of the disease, passing through a period of mild diabetes before insulin replacement therapy was needed (166). Thus GAD-specific islet cell antibodies (that is, β-selective) *per se* do not seem to reflect ongoing β-cell destruction. In support of this possibility are the histological findings of three pancreases that were examined at early necropsy (167). They were obtained from two patients with type 2 and one with type 1 autoimmune polyendocrine syndrome respectively (reviewed in 168), where, even in the latter, GAD antibodies have been reported in the absence of IDDM (169). All three patients had persistent high titers of GAD antibodies but, while alive, did not show any glucose abnormality. When examined with several immunological markers, the islets of these pancreases were clear of any sign of inflammation. Whether GAD antibodies are markers often associated with, but nonspecific for IDDM, and precisely which GAD molecule, either present in the β-cells or in other organs, *e.g.,* brain, elicits the autoimmune response against it, are critical questions that need to be clarified and fully explained.

Antibodies to the "37k Antigen" in the Prediction of IDDM

Of great interest is the report of antibodies immunoprecipitating the islet 37k antigen in IDDM. The data produced so far tend to indicate that these antibodies are more disease specific than 50 kDa and GAD antibodies in pre-IDDM. They were obtained in prospective and cross-sectional studies performed in individuals considered at risk for IDDM, *i.e.,* identical twins (170), first degree relatives of IDDM families (163), and school children (171). They were initially found to be positive for one or more IDDM-related autoantibodies, but the additional presence of antibodies to the 37k antigen was correlated with a more rapid progression to disease. Similarly, in the study of the patients with autoimmune polyendocrinopathy with high titers of GAD antibodies, all patients with these additional specificities manifested IDDM acutely, whereas patients who developed IDDM gradually, with a prolonged period of glucose intolerance, were negative for these antibodies (166). Furthermore, in stiff man syndrome the 37k antigen was found mostly in patients with associated IDDM (166). These findings suggest that antibodies to the 37k antigen may be specific second markers to whole pattern islet cell antibodies for a rapid progression to IDDM.

Cell-Mediated Immune Markers in the Prediction of IDDM

Abnormalities of cell-mediated immunity found in newly diagnosed IDDM patients can also be demonstrated in the prediabetic period. In particular, the quantitative (172) and functional (173) abnormalities of the suppressor/inducer cell subset (CD4$^+$/ 45 RA$^+$) may assist prediction of IDDM. Similarly, low CD4 counts and a persistently low CD4/CD8 ratio have been detected in prediabetic family members (174,175). Furthermore, twin studies have shown a trend to increased numbers of CD5$^+$ B lymphocytes (176) and persistently raised numbers of activated HLA DR$^+$ T cells were found only in the twins who then converted to IDDM (177). In the same group, the presence of activated T cells enhanced the predictive value of islet cell antibodies and insulin autoantibodies.

A defective expression of HLA class I molecules has also been suggested as another marker of pre-IDDM, and the phenomenon has been postulated to play a role in the pathogenesis of the disease (178). Although these data are potentially relevant, they still await confirmation. Pre-IDDM individuals respond to various islet preparations (179) and, as mentioned, both antibodies and T cells react or respond to GAD in the same individuals. However, it has been suggested that a T cell response to GAD could be more predictive than antibodies to the same antigen, at least in first-degree relatives of IDDM patients (180). Independently of this potentially important evidence, it has to be pointed out that cross-sectional studies of cell-mediated immunity are not very useful in predicting the onset of IDDM, as has been shown for the humoral markers, and this is due to the fact that changes in various lymphocyte subsets and their reactivity to islet autoantigens are not very consistent. Repeated testing during a regular follow up has more chance of showing patterns of variability in abnormalities of cell-mediated immunity that are relevant to prediction.

HLA Type and the Prediction of IDDM

The progression to the disease in individuals with autoimmune markers of IDDM is likely to be influenced by factors such as age, environmental exposure, and geographical location (181). Apart from antibodies (reviewed in 182) and changes in cell-mediated immunity, genetic markers also enhance the prediction of IDDM. Genetic markers, in particular those of the major histocompatibility complex, may also be useful in discriminating which ICA-positive individuals will develop IDDM. Not all ICA-positive individuals have the IDDM susceptibility HLA alleles, and selecting those with these genetic markers is likely to assist prediction of disease. The risk conferred by the known disease-associated HLA-DR and DQ alleles has recently been evaluated in two prospective family studies, both of which provided evidence of their utility when used alone or in combination with islet cell antibodies (183,184). Of particular relevance is the additional extent of prediction provided by HLA typing in relatives who have intermediate titers of islet cell antibodies, while in those with high titers of antibodies the additional value for prediction seems limited (reviewed in 145).

Insulin Secretion as Metabolic Marker of the Prediction of IDDM

Among potential metabolic markers of prediction, the most popular is the first-phase insulin response to the intravenous glucose tolerance test (185). Under this stimulating condition, the persistent loss of 1–3 minutes of insulin secretion always precedes the progression to clinical IDDM. However, while this metabolic abnormality is highly predictive in ICA-positive first degree relatives (186), it may not be so in other at-risk groups, such as in adult patients with autoimmune polyendocrinopathy (187).

Combining Markers to Increase Prediction Accuracy

Following a preliminary islet cell antibody screening and quantitative measurement, a quite accurate prediction of IDDM (>80%) can be achieved in unaffected members of IDDM families by using a combination of several, or all, of the above-mentioned markers. However, by limiting the screening to family members, only about 10% of the at-risk population would be identified. For this reason, the same strategy of using multiple tests is even more important in the screening of the general population, in order to circumvent the low predictive value of islet cell antibodies alone expected on the basis of the much lower disease prevalence. In these circumstances, islet cell antibodies and HLA-DQ typing could be used one after the other—it does not matter in which order—thus providing a predictive value similar to that achieved in IDDM families who are tested only for islet cell antibodies. Further use of the remaining markers could enhance risk estimation for future IDDM in the general population to an extent equal to that achieved in relatives of IDDM families (reviewed in 145). We, like others (188,189), do not believe that prediction can be achieved in the general population by screening it with just one marker, for example GAD antibodies, as has recently been claimed (190). Combinations of immune markers will certainly also be useful in predicting which people with type II diabetes will progress faster than others to insulin dependency. So far, islet cell antibodies (191) and GAD antibodies (192) have been tested separately in this population and have identified approximately 15–20% of potential IDDM patients as being positive for one or the other of the markers. Despite important achievements in identifying new antibody/antigen systems in IDDM and pre-IDDM, the work that concentrates on ultimately defining prediction of IDDM with accuracy requires more effort, and any definite conclusion, one way or the other, is premature at this stage.

CONCLUSION

Despite the increasing numbers of autoantigens proposed in IDDM, and the potential of their respective antibodies as predictive markers, several considerations need to be addressed. Standardization of autoantibody measurement is incomplete, especially in relation to the new specificities recently identified, and remains an important goal if these markers are to be used in the prediction of the disease. We need to be reminded that there is a conspicuous lack of evidence for the pathogenic role of these antigens. Nevertheless, recent advances in developing purified antigens and the increased availability of these antigens are likely to provide the means to answer relevant questions in the autoimmune pathogenesis of IDDM and specific tools for its ultimate prevention (reviewed in 193).

ACKNOWLEDGMENTS

The work in London is presently supported by the Autoimmune Diseases Charitable Trust (ADCT), the Local Organized Research Schemes (LORS) the British Diabetic Association, and *Associazione per l'Aiuto ai Giovani Diabetici,* Milan, Italy.

The work in Milan is supported by the Juvenile Diabetes Foundation-International. We are grateful to Laura Roberts and Amanda Payne for patiently editing the manuscript.

REFERENCES

1. Cahill GF, McDevitt HO. Insulin-dependent diabetes mellitus: the initial lesion. *N Engl J Med* 1981; 304: 1454–65.
2. Bottazzo GF. Beta-cell damage in diabetic insulitis: are we approaching the solution? *Diabetologia* 1984; 26: 241–50.
3. Eisenbarth GS. Type 1 diabetes mellitus: a chronic autoimmune disease. *N Engl J Med* 1986; 314: 1360–8.
4. Bottazzo GF. Death of a beta cell: homicide or suicide? *Diab Med* 1986; 3: 119–30.
5. Bosi E, Todd I, Pujol-Borrell R, Bottazzo GF. Mechanisms of autoimmunity: relevance to the pathogenesis of Type 1 (insulin-dependent) diabetes mellitus. *Diabetes Metab Rev* 1987; 3: 893–924.
6. Bach JF. Mechanisms of autoimmunity in insulin-dependent diabetes mellitus. *Clin Exp Immunol* 1988; 72: 1–8.
7. Bottazzo GF. On the honey disease. A dialogue with Socrates. *Diabetes* 1993; 42: 778–800.
8. Gepts W. Pathogenic anatomy of the pancreas in juvenile diabetes mellitus. *Diabetes* 1965; 14: 619–33.
9. Bottazzo GF, Florin-Christensen A, Doniach D. Islet cell antibodies in diabetes mellitus with autoimmune polyendocrine deficiency. *Lancet* 1974; ii: 1279–83.
10. Nerup J, Anderson OO, Bendixen G, Egeverg J, Poulsen JE. Anti-pancreatic cellular hypersensitivity in diabetes mellitus. *Diabetes* 1974; 20: 424–7.
11. Jackson RA, Morris MA, Haynes B, Eisenbarth GS. Increased circulating Ia-antigen bearing T cells in type I diabetes mellitus. *N Engl J Med* 1982; 306: 785–8.
12. Nepom GT. Immunogenetics and IDDM. *Diabetes Rev* 1993; 1: 93–103.
13. Maclaren NK, Riley WJ. Thyroid, gastric and adrenal autoimmunities associated with insulin dependent diabetes mellitus. *Diabetes Care* 1985; 8 (suppl 1): 34–8.
14. Mordes JP, Desemone J, Rossini AA. The BB rat. *Diabetes Metab Rev* 1987; 3: 725–50.
15. Lamperter EF, Signore A, Gale EAM, Pozzilli P. Lessons from the NOD mice for the pathogenesis and immunotherapy of human Type 1 (insulin-dependent) diabetes mellitus. *Diabetologia* 1989; 32: 703–8.
16. Feuren G, Papoz J, Assan R, *et al.*, for the Cyclosporin/Diabetes French Study group. Cyclosporin increases the rate and length of remissions in insulin dependent diabetes of recent onset: results of a multicentre double-blind trial. *Lancet* 1986; ii: 119–24.
17. The Canadian-European randomised control trial group: cyclosporin-induced remission of IDDM after early intervention: association of 1 year of cyclosporin treatment with enhanced insulin secretion. *Diabetes* 1988; 37: 1574–82.
18. Sibley RK, Sutherland DER, Goetz F, Michael AF. Recurrent diabetes mellitus in the pancreas iso- and allograft. A light and electron microscopic and immuno-histochemical analysis. *Lab Invest* 1985; 53: 132–44.
19. Sibley RK, Sutherland DER. Pancreas transplantation: an immunohistologic and histopathologic examination of 100 grafts. *Am J Pathol* 1987; 128: 151–70.
20. Sutherland DER, Gores PF, Farney AC, *et al.* Evolution of kidney, pancreas and islet transplantation for patients with diabetes at the University of Minnesota. *Am Jf Surg* 1993; 166: 456–91.
21. Lendrum R, Walker G, Gamble DR. Islet cell antibodies in juvenile diabetes mellitus of recent onset. *Lancet* 1975; i: 880–2.
22. Lendrum R, Walker IG, Cudworth AG, *et al.* Islet cell antibodies in diabetes mellitus. *Lancet* 1972; ii: 1273–6.
23. Landin-Olsson M, Karlsson A, Dahlquist G, Blom L, Lernmark A, Sundkvist G. Islet cell and other organ-specific autoantibodies in all children developing Type 1 (insulin-dependent) diabetes mellitus in Sweden during one year and in matched control children. *Diabetologia* 1989; 32: 387–95.
24. Bonifacio B, Lernmark A, Dawkins R. Serum exchange and use of dilutions have improved precision and measurement of islet cell antibodies. *J Immunol Methods* 1988; 106: 83–8.

25. Schatz DA, Barrett DJ, Maclaren NK, Riley WJ. Polyclonal nature of islet cell antibodies in insulin-dependent diabetes. *Autoimmunity* 1988; 1: 45–50.
26. Dean BM, Bottazzo GF, Cudworth AG. IgG subclass distribution in organ-specific autoantibodies. The relationship to complement fixing ability. *Clin Exp Immunol* 1983; 52: 61–6.
27. Bruining GJ, Molenaar J, Tuk CW, Lindeman J, Bruining HA, Marner B. Clinical time course and characteristics of islet cell cytoplasmic antibodies in childhood diabetes. *Diabetologia* 1984; 26: 24–9.
28. Bottazzo GF, Dean BM, Gorsuch AN, Cudworth AG, Doniach D. Complement-fixing islet-cell antibodies in Type I diabetes: possible monitors of active beta-cell damage. *Lancet* 1980; i: 668–72.
29. Bottazzo GF, Doniach D. Islet-cell antibodies (ICA) in diabetes mellitus: evidence of an autoantigen common to all the cells in the islet of Langerhans. *Ric Clin Lab* 1978; 8: 29–38.
30. Colman PG, Eisenbarth GS. Immunology of type I diabetes-1987. In: Alberti KGMM, Krall LP, eds. *The diabetes annual 4*. Amsterdam: Elsevier, 1988: 17–45.
31. Nayak RS, Omar MAK, Rabizadeh A, Srikanta S, Eisenbarth GS. "Cytoplasmic" islet cell antibodies: evidence that the target antigen is a sialoglycoconjugate. *Diabetes* 1984; 34: 617–9.
32. Colman PG, Nayak RC, Campbell IL, Eisenbarth GS. Binding of "cytoplasmic" islet cell antibodies is blocked by human pancreatic glycolipid extracts. *Diabetes* 1988; 37: 645–9.
33. Gilliard BK, Thomas JW, Nell LJ, Marcus DM. Antibodies against ganglioside GT3 in the sera of patients with Type I diabetes mellitus. *J Immunol* 1989; 142: 3826–32.
34. Dotta F, Colman PG, Lombardi D, *et al*. Ganglioside expression in human pancreatic islets. *Diabetes* 1989; 38: 1478–83.
35. Zeller CH, Marchase RB. Gangliosides as modulators of cell function. *Am J Physiol* 1992; 262: C1341–55.
36. Cabrera E, Fernandez LE, Carr A, *et al*. Which glycolipids are the autoantigens of cytoplasmic islet cell antibodies? *Acta Diabetol* 1992; 29: 70–4.
37. Buschard K, Josefsen K, Horn T, Fredman P. Sulphatide and sulphatide antibodies in insulin-dependent diabetes mellitus. *Lancet* 1993; 342: 840.
38. Latov NI. Antibodies to glycoconjugates in neurologic disease. *Clin Aspects Autoimmun* 1990; 4: 118–29.
39. Bosi E, Andreotti AC, Girardi AM, Bottazzo GF, Pozza G. The long-term persistence of islet cell antibodies in Type I diabetic patients is unrelated to residual β-cell function. *Diab Nutr Metab* 1991; 4: 319–23.
40. Genovese S, Bonifacio E, McNally JM, *et al*. Distinct cytoplasmic islet cell antibodies with different risks for Type 1 (insulin-dependent) diabetes mellitus. *Diabetologia* 1992; 35: 385–8.
41. Gianani R, Pugliese A, Bonner-Weir S, *et al*. Prognostically significant heterogeneity of cytoplasmic islet cell antibodies in relatives of patients with Type 1 diabetes. *Diabetes* 1992; 41: 347–53.
42. Timsit J, Caillat-Zucman S, Blondel H, Chedin P, Bach JF, Boitard C. Islet cell antibody heterogeneity among Type I (insulin-dependent) diabetic patients. *Diabetologia* 1992; 35: 792–5.
43. Atkinson MA, Kaufman DL, Newman D, Tobin AJ, Maclaren NK. Islet cell cytoplasmic autoantibody reactivity to glutamate decarboxylase in insulin-dependent diabetes. *J Clin Invest* 1993; 91: 350–8.
44. Baekkeskov S, Nielson JH, Marner B, Bilde T, Ludvigsson J, Lernmark A. Autoantibodies in newly diagnosed diabetic children immunoprecipitate human pancreatic islet cell protein. *Nature* 1982; 298: 167–9.
45. Christie M, Landin-Olsson M, Sundkvist G, Dahlquist G, Lernmark A, Baekkeskov S. Antibodies to a Mr 64,000 islet cell protein in Swedish children with newly diagnosed Type 1 (insulin-dependent) diabetes. *Diabetologia* 1988; 31: 597–602.
46. Christie MR, Danetian D, Champagne P, Delovitch TL. Persistence of serum antibodies to 64,000-Mr islet cell protein after onset of Type I diabetes. *Diabetes* 1990; 39: 653–6.
47. Baekkeskov S, Warnock G, Christie M, Rajotte RV, Moss-Larsen P, Fey S. Revelation of specificity of 64K autoantibodies in IDDM serums by high resolution two-dimensional gel electrophoresis: unambiguous identification of 64K target antigen. *Diabetes* 1989; 38: 1133–41.
48. Christie MR, Pipeleers DG, Lernmark A, Baekkeskov S. Cellular and subcellular localisation of a Mr 64,000 protein autoantigen in insulin-dependent diabetes. *J Biol Chem* 1990; 365: 376–81.
49. Solimena M, Folli F, Denis-Domini S, *et al*. Autoantibodies to glutamic acid decarboxylase in a patient with Stiff-man syndrome, epilepsy and Type I diabetes mellitus. *N Engl J Med* 1988; 318: 1012–20.
50. Bosi E, Vicari A, Comi G, *et al*. Association of Stiff-man syndrome and Type I diabetes with islet cell and other autoantibodies. *Arch Neurol* 1988; 45: 246–7.

51. Solimena M, Folli F, Aparisi R, Pozza G, De Camilli P. Autoantibodies to GABA-ergic neurons and pancreatic beta cells in stiff-man syndrome. *N Engl J Med* 1990; 322: 1555–60.
52. Folli F, Solimena M, Cofiell R, *et al*. Breast cancer in stiff-man syndrome patients positive for autoantibodies directed against SyAu, a novel neuronal protein enriched at synapses. *N Engl J Med* 1993; 328: 546–51.
53. Baekkeskov S, Aanstoot HJ, Christgau S, *et al*. Identification of the 64K autoantigen in insulin-dependent diabetes as the GABA-synthesising enzyme glutamic acid decarboxylase. *Nature* 1990; 347: 151–6.
54. Legay F, Pelhare S, Tappaz ML. Phylogenesis of brain glutamic acid decarboxylase from vertebrate: immunochemical studies. *J Neurochem* 1986; 46: 1478–86.
55. Vincent SR, Hokfelt, Wu JY, Elde RP, Morgan IM, Kimmel JR. Immunohistochemical studies of the GABA-system in the pancreas. *Neuroendocrinology* 1983; 36: 197–204.
56. Whelan DT, Scriver CR, Mohyiuddin F: Glutamic acid decarboxylase and gamma-aminobutyric acid in mammalian kidney. *Nature* 1969; 224: 916–7.
57. Erdo SI, Joo F, Wolff JR. Immunohistochemical localisation of glutamic decarboxylase in the rat oviduct and ovary: further evidence for nonneuronal GABA system. *Cell Tiss Res* 1989; 255: 431–4.
58. Persson M, Pello-Huikko M, Meisis M, *et al*. Expression of the neurotransmitter-synthesising enzyme glutamic acid decarboxylase in male germ cell. *Mol Cell Biol* 1990; 10: 4701–11.
59. Kaufman DL, McGinnis JF, Krieger NR, Tobin AM. Brain glutamate decarboxylase cloned in IGT II: fusion protein produces γ-aminobutyric acid. *Science* 1986; 232: 1138–40.
60. Kobayashi Y, Kaufman DL, Tobin AJ. Glutamic acid decarboxylase cDNA: nucleotide sequence encoding an enzymatically active fusion protein. *J Neurosci* 1987; 7: 2768–72.
61. Brilliant MH, Szabo G, Katarova Z, *et al*. Sequences homologous to glutamic acid decarboxylase cDNA are present on mouse chromosomes 2 and 10. *Genomics* 1990; 6: 115–22.
62. Huang WM, Reed-Fourquet L, Wu E, Wu JY. Molecular cloning and amino acid sequence of brain L-glutamic decarboxylase. *Proc Natl Acad Sci USA* 1990; 87: 8491–5.
63. Wyborski RJ, Bond RW, Gottlieb DI. Characterisation of a cDNA coding for rat glutamic acid decarboxylase. *Mol Brain Res* 1990; 8: 193–8.
64. Juben JF, Samama P, Mallet J. Rat brain glutamic acid decarboxylase sequence deduced from a cloned cDNA. *J Neurochem* 1990; 54: 703–5.
65. Erlander MG, Tillakaraine NJK, Feldblum S, Patel N, Tobin AJ. Two genes encode distinct glutamate decarboxylases. *Neuron* 1991; 7: 91–100.
66. Karlssen AF, Hagopian WA, Grubin CE, *et al*. Cloning and primary structure of a human islet isoform of glutamic acid decarboxylase from chromosome 10. *Proc Natl Acad Sci USA* 1991; 88: 8337–41.
67. Kelly C, Carter ND, Johnstone AP, Nussey SS. Cloning of large isoform of human brain glutamic acid decarboxylase. *Lancet* 1991; 338: 1468–9.
68. Giorda R, Pearman M, Tan RC, Vergani D, Trucco M. Glutamic acid decarboxylase expression in islet and brain. *Lancet* 1991; 338: 1469–70.
69. Kaufman DL, Houser CR, Tobin AJ. Two forms of the γ-aminobutyric acid synthetic enzyme glutamic decarboxylase have distinct intraneuronal distributions and cofactor interactions. *J Neurochem* 1991; 56: 720–3.
70. Reets A, Solimena M, Matteoli M, Folli F, Baker R, De Camilli P. GABA and pancreatic β-cells: colocalisation of glutamic acid decarboxylase (*GAD*) and GABA with synaptic-like microvesicles suggests their role in GABA storage and secretion. *EMBO J* 1991; 10: 1275–84.
71. De Camilli P, Jahn R. Pathways to regulated exocytosis in neurons. *Annu Rev Physiol* 1990; 52: 625–45.
72. Sorenson RL, Garry DG, Brette IC. Structural and functional considerations of GABA in islets of Langerhans β-cells and nerves. *Diabetes* 1991; 40: 1365–74.
73. Christgau S, Scherbeck H, Aanstoot HJ, *et al*. Pancreatic β-cells express two autoantigenic forms of glutamic acid decarboxylase: a 65 kDa hydrophilic form and a 64 kDa anaphilic form which can be both membrane bound and soluble. *J Biol Chem* 1991; 266: 257–64.
74. Christie MR, Brown TJ, Cassidy D, Bi MR, Brown TJ, Cassidy D. Binding of anti (insulin-dependent) diabetes patients to glutamic decarboxylase from rat tissues. Evidence for antigenic and non-antigenic forms of the enzyme. *Diabetologia* 1992; 35: 380–4.
75. Hagopian WA, Michelsen B, Karlsen AE, *et al*. Autoantibodies in IDDM primarily recognise the 65,000-M, rather than the 67,000-M, isoform of glutamic acid decarboxylase. *Diabetes* 1993; 42: 631–6.

76. Richter W, Shi Y, Baekkeskov S. Autoreactive epitopes defined by diabetes-associated human monoclonal antibodies are localised in the middle and C-terminal domains of the smaller form of glutamic decarboxylase. *Proc Natl Acad Sci USA* 1993; 90: 2832–6.

77. Martino GV, Tappas M, Braghi S, *et al*. Autoantibodies to glutamic acid decarboxylase (GAD) detected by an immuno-trapping enzyme activity assay: relation to insulin-dependent diabetes mellitus and islet cell antibodies. *J Autoimmunity* 1991; 4: 915–23.

78. Kaufman DL, Erlander MG, Clare-Salzer M, Atkinson MA, MacLaren NK, Tobin AJ. Autoimmunity to two forms of glutamic decarboxylase in insulin-dependent diabetes mellitus. *J Clin Invest* 1992; 89: 283–92.

79. Rowley MJ, Mackay IR, Chen QY, Knowles WJ, Zimmet PZ. Antibodies to glutamic acid decarboxylase discriminate major types of diabetes. *Diabetes* 1992; 41: 548–51.

80. De Alzpurura HJ, Harrison LC, Cram DS. An ELISA for antibodies to recombinant glutamic acid decarboxylase in IDDM. *Diabetes* 1992; 41: 1182–7.

81. Hagopian WA, Karlsen AE, Gottsater A, *et al*. Quantitative assay using recombinant human islet glutamic acid decarboxylase (GAD65) shows that 64k autoantibody positivity at onset predict diabetes Type 1. *J Clin Invest* 1993; 91: 368–74.

82. Schmidli RS, Colman PS, Bonifacio E, Bottazzo GF, Harrison LC, and participating laboratories. High level of concordance between assays for glutamic acid decarboxylase antibodies. *Diabetes* 1994; 43: 1005–9.

83. Christie MR, Vohra G, Champagne P, Daneman D, Delovitch TL. Distinct antibody specificities to a 64-kD islet cell antigen in Type 1 diabetes as revealed by trypsin treatment. *J Exp Med* 1990; 172: 789–95.

84. Christie MR, Hollands JA, Brown TJ, Michelsen BK, Delovitch TL. Detection of pancreatic islet 64,000 Mr autoantigens in insulin-dependent diabetes distinct from glutamate decarboxylase. *J Clin Invest* 1993; 92: 240–8.

85. Palmer JP, Asplin CM, Clemons P, *et al*. Insulin antibodies in insulin-dependent diabetics before insulin treatment. *Science* 1983; 222: 1337–9.

86. Palmer JP. Insulin autoantibodies: their role in the pathogenesis of IDDM. *Diabetes Metab Rev* 1987; 3: 1005–15.

87. Srikanta S, Ricker AT, McCulloch DK, Soeldner JS, Eisenbarth GS, Palmer JP. Autoimmunity to insulin, beta cell dysfunction and development of insulin-dependent diabetes mellitus. *Diabetes* 1986; 39: 139–42.

88. Dean BM, McNally JM, Bonifacio E, *et al*. Comparison of insulin autoantibodies in diabetes related and normal populations by precise displacement ELISA. *Diabetes* 1989; 38: 1275–81.

89. Wilkin TJ, Schoenfeld SL, Diaz JI, Kruse V, Bonifacio E, Palmer JP, and participating laboratories. Systematic variation accounts for much of the differences in insulin autoantibody measurements. *Diabetes* 1989; 38: 172–81.

90. Kuglin B, Kolb H, Greenbaum C, Maclaren NK, Lernmark A, Palmer JP. The Fourth International Workshop on standardisation of insulin autoantibody measurement. *Diabetologia* 1990; 33: 638–9.

91. Sodoyez-Goffaux F, Koch M, Dozio N, Brandenburg D, Sodoyez JC. Advantages and pitfalls of radioimmune and enzyme-linked immunosorbent assays of insulin antibodies. *Diabetologia* 1988; 31: 694–702.

92. Greenbaum CJ, Palmer JP, Kuglin B, Kolb H, and participating laboratories. Insulin autoantibodies measured by RIA methodology are more related to IDDM than those measured by ELISA. *J Clin Endocrinol Metab* 1992; 74: 1040–4.

93. Vardi P, Dib SA, Tuttleman M, *et al*. Competitive insulin autoantibody assay: prospective evaluation of subjects at risk for development of Type 1 diabetes mellitus. *Diabetes* 1987; 36: 1286–91.

94. Vardi P, Ziegler AG, Matthews JH, *et al*. Concentration of insulin-autoantibodies at onset of Type I diabetes—inverse log-linear correlation with age. *Diabetes Care* 1988; 11: 736–9.

95. Kuglin B, Rjasanowski I, Bertrams J, Gries FA, Kolb H, Michaelis D. Antibodies to pro-insulin and insulin as predictive markers of Type 1 diabetes. *Diabetic Med* 1990; 7: 310–14.

96. Castano L, Russo E, Zhou L, Lipes MA, Eisenbarth GS. Identification and cloning of a granule autoantigen (carboxypeptidase-H) associated with Type I diabetes. *J Clin Endocrinol Metab* 1991; 73: 1197–201.

97. Karounos DG, Thomas JW. Recognition of common islet antigen by autoantibodies from NOD mice and humans with IDDM. *Diabetes* 1990; 39: 1085–90.

98. Elias D, Markovits D, Reshef T, Van Der Zee R, Cohen IR. Induction and therapy of autoimmune diabetes in the non-obese diabetic (NOLDI/Lt) mouse by a 65-kDa heat shock protein. *Proc Natl Acad Sci USA* 1990; 87: 1576–90.

99. Jones DB, Hunter RN, Duff GW. Heat-shock protein 65 kD as a β-cell antigen of insulin-dependent diabetes. *Lancet* 1990; 336: 583–5.
100. Kampe O, Velloso L, Andersson A, Karlsson FA. No role for 65kD heatshock protein in diabetes. *Lancet* 1990; 336: 1250.
101. Jones DB, Duff G. Is there no role for heat-shock protein in diabetes? *Lancet* 1991; 337: 115.
102. Johnson JH, Crider BP, McCorki K, Alfrord M, Unger RH. Inhibition of glucose transport into rat islet cells by immunoglobulins from patients with new-onset insulin-dependent diabetes mellitus. *N Engl J Med* 1990; 322: 653–9.
103. Lernmark A, Freedman ZR, Hofman C, *et al.* Islet cell surface antibodies in juvenile diabetes mellitus. *N Engl J Med* 1978; 299: 375–80.
104. Pujol-Borrell R, Khoury EL, Bottazzo GF. Islet cell surface antibodies in type I (insulin-dependent) diabetes mellitus; use of human fetal pancreas cultures as substrate. *Diabetologia* 1982; 22: 89–5.
105. Van de Winkel M, Smets G, Gepts W, Pipeleers DG. Islet cell surface antibodies from insulin-dependent diabetes bind specifically to pancreatic B cells. *J Clin Invest* 1982; 70: 41–9.
106. Vives M, Somoza N, Soldevilla G, *et al.* Re-evaluation of autoantibodies to islet cell membrane in IDDM. Failure to detect islet cell surface antibodies using human islet cells as substrate. *Diabetes* 1992; 41: 1624–31.
107. Boitard C, Sai P, Debray-Sachs M, Assan R, Hamburger J. Anti-pancreatic immunity. *In vitro* studies of cellular and humoral immune reactions directed towards pancreatic islets. *Clin Exp Immunol* 1984; 55: 571–80.
108. Bottazzo GF, Lendrum R. Separate autoantibodies to human pancreatic glucagon and somatostatin cells. *Lancet* 1976; ii: 873–6.
109. Drell DW, Notkins AL. Multiple immunological abnormalities in patients with type I (insulin-dependent) diabetes mellitus. *Diabetologia* 1987; 30: 132–43.
110. Mirakian R, Cudworth AG, Bottazzo GF, Richardson CA, Doniach D. Autoimmunity to anterior pituitary cells and the pathogenesis of type I (insulin-dependent) diabetes mellitus. *Lancet* 1982; ii: 755–9.
111. Vercammen M, Gorus F, Foriers A, *et al.* Cell surface antibodies in type I (insulin-dependent) diabetic patients. I. Presence of immunoglobulins M which bind to rat pituitary cells. *Diabetologia* 1989; 32: 611–7.
112. Serjeantson S, Theophilus J, Zimmet P, Court J, Crossley JR, Eliott RB. Lymphocytotoxic antibodies and histocompatibility antigens in juvenile-onset diabetes mellitus. *Diabetes* 1981; 30: 26–9.
113. Dahlquist G, Savilathi E, Landin-Olsson M. An increased level of antibodies to β-lactoglobulin is a risk determinant for early-onset Type 1 (insulin-dependent) diabetes mellitus independent of islet cell antibodies and early introduction of cow's milk. *Diabetologia* 1992; 35: 980–4.
114. Savilahti E, Saukkonen TT, Virtala ET, Tuomilehto J, Akerblom HK. Increased levels of cow's milk and beta-lactoglobulin antibodies in young children with newly diagnosed IDDM. *Diabetes Care* 1993; 16: 984–9.
115. Karjalainen J, Martin JM, Knip M, *et al.* Evidence for a bovine albumin peptide as a candidate trigger of Type 1 diabetes. *N Engl J Med* 1992; 327: 302–7.
116. Pietropaolo M, Castano L, Babu S, *et al.* Islet cell autoantigen 69kD (ICA69). Molecular cloning and characterisation of a novel diabetes-associated autoantigen. *J Clin Invest* 1993; 92: 359–71.
117. Atkinson MA, Bowman MA, Kao KJ, *et al.* Lack of immune responsiveness to bovine serum albumin in insulin dependent diabetes. *N Engl J Med* 1993; 329: 1853–8.
118. Bosi E, Bonifacio E, Bottazzo GF. Autoantigens in IDDM. *Diabetes Rev* 1993; 1: 204–9.
119. Burroughs AK, Butler P, Sternberg M, Baum H. Molecular mimicry in liver disease. *Nature* 1992; 358: 377–8.
120. Irvine WJ. Immunological aspects of diabetes mellitus: a review. In: Irvine WJ, ed. *Immunology of diabetes*. Edinburgh: Teviot Scientific Publishers, 1980: 1–23.
121. Boitard C, Debray-Sachs M, Pouplard A, *et al.* Lymphocytes from diabetics suppress insulin release *in vitro*. *Diabetologia* 1981; 21: 41–6.
122. Bach J-F. Insulin-dependent diabetes mellitus as an autoimmune disease. *Endocrinol Rev* 1994; 15: 516–42.
123. Harrison LC, DeAizpurua HJ, Loudovaris T, *et al.* Reactivity to human islets and fetal pig proislets by peripheral blood mononuclear cells from subjects with preclinical and clinical insulin-dependent diabetes. *Diabetes* 1991; 40: 1128–33.
124. Honeyman MC, Cram DS, Harrison LC. Transcription factor jun-B is target of autoreactive T-cells in IDDM. *Diabetes* 1993; 42: 626–30.

125. Atkinson MA, Kaufman DL, Campbell L, *et al.* Response of peripheral-blood mononuclear cells to glutamate decarboxylase in insulin-dependent diabetes. *Lancet* 1992; 339: 458–9.
126. Honeyman MC, Cram DS, Harrison LC. Glutamic acid decarboxylase 67-reactive T cells: a marker of insulin-dependent diabetes. *J Exp Med* 1993; 177: 535–40.
127. Lohmann T, Leslie EDG, Hawa M, Geysen M, Rodda S, Londei M. Immunodominant epitopes of glutamic acid decarboxylase 65 and 67 in insulin-dependent diabetes mellitus. *Lancet* 1994; 343: 1607–8.
128. Armstrong NW, Jones DB. Epitopes of GAD 65 in insulin-dependent diabetes mellitus. *Lancet* 1994; 344: 406–7.
129. Atkinson MA, Bowman MA, Campbell L, Darrow BL, Kaufman DL, Maclaren NK. Cellular immunity is a determinant common to glutamate decarboxylase and coxsackie virus in insulin-dependent diabetes. *J Clin Invest* 1994; 94: 2125–29.
130. Bottazzo GF, Pujol-Borrell R, Bonifacio E. The aetiology, genetics and immunology of Type 1 (insulin-dependent) diabetes mellitus. In: Lachmann PJ, Peters DK, Rosen FS, Walport MJ, eds. *Clinical aspects of immunology,* vol 3. Oxford: Blackwell Scientific Publications, 1993: 2009–25.
131. De Berardinis P, Londei M, James RFL, Lake SP, Wise PH, Feldmann M. Do CD4-positive cytotoxic T cells damage islet β-cells in type I diabetes? *Lancet* 1988; ii: 823–4.
132. Van Vilet E, Roep B, Meulenbrock L, Bruining GJ, De Vries RRP. Human T cell clones with specificities for insulinoma cell antigens. *Eur J Immunol* 1989; 19: 213–6.
133. Roep BO, Arden SD, DeVries RP, Hutton JC. T-cell clones from a Type 1 diabetes patient respond to insulin secretory granule proteins. *Nature* 1990; 345: 632–4.
134. Roep BO, Kallan AA, Hazenbos WL, *et al.* T cell reactivity to 38kD insulin secretory granule protein in patients with recent onset type I diabetes. *Lancet* 1991; 337: 1439–41.
135. Bottazzo GF, Dean BM, McNally JM, Mackay EH, Swift PGF, Gamble DR. In situ characterization of autoimmune phenomena and expression of HLA molecules in the pancreas in diabetic insulitis. *N Engl J Med* 1985; 313: 353–60.
136. Bonifacio E, Bottazzo GF. Immunology of IDDM (Type 1 diabetes). Entering the '90's. In: Alberti KGMM, Krall LP, eds. *The diabetes annual 6.* Amsterdam: Elsevier Science Publishing Co, 1991: 20–47.
137. Dawkins RL. Sensitivity and specificity of autoantibody testing. In: Rose NR, Mackay IA, eds. *The autoimmune diseases.* Sydney: Academic Press, 1985: 669–93.
138. Bonifacio E. Where are the T cells? A friendly provocation. *J Endocrinol Invest* 1994; 17: 560–2.
139. Bonifacio E, Bingley P, Shattock M, *et al.* Quantification of islet-cell antibodies and prediction of insulin-dependent diabetes. *Lancet* 1989; 335: 147–9.
140. Gleichmann H, Bottazzo GF. Islet cell and insulin autoantibodies in diabetes. *Immunol Today* 1987; 8: 167–8.
141. Gorsuch AM, Spencer KM, Lister J, *et al.* Evidence for a long pre-diabetic period in Type 1 (insulin-dependent) diabetes mellitus. *Lancet* 1981; ii: 1363–5.
142. Riley WJ, Maclaren NK, Krischer J, *et al.* A prospective study of the development of diabetes in relatives of patients with insulin-dependent diabetes. *N Engl J Med* 1990; 323: 1167–72.
143. Bottazzo GF, Pujol-Borrell R, Gale EAM. Autoimmunity and Type I diabetes: bringing the story up to date. In: Alberti KGMM, Krall LP, eds. *The diabetes annual 3.* Amsterdam: Elsevier Science Publications, 1987: 15–38.
144. Johnstone C, Millward BA, Hoskins P, Leslie RDG, Bottazzo GF, Pyke DA. Islet cell antibodies as predictors of the later development of Type I (insulin-dependent) diabetes. A study in identical twins. *Diabetologia* 1989; 32: 382–6.
145. Bingley PJ, Bonifacio E, Gale EAM. Can we really predict IDDM? *Diabetes* 1993; 42: 213–20.
146. Bingley PJ, Bonifacio E, Shattock M, *et al.* Can islet cell antibodies predict insulin-dependent diabetes in the general population? *Diabetes Care* 1993; 16: 45–50.
147. Green A, Gale EAM, Patterson CC, for the EURODIAB ACE Study Group. Incidence of childhood-onset insulin-dependent-diabetes mellitus: EURODIAB ACE Study. *Lancet* 1992; 339: 905–9.
148. Karjalainen JK. Islet cell antibodies as predictive markers for IDDM in children with high background incidence of disease. *Diabetes* 1990; 39: 1144–50.
149. Loviselli A, Shattock M, Cambosu MA, *et al.* Prevalenza di anticorpi antiisola pancreatica (ICA) in 6463 bambini della scuola dell'obbligo in Sardegna. *Il Diabete* 1994; (Suppl 1): 207A.
150. Bingley PJ, Gale EAM. The incidence of insulin-dependent diabetes in England: a study in the Oxford region 1985–1986. *BMJ* 1989; 289: 558–60.
151. Bottazzo GF, Genovese S, Bosi E, Dean BM, Christie MR, Bonifacio E. Novel considerations on

the antibody/antigen system in Type 1 (insulin-dependent) diabetes mellitus. *Ann Med* 1991; 23: 453–61.

152. Ziegler AG, Zigler R, Vardi P, Jackson RA, Soeldner JS, Eisenbarth GS. Life-table analysis of progression to diabetes of anti-insulin autoantibody-positive relatives of individuals with Type 1 diabetes. *Diabetes* 1989; 38: 1320–5.

153. Ziegler R, Alper CA, Awdeh ZL, *et al.* Specific association of HLA-DR4 with increased prevalence and level of insulin autoantibodies in first degree relatives of Type I diabetes. *Diabetes* 1991; 40: 709–14.

154. Ziegler AG, Hillebrand B, Rabl W, *et al.* On the appearance of islet associated autoimmunity in offspring of diabetic mothers: a prospective study from birth. *Diabetologia* 1993; 36: 402–8.

155. Baekkeskov S, Landin M, Kristensen JK, *et al.* Antibodies to a 64000 Mr human islet cell protein precede the clinical onset of insulin-dependent diabetes. *J Clin Invest* 1987; 79: 926–34.

156. Atkinson MA, Maclaren NK, Scharp DW, Lacy PE, Riley WJ. 64,000 Mr autoantibodies as predictors of insulin-dependent diabetes. *Lancet* 1990; 335: 1357–60.

157. De Aizpurua HJ, Wilson Y, Harrison LC. Glutamic acid decarboxylase (GAD) autoantibodies in pre-clinical insulin-dependent diabetes. *Proc Natl Acad Sci USA* 1992; 89: 9841–5

158. Solimena M, De Camilli P. Autoimmunity to glutamic acid decarboxylase (GAD) in Stiff-man syndrome and insulin dependent diabetes mellitus. *Trends Neurosci* 1991; 14: 452–7.

159. Grubin CE, Daniels T, Toivola B, *et al.* A novel radiobinding assay to determine diagnostic accuracy of isoform-specific glutamic acid decarboxylase antibodies in childhood IDDM. *Diabetologia* 1994; 37: 344–50.

160. Petersen JS, Hejnaes KR, Moody A, *et al.* Detection of GAD65 antibodies in diabetes and other autoimmune diseases using a simple radioligand assay. *Diabetes* 1994; 43: 459–67.

161. Thivolet CH, Tappaz M, Durand A, *et al.* Glutamic acid decarboxylase (GAD) autoantibodies are additional predictive markers of Type 1 (insulin-dependent) diabetes mellitus in high risk individuals. *Diabetologia* 1992; 35: 570–6.

162. Chen Q-Y, Rowley MJ, Byrne GC, *et al.* Antibodies to glutamic acid decarboxylase in Australian children with insulin-dependent diabetes mellitus and their first-degree relatives. *Pediatr Res* 1993; 34: 785–90.

163. Bingley PJ, Christie MR, Bonifacio E, *et al.* Combined analysis of autoantibodies improves prediction of insulin dependent diabetes in islet cell antibody positive relatives. *Diabetes* 1994; 43: 1304–10.

164. Bosi E, Becker F, Bonifacio E, *et al.* Progression to Type I (insulin-dependent) diabetes in autoimmune endocrine patients with islet cell antibodies. *Diabetes* 1991; 40: 977–84.

165. Bonifacio E, Genovese S, Stephens H, *et al.* Autoantibodies to glutamic acid decarboxylase vary in their MHC Class II allele associations. (Abstract) *Diabetologia* 1992; 35 (suppl 1), A50.

166. Christie MR, Genovese S, Cassidy D, *et al.* Antibodies to islet 37k-antigen, but not to glutamate decarboxylase, discriminate rapid progression to insulin-dependent diabetes mellitus in endocrine autoimmunity. *Diabetes* 1994; 43: 1254–59.

167. Wagner R, McNally JM, Bonifacio E, *et al.* Lack of immunohistological changes in the islets of non-diabetic autoimmune polyendocrine patients with β-selective GAD-specific islet cell antibodies. *Diabetes* 1994; 43: 851–6.

168. Bottazzo GF, Mirakian R, Drexhage HA. Adrenalitis, oophoritis and autoimmune polyglandular disease. In: Rich RR, ed. *Clinical immunology: principles and practice.* St Louis: CV Mosby (in press).

169. Velloso LA, Winqvist O, Gustafsson J, Kampe O, Karlsson FA. Autoantibodies against a novel 51 kDa islet antigen and glutamate decarboxylase isoforms in autoimmune polyendocrine syndrome Type 1. *Diabetologia* 1994; 37: 61–9.

170. Christie MR, Tun RYM, Lo SSS, *et al.* Antibodies to glutamic acid decarboxylase and tryptic fragments of islet 64kD antigen as distinct markers for the development of insulin-dependent diabetes: studies with identical twins. *Diabetes* 1992; 41: 782–7.

171. Genovese S, Bingley PJ, Christie MR, *et al.* Combined analysis of IDDM-related autoantibodies in healthy school children. *Lancet* 1994; 344: 756.

172. Faustman D, Schoenfeld D, Ziegler R. T lymphocyte changes linked to autoantibodies: association of insulin antibodies with DC4+/CD45R+ lymphocyte subpopulation in pre-diabetic subjects. *Diabetes* 1991; 40: 590–7.

173. Schatz DA, Riley WJ, Maclaren NK, Barrett DJ. Defective inducer T cell function before the onset of insulin-dependent diabetes mellitus. *J Autoimmun* 1991; 4: 125–36.

174. Al Sakkaf L, Pozzilli P, Tarn AC, Schwartz G, Gale EAM, Bottazzo GF. Persistent reduction of

CD4/CD8 ratio and T cell activation before the onset of type 1 (insulin-dependent) diabetes. *Diabetologia* 1989; 32: 322–5.

175. Al-Sakkaf L, Pozzilli P, Bingley PJ, *et al*. Early T-cell defects in pre-type1 diabetes. *Acta Diabetol* 1992; 28: 189–92.

176. Smerdon RA, Peakman M, Hussain MJ, *et al*. CD5$^+$ B-cells at the onset of Type 1 diabetes and in the prediabetic period. *Diabetes Care* 1994; 17: 657–64.

177. Tun RYM, Peakman M, Alviggi L, *et al*. Importance of persistent cellular and humoral immune changes before diabetes develops: prospective study of identical twins. *BMJ* 1994; 308: 1063–8.

178. Faustman D, Li X, Lin HY, *et al*. Linkage of faulty major histocompatibility complex Class I to autoimmune diabetes. *Science* 1991; 254: 1756–61.

179. Harrison LC, Chu XS, DeAizpurua HJ, Graham M, Honeyman MC, Colman PG. Islets reactive T-cells are a marker of preclinical insulin-dependent diabetes. *J Clin Invest* 1992; 89: 1161–5.

180. Harrison LC, Honeyman MC, de Aizpurua HJ, *et al*. Inverse relation between humoral and cellular immunity to glutamic acid decarboxylase in subjects at risk of insulin-dependent diabetes. *Lancet* 1993; 341: 1365–9.

181. Leiter EH. The role of environmental factors in modulating insulin-dependent diabetes. In: de Vries RRP, Cohen IR, van Rood JJ, eds. *The role of micro-organisms in non-infectious disease*. 14th Argenteuil Symposium, Brussels. Berlin: Springer-Verlag, 1990: 39–54.

182. Harrison LC. Islet cell antigens in insulin-dependent diabetics. Pandora's box revisited. *Immunol Today* 1992; 13: 348–52.

183. Deschamps J, Boitard C, Hors J, *et al*. Life-table analysis of the risk of Type 1 (insulin-dependent) diabetes in siblings according to islet cell antibodies and HLA markers. An 8 year prospective study. *Diabetologia* 1992; 35: 951–7.

184. Lipton RB, La Porte RE, Dorman JS, Riley WJ, Trucco M, Becker DJ. A combination of HLA-DQ-β non-ASP-57 homozygosity and positive islet cell antibody (ICA) assay predicts insulin dependent diabetes in relatives of children with IDDM. (Abstract) *Diabetes* 1991; 40 (suppl 1): 151A.

185. Srikanta S, Ganda OP, Gleason RE, Jackson RA, Soeldner JS, Eisenbarth GS. Pre-type I diabetes: linear loss of β-cell response to intravenous glucose. *Diabetes* 1984; 33: 717–20.

186. Vardi P, Crisà L, Jackson RA. Predictive value of intravenous glucose tolerance test insulin secretion less than or greater than the first percentile in islet cell antibody positive relatives of Type 1 (insulin-dependent) diabetic patients. *Diabetologia* 1991; 34: 93–102.

187. Wagner R, Genovese S, Bosi E, *et al*. Slow metabolic deterioration towards diabetes in islet cell antibody positive patients with autoimmune polyendocrine disease. *Diabetologia* 1994; 37: 365–71.

188. Palmer JP. What is the best way to predict IDDM? *Lancet* 1994; 343: 1377–8.

189. Bingley PJ, Bonifacio E, Gale EAM. Antibodies to glutamic acid decarboxylase as predictors of insulin-dependent diabetes mellitus. *Lancet* 1994; 344: 266.

190. Tuomilehto J, Zimmet P, Mackay IR, *et al*. Antibodies to glutamic acid decarboxylase as predictors of insulin-dependent diabetes mellitus before clinical onset of disease. *Lancet* 1994; 343: 1383–5.

191. Groop L, Bottazzo GF, Doniach D. Islet cell antibodies identify latent Type I diabetes in patients aged 35–75 years at diagnosis. *Diabetes* 1986; 35: 237–42.

192. Tuomi T, Groop LC, Zimmet PZ, Rowley MJ, Knowley W, Mackay JR. Antibodies to glutamic acid decarboxylase reveal latent autoimmune diabetes mellitus in adults with a non-insulin dependent onset of disease. *Diabetes* 1993; 42: 359–62.

193. Bosi E, Bottazzo GF. Autoimmunity in insulin-dependent diabetes mellitus: implications for prediction and therapy. *Clin Immunother* 1995; 3: 125–35.

DISCUSSION

Dr. Swift: You mentioned in one part of your talk that diabetes mellitus has a long latency period, but 25% of children develop diabetes before the age of 5 years. Of course diabetes in the first year of life is very rare indeed and probably has a different etiology, but what about those children aged between 1 and 2 who develop diabetes?

Dr. Bottazzo: I have shown that the peak of IDDM is increased at 5 years, so there appears to be a trend toward onset of the disease at a younger age. The latency period thus seems to be getting shorter in this young age group.

Dr. Swift: Is the age group distribution similar in Sardinia, and is there a switch from older presentation of diabetes to the younger age groups?

Dr. Bottazzo: We have not fully analyzed all the epidemiological data yet. The only thing I can tell you is that males are more affected than females at the 14-year peak of age on the Island, a trend generally observed in IDDM in all the countries in which this particular parameter has been analyzed.

Dr. Swift: Are we seeing a real increase in the overall incidence and prevalence of diabetes internationally or is there a switch from an older age group to a younger age group?

Dr. Bottazzo: This is an important question. Preliminary data from Kuwait suggest that the incidence of IDDM has increased there from 9.5 per 100,000 in 1987 to 11 per 100,000 in 1992–1993, so something is changing in an apparently "cold" area for IDDM. In the Mediterranean area, even if we still maintain overall a low incidence of the disease and even if a different age range of affected patients is maintained, there has definitely been a cumulative increase of IDDM in the last twenty years. However, this increase was not so impressive as in Finland and Sardinia.

Dr. Bartsokas: We should note here that the incidence rates previously reported as low from certain Eastern European countries did not represent the true figures, because, due to lack of insulin, many cases of insulin-dependent diabetes were lost. It is expected, however, that through participation in the EURODIAB project and the assistance of WHO/EUROPE offering better care in these countries, the figures obtained presently are more accurate.

Dr. Drash: The issue of the age of onset is presently unclear. Certainly in the Pittsburgh data we are seeing younger children, that is, statistically younger than we did 10 years ago, and in my discussions with friends around the world many are describing the same phenomenon, but I have seen no analysis. However, I think that it is correct that we are seeing more patients presenting in an earlier age group.

Dr. Otten: We find only 75–80% islet cell antibody (ICA) positivity at the time of diagnosis and before treatment is started. You produced similar figures. What happened to the other 20–25%? We looked to see if there were a higher percentage of ICA positivity in older children, but in our group there was no difference. We followed 60 children over 4 years and did ICA estimations twice a year. The young ones with onset between 5 and 8 years lost their ICA positivity to a great extent within the first 2 years, but positivity in the older ones persisted at around 60%. I don't have any explanation for this.

Dr. Bottazzo: These 20–25% of ICA-negative IDDM patients at diagnosis have always been present in all the series published so far, no matter how sensitive was the method for the detection of these antibodies. However, if one follows first-degree relatives of IDDM families, the ones who become diabetic without being ICA positive are the exception. So, at least in susceptible, first-degree relatives of IDDM children, one can say that the majority at diagnosis are ICA positive. What we don't know is the situation in the so-called "sporadic" cases, the ones without a family history of the disease and that are picked up from surveys of healthy school children. Among the first 1142 school children we have followed in Sardinia, five have become diabetic, and all were ICA positive. However, I cannot exclude the possibility that there may be a small proportion of cases that are not autoimmune in nature.

Dr. Beauvais: What do you think about the proposed treatment of prediabetes with insulin?

Dr. Bottazzo: Everyone quotes the animal studies to support intervention trials in prediabetes in humans. However, even if animal studies are very instructive, we are a long way from being able to extrapolate the data obtained in them and apply them to the human situation. Indeed, insulin has worked in the NOD mouse when injected in the prediabetic period, reducing the appearance of diabetes in these animals but, let me tell you, everything else has worked in the NOD mouse too.

Dr. Crofford: What kind of rules do you use to classify a sporadic case as opposed to a familial case, or whether the family history is inadequate or incorrect? How do you decide whether it is just a sporadic case or a familial case with an incomplete family history?

Dr. Bottazzo: In our Sardinia-IDDM study, the school children are always interviewed by a doctor, using a questionnaire. So, the questionnaire is filled out properly by a competent person who asks the child if there is anybody with diabetes, and with which type of diabetes, in the family. Of course, a 10-year-old child may not have any idea whether there is diabetes, or which type of diabetes, in the family. It is because of this possibility that the questionnaire is always validated by interviewing either the mother or the father.

Dr. Marliss: Don't you think it is possible that we are dealing with a number of different diseases? Why may it not be a different disease in children under the age of 5. Clearly the rate of progression and the presence or absence of antibodies are different in this subset. Maybe it is also a different disease in twins or multiplex families than it is in sporadic cases. Perhaps we are looking at the whole bunch of different pathophysiologic mechanisms and that we are confusing ourselves by trying to fit them all into one condition.

Dr. Bottazzo: If anybody is interested in the 20% of cases who are found to be ICA negative at diagnosis, then let them concentrate on them. I prefer to concentrate on the 80% who are ICA positive. I, personally, no longer believe that IDDM is a multifactorial disease. If one goes back and reads the pathology books of 30 or 40 years ago on the ethiopathogenesis of hepatitis and polio, when the viruses causing the corresponding disease were not yet discovered, one can see the type of "fantasy and imagination" indulged in by our colleagues at that time, just as we do now when we write our reviews on the pathogenesis of IDDM. As you know, it ultimately turned out that one virus was the causative agent for each of the two diseases; and, even if it is true to say that there are several variants of the hepatitis virus, but all belonging to the same family. I cannot believe that in Sardinia and in Finland, two isolated countries that have been genetically different for centuries, several distinct causative agents of IDDM should come into the story. I believe that a single putative agent must play a part in cause and effect in the ultimate damage of the islet beta cells.

Diabetes, edited by Richard M. Cowett,
Nestlé Nutrition Workshop Series,
Vol. 35. Nestec Ltd.,
Vevey/Raven Press, Ltd., New York © 1995.

Can We Detect and Can We Treat Subjects at High Risk of Type 1, Insulin-Dependent Diabetes Mellitus?

Roger Assan, Etienne Larger and *José Timsit

*Diabetes Department, Hôpital Bichat, Paris, France, and *Clinical Immunology, Hôpital Necker, Paris, France*

Until recently, the diagnosis of type 1 (insulin-dependent) diabetes mellitus (IDDM) was simple. Hyperglycemia has always been the gold standard for the diagnosis of diabetes, and insulin dependency is usually easy to identify from simple clinical and metabolic parameters. When diagnosed at that stage of the disease, patients are condemned to daily insulin therapy, indefinitely prolonged, and to the long-term serious complications (retinal, renal, etc.) of chronic hyperglycemia. Intensive insulin therapy designed to normalize blood glucose values has been shown to defer the onset of these complications (1), but it adds an additional burden of discomfort to the patient's daily life. For these reasons, other therapeutic avenues have been intensively explored over the past 10–15 years.

Type 1 diabetes is the result of progressive autoimmune destruction of the β cells of the islets of Langerhans that develops over the course of years before the overt clinical onset of IDDM (2). The autoimmune character of IDDM has been strongly suggested by its relatively frequent association with polyendocrine and nonendocrine tissue-specific autoimmune diseases by the presence of circulating antibodies directed against the islet cells and demonstrable at the clinical onset of the disease, and by the detection of insulitis in recent-onset diabetic subjects. Definite proof of the autoimmune nature of the disease, and of the predominant role of T lymphocytes in this process, has been provided by cyclosporin-A-induced remissions from insulin dependency. Finally, the nonobese diabetic (NOD) mouse strain, and the BB rat strain are animal models of autoimmune insulin-dependent diabetes, in many ways similar to the human IDDM, and particularly useful for the study of its pathophysiology and for experimental therapeutic trials (2). In human subjects, as well as in animal models, a long period of latency precedes the clinical onset. It has become increasingly apparent that more than 80% of the normal insulin secretory capacity is lost during this latent period, before the clinical onset of disease. Early immunosuppressive trials, and to some extent intensified insulin therapy (when started early), can suspend the β-cell destruction process and induce transient remissions from insulin dependency but, to date, no definitive cure for the disease has been obtained. Other means are therefore needed.

Newer, nontoxic immuno-interventions, particularly those based on the concept of tolerogenesis, are emerging and may soon be available for clinical use. For this reason diabetologists and practitioners (particularly pediatricians) are confronted with the problem of identifying people at risk of IDDM, but not yet diabetic, in view of the potential for preventive treatment.

The aim of the present review is to consider: 1. the diagnostic tools for "pretype 1 diabetes," and 2. the new potential therapies, in their present state.

DIAGNOSIS OF PRETYPE 1 DIABETES

The initial contribution of the clinician, albeit limited, is not negligible. When type 1 diabetes is suspected in a family or an individual subject because of transient hyperglycemia, one must not be fooled by other hyperglycemic syndromes such as type 2 (maturity onset) diabetes, MODY (maturity onset diabetes in the young), transient hyperglycemia, and insulin dependency in non-Caucasian adolescents, and so on. This is not a purely academic exercise; correct diagnosis is essential before considering the use of immunosuppressive treatment.

Pretype 1 subjects are defined by the concomitant presence of (a) *normal* blood glucose values, a *normal* oral glucose tolerance test (OGTT), and a decreased β-cell secretory response to intravenous glucose, particularly the early phase of the response (sum of plasma insulin levels at 1 minute and 3 minutes after an intravenous glucose load of 0.5 g/kg, given under well defined conditions); and (b) the presence of circulating antibodies directed at the islet cells (ICA). Most Caucasians carry the (HLA) risk alleles DR3 or DR4, or both.

Pretype 1 subjects differ from "pre-clinical" type 1 patients, who present with abnormal glucose tolerance (abnormal OGTT and excessive fasting and postprandial blood glucose levels), corresponding to a more pronounced deterioration of islet β-cell function.

Immunologic Indices: Islet Cell Antibodies

Islet cell antibodies (ICA), as detected by indirect fluorescence on human group O pancreatic sections, were described nearly a quarter century ago. They remain the cornerstone of the identification of the immunologic nature of prediabetes and recent-onset diabetes in everyday clinical practice (3). This is not the place to discuss the technical details of the detection of islet cell antibodies by complement fixation (CF-ICA), or the increased sensitivity that can be obtained by the addition of aprotinine, or the significance of antibodies that are restricted, or not, to the β cells.

However it is of prime importance to note that islet cell antibodies must: 1. be detected by a rigorous and well-defined technique, with constant reference to quality controls; 2. be quantified by serial dilution and expressed as JDF units; and 3. be serially reassessed. High titers of islet cell antibodies have a prognostic significance and herald the imminent onset of overt IDDM. Seroconversion (from negativity to positivity) has been observed in some instances. Fluctuations in titer (and in positivity) have also been observed in a few cases.

Two problems still remain, however. 1. The exact nature of the β-cell antigen(s) that account for antibody binding to the islets is not known. A multiplicity of chemically defined antigens has been described (Table 1) that include β cell secretory products, membrane proteins and glycolipids, structural proteins, and protein fragments. However, none of these fulfill the criteria of a primary antigen, responsible for triggering the autoimmune cellular process, particularly T cell dependency. 2. The second problem consists of the absence, at present, of an *in vitro* T cell test for the diagnosis of an autoimmune process that appears to be T cell mediated, rather than antibody mediated.

These problems are likely to be resolved in the near future in view of the identification of the 65 kDa and 67 kDa antigens to glutamic acid decarboxylase (GAD) (4) and the description, in the NOD model of proliferative Th1 lymphocyte responses *in vitro,* of GAD epitopes (5). Briefly, lymphocytes from NOD mice, when incubated *in vitro* with various GAD epitopes, develop a proliferative response as early as the third week of age. The earliest stimulatory peptide is the 509–528 GAD sequence, proliferative responses to other epitopes being recruited later on. Some peptides not structurally related to GAD induce no reaction, and the lymphocytes from other nondiabetic mouse strains do not respond to GAD epitopes. Early postnatal injections of GAD 65 into the thymus of NOD mice "tolerize" the animals specifically to this peptide; in these animals the prevalence of diabetes is decreased by 60%, and the onset (in those that develop the disease) is also significantly delayed (6).

TABLE 1. *Target autoantigens in type 1 (insulin-dependent) diabetes mellitus*

Insulin, proinsulin
Glycolipids, ganglioside GT3
64kDa antigen, glutamic acid decarboxylase
Carboxypeptidase H, PM-1, polar antigen
P-69, ABBOS
38-kDa secretory granule membrane component
Peripherin
Heat shock proteins 65 and 60
Insulin receptor
Endocrine cell antigen
Tubulin, actin, reticulin
Nuclear antigens (ssDNA, ssRNA)

B Cell Functional Defect: The [1' + 3'] Insulin Peak

The normal (physiological) β-cell secretory response to an intravenous glucose challenge (IVGTT) is biphasic, with an early peak of secretion, followed by a transient decrease, and then by a secondary sustained insulin secretory response. In pretype 1 subjects, the early phase of secretion is decreased, and this alteration can precede by several years the onset of diabetes. A progressive loss of the early secretion peak during the prediabetic period has been observed, and a linear biparametric mathematic expression of this loss has been tentatively proposed by Eisenbarth *et al.* (7). If verified in all cases, this equation might allow an exact prediction of the onset of insulin dependency. By and large, the [1 + 3] minute insulin secretory response is above 50 μU/ml in the normal individual (islet cell antibody negative, not a relative of a patient with IDDM); it is lower than 25 μU/ml in prediabetic subjects who later on developed diabetes (8). The predictive value of the IVGTT is somewhat diminished by some interindividual and intraindividual variations. Mean [1 + 3] insulin values increase from infancy to puberty, possibly because of maturation of β-cell function during the first postnatal years, and because of insulin resistance of hormonal origin during puberty (9). A wide scattering of values in normal nonprediabetic individuals is observed. Obesity can be present in prediabetic children, which generates insulin resistance and increases the plasma insulin concentrations. Stress and the nutritional state at the time of the test are other factors in the response variation. At recruitment of subjects for study, two successive intravenous glucose tolerance tests must be performed, and, if the results are discordant, a third one should be done. It has been shown that the predictive efficiency of low first-phase insulin values is better when cross-checked by islet cell antibody and genetic determinations.

Genetic Typing

IDDM has long been known to be associated with particular histocompatibility leukocyte antigen (HLA) alleles and there is substantial evidence, from family studies, that the major loci that confer disease susceptibility are found on the class II HLA region of the major histocompatibility complex (MHC) (10), that is, HLA DRB1, DQA1, and DQB1. These genes code for HLA molecules expressed at the surface of macrophages and other antigen presenting cells that present antigens to the T $CD4^+$ cells. Therefore, these molecules are not only markers associated with the disease, but are functionally significant by reason of their ability to bind pathogenic antigens and transfer a message to the T cells. Their role is also essential in the thymic selection of the T lymphocyte repertoire. We have studied HLA class II DRB1, DQA1 and DQB1 alleles in 402 type 1 diabetic patients and in 405 healthy controls (all Caucasian), using oligonucleotide typing after gene amplification (11). Alleles DRB1*03, DRB1*04, DQB1*0201, DQB1*0302, DQA1*0301, and DQA1*0501 were indeed enriched in diabetics and the highest relative risk was observed in patients carrying the DRB1*03, DQB1*0201 and DRB1*0402 or DRB1*0405-DQB1*0302 haplotypes. However, none of these alleles, or specific residues, could alone account for the susceptibility to IDDM. Furthermore, there were major differences in HLA class II gene profiles according to the age of onset. Patients with onset after 15 years (n = 290) showed a significantly higher percentage of non-DR3/non-DR4 genotypes than those with childhood onset (n = 112) and a lower percentage of DR3/4 genotypes. These non-DR3/non-DR4 patients, although presenting clinically as IDDM type 1 showed a lower frequency of islet cell antibodies at diagnosis and a significantly milder initial insulin deficiency. These subjects probably represent a particular subset of IDDM patients whose frequency increases with age. The data confirm the genetic heterogeneity of IDDM and emphasize the need for caution in extrapolating to adult patients the genetic concepts derived from childhood IDDM.

The highest risk for developing IDDM was found in heterozygous individuals carrying the DR3-DQB1*0201 haplotype together with the DRB1*0402 or 0405-DQB1*0202 haplotype. Although this genotype, which occurred in none of the healthy controls, was present in only 8.3% of the IDDM patients, it provided a relative risk of 40.05. Thus this haplotype combination appears to be relatively specific but poorly sensitive as a screening test for genetic predisposition to IDDM.

The distribution of DPB alleles was not significantly different among diabetics and controls. However, DPB1*0301 allele was enriched in DR3 and DR4 diabetic patients and was more frequent in type 1a than in type 1b patients.

Genetic polymorphism affects other loci contributing to the immune system: genes coding for the digestion and transport of antigens within macrophages (LMP and TAP loci), for some effector molecules such as tumor necrosis factor, and for the DNA "boxes" that regulate the expression of the MHC genes. Owing to the presence of some linkage disequilibria, one can infer the allelic profile of other polymorphic genes from HLA-DR and/or DQ typing.

When only the main HLA-DR and DQ markers are determined when screening for a predisposition to diabetes in the genetic background, a compromise exists between maximum sensitivity (87%), as obtained by the HLA DR3 or DR4 genotype, and maximum specificity, as obtained by the HLA DQB Asp $-/-$ and HLA-DRA Arg $+/+$ genotypes (100%), but at the price of missing 75% of the subjects at risk (Table 2).

TABLE 2. *Sensitivity/specificity of the main HLA markers*

Markers	Sensitivity (%)	Specificity (%)
DR3, or DR4	87	64
DQB57 asp $^{--}$	74	75
DQA52 arg $^{++}$	68	77
DQB asp $^{--}$/DQA arg $^{++}$	52	94
DR3/DR4	31	95
DQB 2/3; DQA 3/4.1	25	100

TABLE 3. *ICA positivity in 597 siblings of diabetic children, according to HLA phenotype of the proband and the number of haplotypes shares with the proband*

		HLA phenotype of the proband				
		DR3m/X* (%)	DR4/Y* (%)	DR*/4 (%)	DRX/Y* (%)	All (%)
No haplotype	(n = 144)	0	0	0	0	0
1 haplotype	(n = 305)	2.6	7.4	23	0	5.6
2 haplotypes	(n = 148)	2.4	2.2	19	11	8.8

* X, any haplotype except DR3; Y, any haplotype except DR4

Some type 1 diabetic subjects have neither the DR3 nor the DR4 alleles. The "diabetogenic gene" is still to be identified, and some non-HLA genes must contribute to the genetic predisposition.

Cross-check of Immunologic and HLA Markers

Among 597 siblings of type 1 diabetic children studied at the Necker hospital, the distribution of HLA haplotypes respected Mendelian laws: 25% were HLA nonidentical (no haplotype in common with the proband), 50% were HLA haplo-identical (1 haplotype shared with the proband), and 25% were HLA identical with the proband. Islet cell antibody positivity was strongly linked with sharing the HLA haplotype: none of the HLA nonidentical siblings were islet cell antibody positive. Positivity for islet cell antibodies increased to 5.6% of HLA haplo-identical and 8.8% of HLA identical siblings (Table 3). The link was even stronger if the HLA phenotype of the proband was HLA DR3 and DR4: 23% of HLA haplo-identical and 19% of HLA identical siblings of DR3 and DR4 patients were islet cell antibody positive, the risk of developing diabetes being 70% after 8 years in these individuals. This uneven distribution of risk in siblings according to HLA genotype and HLA genotype sharing with the proband underlines the functional importance of HLA molecules in the development of the disease (12).

ORAL TOLEROGENESIS: FACTS AND PERSPECTIVES

The intestinal epithelium is not an impermeable barrier to dietary macromolecules. However, in most individuals the presence of dietary proteins in the blood stream causes no problems. Moreover, feeding on animal protein antigen results in specific unresponsiveness to the same antigen given parenterally (13). This phenomenon, termed *oral tolerance,* is to some extent understood. Cells recovered from Peyer's patches and from the mesenteric lymph nodes following oral ingestion of an antigen and then transferred to syngeneic recipients cause a marked suppression of systemic T cell and β-cell responses to subsequent parenteral immunization with the same antigen. In mice, the particular cells that transfer nonresponsiveness bear the surface markers Thy1 and CD8, which used to be considered characteristic of suppressor T cells.

Oral tolerance has been used as an experimental means of subverting autoimmune responses. Thus feeding animals myelin basic protein (MBP) or proteolipid protein (PLP) suppresses the development of experimental autoimmune encephalitis, a condition that is induced by injecting rats with MBP or PLP and that serves as a model for multiple sclerosis. Feeding type II collagen prevents collagen-induced arthritis, an animal model of rheumatoid arthritis. Indeed, oral tolerance to autoantigens is a general phenomenon: feeding S antigen suppresses experimental uveitis; feeding glutamate decarboxylase or insulin suppresses spontaneous diabetes in NOD mice; feeding acetyl choline receptor inhibits experimental myasthenia gravis; and feeding thyroglobulin suppresses experimental thyroiditis.

The therapeutic efficacy of oral tolerance was first assessed clinically in multiple sclerosis, in a double-blind pilot trial of feeding patients with bovine myelin (300 mg) daily for one year. Although patients fed myelin had fewer major attacks than those fed placebo, the results did not achieve statistical significance. The efficacy of oral tolerance as a treatment for autoimmune disease was, however, confirmed by the results of a recent double-blind trial on the effects on severe active rheumatoid arthritis of feeding small amounts (0.5–1.0 mg per day) of type II chicken collagen for one year. In the patients fed collagen, there was a significant decrease in the number of swollen joints, in the degree of swelling, in the number of tender joints, and in the amount of pain. Importantly, all patients were taken off steroids and other immunosuppressive agents before the start of treatment. This study therefore establishes the efficacy of oral tolerance as a therapy in autoimmune disease. Because of the innocuous nontoxic nature of the treatment, it might be preferable to conventional immunosuppression or it might form an important adjunct.

Immunohistochemical staining for cytokines in the brains of rats with acute experimental allergic encephalomyelitis (EAE) reveals that, during active disease, cells staining for IL-2 and interferon-Y are prominent in the lesions. These cytokines, which are made by $CD4^+$ Th1 subset helper T cells, are strongly pro-inflammatory. During the recovery phase of EAE, cells staining for transforming growth factor α and interleukin-4 are prominent: these cytokines suppress Th1 responses and may be important in the resolution of the lesions. In the brains of animals fed myelin basic protein, by contrast, inflammation is low after subsequent immunization with this antigen, and there are few IL-2 and interferon-Y containing cells, but cells containing TGF13 are prominent. Finally, treating rats with antiserum to TGF13 abrogates the protective effects of oral feeding with myelin basic protein, and in fact makes the lesions worse.

Thus it would appear that feeding myelin basic protein induces the production of regulatory $CD8^+$ cells that inhibit encephalogenic Th1 $CD4^+$ T cells by producing TGFβ, and perhaps other downregulatory cytokines such as interleukin-4 and interleukin-10. Rats fed ovalbumin and then immunized with ovalbumin mixed with myelin basic protein do not develop EAE, unlike rats immunized with myelin basic protein alone. Since ovalbumin is unlikely to be present in the central nervous tissues but will be present in the draining lymph nodes, *bystander suppression* must be occurring at this site. This proposal is consistent with data showing that CD8$^+$ cells do not appear to be important in recovery from EAE but are important in resistance to subsequent EAE induction.

The concept of tolerogenesis is currently being tried in the NOD mouse model of autoimmune diabetes (14). In mice fed insulin by gastric tubing from the fifth week of life, the incidence of diabetes is significantly reduced over one year and lymphocytic infiltration in the islets is curtailed. Furthermore, splenic T cells from animals orally treated with insulin adoptively transfer protection against diabetes, showing that oral insulin administration generates active cellular mechanisms that suppress disease (14).

These results raise the possibility that the oral administration of insulin or other pancreatic autoantigens (glutamic acid decarboxylase?) may provide a new approach for the prevention of IDDM. Several trials in human pretype 1 subjects are presently being prepared along these lines.

REFERENCES

1. Lasker RD. The Diabetes Control and Complication Trial. *N Engl J Med* 1993: 329: 1035–6.
2. Castano L, Eisenbarth GS. Type 1 diabetes: a chronic autoimmune disease of human, mouse and rat. *Annu Rev Immunol* 1990; 8: 647–79.
3. Riley WJ, Maclaren NK, Krischer J, *et al*. A prospective study of the development of diabetes in relatives of patients with insulin-dependent diabetes. *N Engl J Med* 1990; 323: 1167–72.
4. Baekkeskov S, Aanstoot HJ, Christgau S, *et al*. Identification of the 64 k autoantigen in insulin-dependent diabetes as the GABA synthesizing enzyme glutamic acid decarboxylase. *Nature* 1990; 347: 151–6.
5. Kaufman DL, Clare-Salzler M, Tian J, *et al*. Spontaneous loss of T-cell tolerance to glutamic acid decarboxylase in murine IDDM. *Nature* 1993; 366: 69–72.
6. Tisch R, Yang XD, Singer SM, *et al*. Immune response to glutamic acid decarboxylase correlates with insulitis in non-obese diabetic mice. *Nature* 1993; 366: 72–5.
7. Bleich D, Jackson RA, Soeldner JS, Eisenbarth GS. Analysis of metabolic progression to type 1 diabetes in ICA-positive relatives of patients with type I diabetes. *Diabetes Care* 1990; 13: 111–8.
8. Rayman G, Clark P, Schneider AE, Hales CN. The first phase insulin response to intravenous glucose is highly reproducible. *Diabetologia* 1990; 33: 631–4.
9. Palmer JP, McCulloch DK. Perspective in diabetes. Prediction and prevention of IDDM-1991. *Diabetes* 1991; 40: 943–7.
10. Todd JA. Genetic control of autoimmunity in type 1 diabetes. *Imunol Today* 1990; 11: 122–9.
11. Caillat-Zucman S, Garchon HJ, Timsit J, *et al*. Age-dependent HLA genetic heterogeneity of type 1 insulin-dependent diabetes mellitus. *J Clin Invest* 1992; 90: 2242–50.
12. Deschamps I, Boitard C, Hors J, *et al*. Life table analysis of the risk of type 1 (insulin-dependent) diabetes mellitus in siblings according to islet cell antibodies and HLA markers. An 8-year prospective study. *Diabetologia* 1992; 35: 951–7.
13. McDonald TT. Eating your ways toward immunosuppression. *Curr Biol* 1994; 4: 178–81.
14. Zhang ZJ, Davidson L, Eisenbarth G, and Weiner HL. Suppression of diabetes in nonobese diabetic mice by oral administration of porcine insulin. *Proc Natl Acad Sci USA* 1991; 88: 10252–6.

DISCUSSION

Dr. Bottazzo: A recent paper published in *Clinical and Experimental Immunology* by the Uppsala group (1) showed that pre-IDDM and overtly diabetic NOD mice do not produce autoantibodies to glutamic acid decarboxylase (GAD), nor could the Authors find GAD_{65}, in mouse islets in general. So, it is not easy to interpret the data you have just quoted and which appeared in the two papers recently published in *Nature* (2,3). There the authors have detected instead autoantibodies to GAD_{65} in pre-IDDM NOD mice. However, one can always argue that a T cell response to GAD_{65} might be more relevant than antibodies to the enzyme in these pre-IDDM mice, as indeed it was also shown by the same two groups (2,3). However, could you tell us how the T cells of the mice can exert their direct pathogenetic role against β cells, if GAD_{65} is not expressed in them? Let me add something else. Close to the time of the publication of the two reports in *Nature,* another paper appeared in *Diabetes* that showed that the first response of T cells in the pre-IDDM NOD mice is to a crude homogenate of islets, and this precedes their response to GAD (4). So, even if everybody tends to believe that GAD is the ultimate solution to the problem of IDDM (and I have expressed my scepticism on this general opinion during my presentation), I think we need a much more critical evaluation of the data and compare them with what is actively going on in human IDDM, before concluding that this is indeed the case.

Dr. Assan: You have yourself underlined the fact that sequence similarities do exist between GAD and some exogenous antigens. One may well be exposed to a foreign antigen and then respond to GAD. I am aware of what you are saying, but a very attractive concept for me was that of a progressive recruitment accounting for the variety of antibodies. Maybe GAD is not the genuine primary antigen, but would you agree that it comes near to it?

Dr. Bottazzo: Maybe. However, I believe that all the effort has to be placed in identifying the islet autoantigen that initiates the whole process and the subsequent cascade of events leading to β-cell destruction. To reiterate what I said before, the main question remains: can we fully extrapolate data from the NOD mice to the human situation? We are now in the process of testing 10,000 Sardinian school children for GAD antibodies. In addition, cord blood will be collected from 15,000 newborns, and these infants will be followed yearly and bled for at least 5 years. The main aim behind this project is to find out which of the IDDM-related markers appears first, second, third, and so on. This is the only way to clarify the temporal appearance of the known autoantibodies in human pre-IDDM.

Dr. Drash: What about some of the practical aspects of the protocols that are now being worked out? A very specific point has been raised about the possible loss of those extraordinarily valuable but rare individuals, the first-degree relatives at high risk. It is going to take many thousands of cases by everybody's calculations to obtain the necessary 300 or 400 to do the study. If that resource is wasted, it will be years before it can be recovered. This is an issue that needs to be taken into consideration right now, not later on. Is the insulin protocol the right one for now? I don't know how things have gone as far as they have. It is absolutely clear that FDA regulations require that new drugs or new treatments be proved to be safe and effective in adults before they are used on children, and if that rule is properly applied then the study can go forward only with young adults. The likelihood of these people developing diabetes is 50% or less than 50% of that in children under 10 or 12. I am concerned that we are moving into an area that ought to involve the FDA. This is a study that requires two injections of human insulin a day, a total dose of 0.3 units per kg, which is not an insignificant dose by any means, plus two or three hospital admissions a year for, I think, 2 or 3 days of continuous high dose intravenous insulin. This is not a benign procedure and I have some real concerns about whether it is an appropriate thing to do at this point.

Dr. Assan: I share your concern. There are not only theoretical difficulties but also practical clinical difficulties, for example the choice of control. However, it is no good just contemplating things and waiting for the perfect hypothesis. Nothing would ever get done.

Dr. Bergman: If you were able to assess insulin sensitivity, even if it is in the normal range, would you not have a more accurate predictor of β-cell function and therefore of the eventual development of type 1 diabetes?

Dr. Assan: I am aware that people such as MacLaren and Atkinson use the so-called minimal model of Cobelli that requires a large number of samplings, mathematical treatment, and so on, but I am not sure it gives more precise results than the glucose clamp.

Dr. Marliss: What have we learned so far about the pathophysiology of type 1 diabetes from transgenic experiments? These have not been mentioned at all. A multitude of genes have been introduced into β cells, certain of which have resulted in what looks like insulitis with or without β-cell destruction, while others have resulted in loss of β cells without any apparent evidence of cell-mediated immune response. We should see what can we pull out of all of this which might be of some value in our understanding of the disease, and potentially even for interventions.

Dr. Hoet: This may or may not be relevant, but I should like to note our latest observation that concentrates on nonspecific rather than specific immune reactions. We have been studying the effects of lysosyme, which appears immediately after any type of infection. We wanted to see if human lysosyme was able to counteract, at least *in vitro,* the effect of interleukin-1 on neonatal β cells. We found that if you put lysosyme A_2 into the culture before the interleukin-1 you can stop the destructive effect of interleukin-1. I wonder if we should not look at the possible preventive effects of nonspecific immune reactions in diabetes.

REFERENCES

1. Velloso LA, Eizirik DL, Karlsson FA, Kampe O. Absence of autoantibodies against glutamate decarboxylase (GAD) in the non-obese diabetic (NOD) mouse and low expression of the enzyme in mouse islets. *Clin Exp Immunol* 1994; 96: 129–37.
2. Kaufman DL, Clare-Salzler M, Tian J, *et al.* Spontaneous loss of T-cell tolerance to glutamic acid decarboxylase in murine insulin-dependent diabetes. *Nature* 1993; 366: 69–72.
3. Tisch R, Yang XD, Singer SM, Liblau RS, Fugger L, McDevitt HO. Immune response to glutamic acid decarboxylase correlates with insulitis in non-obese diabetic mice. *Nature* 1993; 377: 72–5.
4. Gelber C, Paborsky L, Singer S, *et al.* Isolation of non-obese diabetic mouse T-cells that recognise novel autoantigens involved in the early events of diabetes. *Diabetes* 1994; 43: 33–9.

Diabetes, edited by Richard M. Cowett,
Nestlé Nutrition Workshop Series,
Vol. 35. Nestec Ltd.,
Vevey/Raven Press, Ltd., New York © 1995.

The Epidemiology of Non-Insulin-Dependent Diabetes Mellitus

John H. Fuller

University College of London Medical School, 1–19, Torrington Place, London WC1E 6BT England

Studies of the prevalence of diabetes in the population can serve several useful purposes. They can provide information vital to the rational planning of health services for diabetic patients, they can explore hypotheses about risk factors for the disease and possible causal mechanisms, and finally they can provide estimates of the impact of the disease on the health of the population.

METHODOLOGICAL ISSUES

A major development in diabetes epidemiology has been the adoption of standardized diagnostic criteria as recommended by the World Health Organization (WHO) (1) and the National Diabetes Data Group (NDDG) (2). As discussed by Zimmet (3), the interpretation of the results of diabetes prevalence studies carried out before the adoption of the WHO criteria was complicated by the use of different glucose loads in the oral glucose tolerance test (OGTT), a range of differing diagnostic criteria, and varying use of blood or plasma for glucose measurements derived from venous or capillary blood sampling.

Following the WHO and NDDG recommendations, it is generally agreed that, for epidemiological studies, a whole blood plasma glucose value 2 hours after a 75-g oral glucose load is the most satisfactory measure of glucose tolerance, with high specificity and a greater sensitivity than the corresponding fasting blood glucose value. For 2-hour venous plasma glucose concentrations, the WHO diagnostic criteria are: diabetes ≥ 11.1 mM/l, impaired glucose tolerance ≥ 7.8 and < 11.1 mM/l, and normal < 7.8 mM/l. There are corresponding values for venous whole blood and capillary plasma and whole blood samples (4). Although now regarded as the gold standard for studies of diabetes prevalence, the 2-hour blood glucose measurement during an OGTT has several disadvantages. The 2-hour value has poor within-person reproducibility (5), OGTTs are costly to administer, and they are time consuming and uncomfortable for the subject. Consequently, some have recommended the use of a fasting plasma glucose cut-off of 7.0 mM/l, which, in Pacific populations at least, provides an estimate of prevalence equivalent to that based on a 2-hour value (6).

When the purpose of the study is to predict those individuals at risk of developing diabetic complications, studies in the Pima Indians have indicated that a single measurement of glycated hemoglobin may have an equivalent predictive power to a fasting or 2-hour blood glucose measurement in the prediction of diabetic nephropathy or retinopathy (7). The glycated hemoglobin test has several advantages over the OGTT, which is often criticized for being unphysiological. It requires just one venepuncture, it can be performed at any time of the day, it is reliable and repeatable (8), it does not alter appreciably with age (9), and it is a valid marker of chronic hyperglycemia. Since the current WHO diagnostic criteria are based on the ability of the 2-hour blood glucose to predict complications (1), then it is likely that this role may eventually be taken over by glycated hemoglobin in view of its distinct advantages for clinical and epidemiological studies.

As far as the practical details of organizing field surveys of diabetes and other noncommunicable diseases are concerned, Dowse and Zimmet have drawn upon their extensive experience to produce a valuable model protocol that can be adapted to various research environments (10). This model protocol gives advice on sampling techniques, survey procedures, laboratory methods, and quality control schemes for use in surveys carried out in a variety of settings.

THE PREVALENCE OF NON-INSULIN-DEPENDENT DIABETES MELLITUS (NIDDM)

Agreement on the WHO standardized criteria for the diagnosis of diabetes mellitus and impaired glucose tolerance has now made possible a valid comparison of estimates of the prevalence of these conditions throughout the world. In most populations, diabetes prevalence is strongly age related, and a major difficulty of previous comparisons (3) has been the varying population age ranges studied. King, Rewers, and the WHO ad hoc Diabetes Reporting Group have tackled this problem by carrying out age standardization on raw data from 75 population surveys in 32 countries for subjects in the age range 30–64 years (11).

As expected from previous studies, the highest prevalences of diabetes were found in the Pima/Papago Indians of Arizona, USA (50%) and the Micronesian population on the Pacific island of Nauru (41%). Some Arab, migrant Asian Indian, Chinese, and Hispanic American populations were also at moderately high risk with prevalences from 14–20%. Lower prevalences were found in five European populations (from Italy [two studies], Malta, Poland, and Russia) varying from 3–10%, but this study highlighted the relative lack of comparable data on diabetes prevalence in Europe.

Pozza *et al.* (12) have carried out a review of European prevalence studies going back to the 1960s. They made adjustments in prevalence, taking into account the various diagnostic criteria used in the earlier studies and found the highest European prevalence to be about 30% in Finland for the age range 65–84 years. A further

TABLE 1. *Prevalence of diabetes mellitus (percentage of population) in European populations*[a]

Population	Men		Women	
	Rate	95% CI	Rate	95% CI
Islington, UK (1986)				
40–69 years	1.8		1.5	
70+ years	4.7		6.3	
Finland (1986)				
65–84 years				
East	29.6		—	
West	29.8		—	
W. London, UK (1991)				
40–69 years				
European	4.8	3.7–5.8	2.3	
South Asian	19.6	17.5–21.7	16.1	11.7–20.5
Afro-Caribbean	14.6	9.6–19.5	—	
Coventry, UK (1992)				
20+ years				
Punjabi Sikh	8.9	7.2–11.0	7.5	6.0–9.4
Pakistani Muslim	9.1	6.7–12.0	10.3	7.8–13.3
Gujarati Muslim	16.0	10.7–22.8	20.4	14.4–28.3
Gujarati Hindu	8.4	5.7–12.0	8.8	6.2–12.2
Punjabi Hindu	11.3	7.4–17.1	11.6	7.7–17.4
London, UK (1993)				
40–64 years				
European	6.5	5.0–8.0	4.0	2.7–5.3
Afro-Caribbean	12.9	10.4–15.4	17.7	25.4–35.0
Sanza, Italy (1982)				
30–64 years	8.1	5.0–10.4	5.5	3.1–7.3
Laurino, Italy (1978)				
30–64 years	11.4	5.9–15.6	13.0	6.2–13.3
Malta (1981)				
30–64 years	8.6	5.9–9.6	10.1	8.0–11.4
Wroclaw, Poland (1986)				
30–64 years	4.1	2.4–4.6	3.7	2.5–4.6
Novosibirsk, Russia (1988)				
30–64 years	2.1	0.9–2.7	4.0	2.3–4.9

[a] From King H, Rewers M, WHO Ad Hoc Diabetes Reporting Group. Global estimates for prevalence of diabetes mellitus and impaired glucose tolerance. *Diabetes Care* 1993; 16:157–77; Pozza G, Garancini P, Gallus G. Prevalence and incidence of NIDDM. In: Williams R, Papoz L, Fuller J, eds. *Diabetes in Europe.* London: John Libbey, 1994:21–38.

summary of European studies is shown in Table 1, emphasizing the high diabetes rates in the South Asian and Afro-Caribbean ethnic minorities in the United Kingdom (13,14).

The study of King *et al.* (11) also included an analysis of the proportion of previously undiagnosed diabetes in the various world populations. The proportion of unknown cases was up 100% in some Pacific populations and was about 50% for European and American communities. In view of this significantly high proportion of unknown cases of diabetes in many communities, estimates of diabetes prevalence based on known cases of the disease will almost always be underestimates. Pozza *et al.* (12) have reviewed the European data on prevalence estimates derived from population-based diabetes registers. The most extensive national register of this type was the one held in the former German Democratic Republic (GDR), which gave a prevalence estimate of 3.2% for drug-treated patients in 1984. Although they underestimate "true" diabetes, registers may be the only practical and economical way of monitoring trends in diabetes worldwide, and their accuracy may be improved by the use of the capture-recapture technique (15).

THE INCIDENCE OF NIDDM

Population-based estimates of NIDDM incidence are hard to obtain because of the difficulty in ascertaining the occurrence of the disease without costly repetitive OGTT screening in the community. A study in three communities in Minnesota, USA, gave an incidence of 1.17 per 1000 person-years (16) whereas incidence estimates for the Pima Indians are nearly 20 times higher (18.5 per 1000 person-years).

IMPAIRED GLUCOSE TOLERANCE

Global estimates for the prevalence of impaired glucose tolerance indicate a low prevalence (<3%) in some Chinese, traditional Native American, and Pacific island populations (11). The highest estimates were found in female Muslim Asian Indians in Tanzania (32%) and in urban male Micronesians in Kiribati (28%).

RISK FACTORS FOR NIDDM

Genetic Susceptibility

Zimmet *et al.* (17) have reviewed the evidence for a strong genetic basis of NIDDM including a 58–90% concordance for the condition in identical twins, a declining prevalence in some populations with an increasing proportion of Caucasoid genetic admixture, and evidence from pedigree studies in Nauruans and Pima Indians of an autosomal dominant pattern of inheritance. The search is now on for the genes associated with an increased susceptibility to NIDDM.

Environmental Determinants of NIDDM

There is increasing evidence for the critical involvement of insulin resistance and impaired glucose secretory function in the aetiology of NIDDM (18). In several high-risk populations, hyperinsulinemia has been shown to predict the subsequent development of impaired glucose tolerance and NIDDM (19,20). The detailed mechanism of this process are discussed elsewhere in this volume. These theories of the pathogenesis of NIDDM have to be consistent with the lifestyle characteristics that have been shown in epidemiological studies to be risk factors for NIDDM, that is, obesity, central body fat distribution, and lack of exercise (17).

Early Life Experience and Adult Non-Insulin-Dependent Diabetes Mellitus

Barker and his colleagues from Southhampton, UK, have suggested that the risk of cardiovascular and other chronic diseases in adult life may be determined (at least in part) by a "programmed" effect of interference with early growth and development during fetal life and infancy. This group has studied the relationship of the degree of glucose intolerance to birthweight and weight at 1 year in 468 men born and still living in the county of Hertfordshire, UK (21). They found that the proportion of men with glucose intolerance or NIDDM varied inversely with birthweight and weight at 1 year. This has led to the hypothesis that poor nutrition in fetal and early infant life may be detrimental to the development and function of the β cells of the islets of Langerhans, thus predisposing to the later development of NIDDM.

These findings are beginning to be confirmed in other epidemiological studies, including those of the Pima Indians (7) and promise to advance our knowledge of the pathogenesis of NIDDM.

CONCLUSION

In this review of the epidemiology of NIDDM, methodological issues are discussed with particular reference to the generally accepted World Health Organization recommendations on the diagnostic criteria for diabetes mellitus. The relative merits of the 2-hour post-load blood glucose measurement *versus* fasting values and measures of glycated hemoglobin are discussed. An overview of the worldwide prevalence of NIDDM and impaired glucose tolerance is given and more recent data on the frequency of NIDDM in Europe are discussed. The genetic and lifestyle factors related to the risk of developing NIDDM, including insulin resistance, obesity, body fat distribution, and physical inactivity, are presented.

REFERENCES

1. World Health Organization. *WHO Expert Committee on Diabetes Mellitus*. Geneva: Tech Rep Ser, 1980.
2. National Diabetes Data Group. Classification and diagnosis of diabetes mellitus and other categories of glucose intolerance. *Diabetes* 1979; 28: 1039–57.
3. Zimmet P. Type 2 (non insulin dependent) diabetes—an epidemiological overview. *Diabetologia* 1982; 22: 399–411.
4. World Health Organization. *Diabetes mellitus: report of a study group*. Geneva: Tech Rep Ser, 1985.
5. Ganda OP, Day JL, Soeldner JS, Connon JJ, Gleason RE. Reproducibility and comparative analysis of repeated intravenous and oral glucose tolerance tests. *Diabetes* 1978; 27: 715–25.
6. Finch CF, Zimmet PZ, Alberti KGMM. Determining diabetes prevalence: a rational basis for the use of fasting plasma glucose concentrations? *Diabetic Med* 1990; 7: 603–10.
7. McCance DR, Hanson RL, Charles MA, *et al.* Comparison of tests for glycated haemoglobin and

fasting and two hour plasma glucose concentrations as diagnostic methods for diabetes. *BMJ* 1994; 308: 1323–8.

8. Jovanovic L, Peterson CM. The clinical utility of glycosylated hemoglobin. *Am J Med* 1981; 70: 331–8.

9. Verillo AT, Ade T, Golia R, Nunziata V. The relationship between glycosylated haemoglobin levels and various degrees of glucose intolerance. *Diabetologia* 1983; 24: 391–3.

10. Dowse GK, Zimmet P. A model protocol for diabetes and other noncommunicable disease field surveys. *World Health Stat Q* 1992; 45: 360–9.

11. King H, Rewers M, WHO Ad Hoc Diabetes Reporting Group. Global estimates for prevalence of diabetes mellitus and impaired glucose tolerance. *Diabetes Care* 1993; 16: 157–77.

12. Pozza G, Garancini P, Gallus G. Prevalence and incidence of NIDDM. In: Williams R, Papoz L, Fuller J, eds. *Diabetes in Europe*. London: John Libbey, 1994: 21–38.

13. McKeigue PM, Shah B, Marmot MG. Relation of central obesity and insulin resistance with high diabetes prevalence and cardiovascular risk in South Asians. *Lancet* 1991; 337: 382–6.

14. Chaturvedi N, McKeigue PM, Marmot MG. Resting and ambulatory blood pressure differences in Afro-Caribbeans and Europeans. *Hypertension* 1993; 22: 90–6.

15. LaPorte RE, McCarthy D, Bruno G, Tajima N, Baba S. Counting diabetes in the next millennium. *Diabetes Care* 1993; 16: 528–34.

16. King H, Zimmet P. Trends in the prevalence and incidence of diabetes: non-insulin-dependent diabetes mellitus. *World Health Stat Q* 1988; 41: 190–6.

17. Zimmet P, Dowse G, Kriska A, Serjeantson S. Current perspectives in the epidemiology of non-insulin dependent (Type II) diabetes mellitus. *Diabetes Nutr Metab* 1990; 3 (suppl 1): 3–15.

18. Reaven GM. Role of insulin resistance in human disease. *Diabetes* 1988; 37: 1595–607.

19. Saad MF, Knowler WC, Pettitt DJ, Nelson RG, Mott DM, Bennett PH. The natural history of impaired glucose tolerance in the Pima Indians. *N Engl J Med* 1988; 319: 1500–6.

20. Haffner SM, Stern MP, Hazuda HP, Pugh JA, Patterson JK. Hyperinsulinemia in a population at high risk for non-insulin-dependent diabetes mellitus. *N Engl J Med* 1986; 315: 220–4.

21. Barker BJP, Hales CN, Fall CHD, Osmond C, Phipps K, Clark PMS. Type 2 (non-insulin-dependent) diabetes mellitus, hypertension and hyperlipidaemia (syndrome X): relation to reduced fetal growth. *Diabetologia* 1993; 36: 62–7.

DISCUSSION

Dr. Nattrass: The ascertainment of cause of death is of course extremely tricky. It is widely held that cardiovascular disease is a major cause of death in diabetes and I wonder whether that in turn biases people toward putting down cardiovascular disease as the cause of death when it is not clear what the cause actually was.

Dr. Fuller: I fully accept the problems of assigning cause of death. Most of these analyses have been done by looking at all-cause mortality so one is not really concerned about the actual cause of death. This is what we did in our comparisons with the general population, and one can derive some significant conclusions from such data. So far as specific causes of death are concerned, this is a very difficult area. For example what do you do about the diabetic patient who is on renal dialysis, in renal failure, and who dies from myocardial infarction? What should one put down as the underlying cause of death in such a case? In the WHO system, I think it would be myocardial infarction. However, in practice we look at all the causes written on the death certificates rather than at the data published by the WHO, which are based upon the so-called underlying cause of death and are not really worthwhile as far as the diabetic patient is concerned. You have to look at all the information.

Dr. Nattrass: There must be some causes of death that don't appear very often in the diabetic population, and I wonder what they are. Is the diabetic population protected from some causes of death?

Dr. Fuller: You probably mean are they less likely to get cancer, for instance, but all the studies of cancer in diabetes are confounded by the problem of the way the cause of death was assigned, because if you have an excess proportion with one particular cause of death you are going to get a reduction in another cause.

Dr. Katsilambros: We had the opportunity to show in large groups of normal young Greek men and women a significant positive correlation between the waist-hip ratio (WHR) and different risk factors for coronary heart disease including blood pressure, total cholesterol, and negative correlations with HDL cholesterol. However, blood glucose, at least the fasting value, did not correlate with WHR. My question refers to the possible quantitative differences in WHR among the sexes. Are you aware of any paper describing differences among the sexes concerning the relative effect of WHR on the frequency of diabetes mellitus? The papers I am aware of combine the data from men and women.

Dr. Fuller: As you say, most studies do not separate the genders when they examine these relationships. There is obviously a big difference in the shape of men and women, but I am not sufficiently familiar with the literature relating, for instance, sex hormone data to waist-hip ratio. I am sure that there are other people in the group with more information on this.

Dr. Katsilambros: We did a study of androgens in young women. We found that the higher the waist-hip ratio in these women, the higher the androgens of any kind.

Dr. Drash: I should like to comment on a specific population group from Haiti. I have had the opportunity to spend a great deal of time in Haiti over the years. There have been no studies to my knowledge among the Haitians and my observations are anecdotal but have been discussed with many Haitian and non-Haitian physicians working in the country. First of all, you simply don't see obesity in Haiti because of general malnutrition. Secondly, diabetes is almost nonexistent, but hypertension is very common and therefore cerebral hemorrhage is one of the major causes of death. This would seem to me a very important group to study from the point of view of the whole concept of syndrome X. They have bad hypertension and bad cerebral vascular disease, but they don't have coronary heart disease for the most part, and they have very little diabetes.

Dr. Fuller: I am not familiar with the area but do they have a high sodium intake?

Dr. Drash: They have very high sodium intake. They also have a very high sugar intake but their overall energy intake is deficient.

Dr. Bergman: I would like to ask a question about the low birthweight data from the United Kingdom study. Has it been studied whether women with low birthweight children overfeed them in early life? It seems reasonable that this could happen.

Dr. Hoet: I can answer Dr. Bergman's question on the Barker data. The low birthweight infants in his study were under 8 kg in weight at 1 year of age so early overfeeding definitely did not occur. What we know from animal experiments is that growth-retarded animals reared to adult life will become obese. So there is a relation between intrauterine growth retardation and obesity later in life.

Dr. Catalano: We have done a longitudinal study on infants of diabetic women compared with a control group. The preliminary data for the first year of life show that there is catch-up growth in the smaller babies until they get to about one year of age but there is no excess growth in the babies of the women who have had gestational diabetes. So there may be some catch-up but there does not appear to be excessive growth by one year of age.

Dr. Hoet: How do you explain that the latest data of Paul Zimmet, showing that the incidence or prevalence of diabetes is now decreasing rather than increasing, even though food intakes are high? His sample of relatively young Nauruans have actually become more obese, and therefore they should now have a higher prevalence of diabetes; in fact the incidence is getting less. This is not a cohort effect.

Dr. Fuller: As has been said before, NIDDM is a multifactorial disease. There must be other factors involved apart from obesity.

Diabetes, edited by Richard M. Cowett,
Nestlé Nutrition Workshop Series,
Vol. 35. Nestec Ltd.,
Vevey/Raven Press, Ltd., New York © 1995.

Pathogenesis of Non-Insulin-Dependent Diabetes Mellitus

Richard N. Bergman and Marilyn Ader

*Department of Physiology and Biophysics, University of Southern California School of
Medicine, 1333 San Pablo St., MMR 626, Los Angeles CA 90033, USA*

Non-insulin dependent diabetes is a cause of rising morbidity and mortality in developed countries. In the United States, it is estimated that there are 14 million NIDDM cases (7% of the population), approximately half of whom remain undiagnosed. The prevalence of the disease is increasing due to the increasing proportion in the U.S. population of ethnic groups at particular risk, including Latinos from Mexico and Central America, and African Americans. Since NIDDM is associated with a major risk of complications, including blindness, kidney disease, and cardiovascular disease, it is clear that understanding the factors in the etiology of this disease could have a significant impact in improving the health of the U.S. population as a whole. Such understanding would have similar advantages for other Western and Westernized countries where NIDDM is a major health problem.

Understanding the natural history of NIDDM has become increasingly important in view of the recent revolution in molecular genetics. The elucidation of the mutations causing monogenic diseases such as cystic fibrosis (1) has kindled hope that in the future the genes responsible for polygenic diseases, of which NIDDM is one of the most prominent, will be identified. While mutations have been discovered in a few families with some diabetes phenotypes, including maturity onset diabetes of the young (MODY) (2,3), progress in elucidating the underlying genetics of "garden-variety" NIDDM has been frustrating. While initial efforts exploited the concept of candidate genes, including insulin (4), insulin receptor (5,6), and β-cell glucokinase (7), a disappointing lack of success with this approach has led to a consensus that it would be more profitable to examine the human genome.

The standard approach to identifying the gene for a disease is to compare genomes of afflicted and nonafflicted individuals. One of the conundrums of NIDDM genetics is the difficulty of separating not-at-risk individuals from those who do not yet have the disease, but will later get it. One approach is to study older individuals. Unfortunately, however, in the elderly population a significant number of individuals with NIDDM have perished prematurely. This difficulty leads to the need to identify individuals who are at high risk for NIDDM before the disease presents. In other words, it is important to understand the phenotypic characteristics that will lead to

NIDDM, so that the genetics of at-high-risk individuals may be characterized. This requires understanding of the natural history of the disease.

FASTING CONDITIONS

To review the pathogenesis, of NIDDM it is useful to consider the regulation of the fasting blood glucose concentration. It is commonly believed that the blood sugar is determined by a combination of the insulin secretory function of the β cells of the pancreas and the ability of insulin to stimulate glucose utilization. However, the situation is somewhat more complex (Fig. 1). Under fasting conditions, despite the apparent rock-solid stability of the blood glucose concentration in normal individuals (8), the glucose in the extracellular fluid is turning over rather rapidly, replacing half the extracellular glucose every 45 minutes. Thus an exquisite balance is maintained between the rate of glucose production, primarily by the liver, and the rate of glucose utilization. It is commonly held that the balance between glucose output and uptake is determined by the action of the basal insulin concentration. Insulin is seen to restrain glucose output by the liver and to control fasting extrahepatic glucose utilization. However, this conception is oversimplified. It is important to remember that

RESTORATIVE EVENTS AFTER GLUCOSE

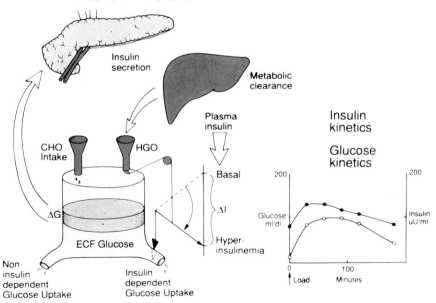

FIG. 1. Schematic representation of the metabolic events stimulated by carbohydrate ingestion. In the fasting state, glucose uptake is primarily independent of insulin. Glucose ingestion raises extracellular fluid (ECF) glucose and prompts secretion of insulin, which acts to normalize glycemia by enhancing insulin-dependent glucose disposal and inhibiting hepatic glucose output (HGO). Reproduced from Bergman RN (15).

about 75% of the glucose utilization by fasting tissues is by insulin-insensitive tissues. Thus an important factor in the establishment of basal glycemia is the ability of glucose *per se* to control its own uptake by insulin-insensitive tissues (brain, gut, red blood cells, adrenal medulla). [We have termed the effect of glucose in enhancing its own uptake *glucose effectiveness* (9).] Second, insulin may not be the primary signal regulating hepatic glucose production in the fasting state. Therefore, while insulin secretion and insulin sensitivity are no doubt important in determining fasting carbohydrate metabolism, other factors not yet clearly elucidated may well come into play.

CARBOHYDRATE INTAKE

Upon ingestion of carbohydrate, insulin secretion and insulin action together determine the efficiency with which the organism can dispose of glucose in the blood. Normally glucose interacts with gastrointestinal factors, probably GLP-1 (glucagon-like peptide 1), to mount a rapid and profound insulin response. The insulin mobilizes glucose transporters that allow a massive outpouring of glucose from the extracellular space into insulin-sensitive cells. However, due to the rise in glucose, glucose effectiveness also plays a role in determining the rate of glucose disposal (glucose tolerance), and this role is proportionately greater in conditions of impaired glucose tolerance and NIDDM. It cannot be disputed that resistance to the action of insulin on glucose uptake by insulin-sensitive cells is an important factor in NIDDM, and it is probably important in the preclinical phase of the disease (10).

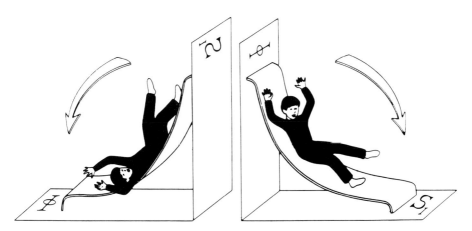

FIG. 2. Cartoon illustrating the reciprocal relationship between insulin sensitivity (S_1) and insulin secretory function (Φ) in the maintenance of normal glucose tolerance. In the individual on the right, normal variations in insulin sensitivity are adequately compensated for by reciprocal changes in β-cell function. In contrast, the individual on the left, perhaps due to a latent β-cell defect, is unable to compensate appropriately, and appears to fall off the slide depicting the hyperbolic curve of glucose tolerance (See Eq. 1 in text). Reproduced from Bergman RN (15).

Insulin sensitivity is determined by genetic as well as environmental factors. Under normal conditions, increasing adiposity, reduced physical activity, and high fat feeding will all induce insulin resistance (11–13), while insulin sensitivity will increase with weight loss, exercise training, and high carbohydrate diets. It is to be expected that these changes would have a comparable effect on glucose tolerance. However, the glucose tolerance is normally regulated in such a way as to counteract alterations in insulin sensitivity. This tendency can be represented as the hyperbolic law of glucose regulation, proposed by us in the 1980s (Fig. 2) (14,15) and recently confirmed by Kahn *et al.* (16):

$$\text{Insulin secretion} \times \text{insulin sensitivity} = \text{a constant} \qquad [\text{Eq. 1}]$$

The significance of this relationship is that an environmental change in insulin sensitivity will result in an equal and opposite change in β-cell sensitivity to glucose. The increased β-cell sensitivity will, in turn, minimize the relative glucose intolerance that would otherwise be observed in a relatively insulin-resistant state.

The propensity of normal individuals to mount a compensatory increase in β-cell responsiveness can be seen clearly in pregnancy. As insulin resistance progresses with gestation, the compensatory, and appropriate, increment in β-cell sensitivity

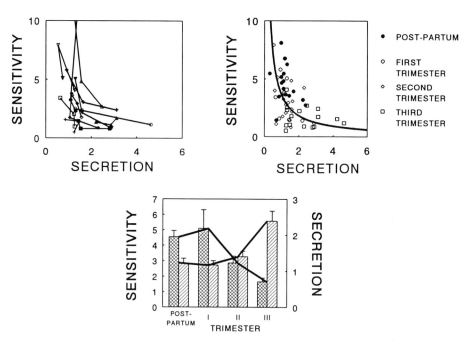

FIG. 3. Reciprocal relationship between insulin sensitivity and insulin secretion observed during and after pregnancy. As gestation proceeds, insulin sensitivity decreases, and secretion is enhanced (*top left*), and this compensation can be described by a hyperbolic curve (*top right*). Interestingly, these metabolic changes in sensitivity (*hatched bars*) and secretion (*striped bars*) are not evident until the second trimester of pregnancy (*bottom*).

can be seen (Fig. 3). Clearly, the absence of such an appropriate increase (*i.e.,* one defined by Equation 1) may be indicative of relative β-cell failure.

SIGNIFICANCE OF THE HYPERBOLIC LAW

The natural propensity of the β cell to compensate for insulin resistance, as represented in the hyperbolic law, tends to obscure subtle but real changes in the function of cells, which might portend the development of NIDDM. Thus if the β cells were unable to increase their relative gain (*i.e.,* the ratio of insulin secreted to glucose stimulus), a small decline in insulin sensitivity would be reflected in a similar derangement in glucose tolerance. However, the compensatory increase in β-cell gain acts to compensate for and thus reduce any reduction in tolerance. Therefore, to elucidate early but subtle changes in metabolic control, it is necessary to measure not only glucose tolerance, but also insulin sensitivity and β-cell responsiveness directly. Early defects in β-cell function, in this context, can be a reduced relative compensation for insulin resistance, or

$$\text{Insulin secretion} \times \text{insulin sensitivity} < \text{constant} \qquad \text{[Eq. 2]}$$

It is the hyperbolic relationship that tends to hide subtle changes in metabolic function. Thus to understand the pathogenesis of glucose tolerance as it develops, it is necessary to follow not only basal glucose turnover and glucose tolerance, but also the factors that determine them. Basal glucose turnover is determined by the rate of glucose production and utilization. The latter factors are established by peripheral insulin sensitivity, "insulin sensitivity of the liver," and glucose effectiveness. The exquisite interaction of these factors to determine glycemia has been discussed eloquently by Porte (17).

SEQUENCE OF EVENTS

Overt NIDDM

One approach to understanding the sequence of events leading to NIDDM has been to study the overt state of type 2 diabetes. NIDDM is associated with severe insulin resistance (18) as well as severely depressed β-cell function. The degree of resistance in NIDDM is profound; however, there remain difficulties in the exact quantification of the reduction in insulin sensitivity in this state. Glucose clamps reveal that insulin sensitivity is reduced by approximately 70% compared with normal subjects and by 28% compared to the obese. The difficulty in making this quantitative comparison results from the fact that glucose utilization during clamps depends on the prevailing blood glucose level. Clamps done in NIDDM must either be under fasting hyperglycemic conditions (*isoglycemic clamps),* or they must follow prenormalization of blood glucose, which can be achieved by slow overnight insulin infusion (19,20), or acutely by a more rapid insulin infusion (21,22). There is evidence that preinfusion with insulin may increase insulin sensitivity (23), leading to an underestimation of insulin resistance in NIDDM. Some investigators have recommended the use of glucose clearance (the glucose utilization rate divided by the prevailing glucose concentration during the clamp study) to normalize utilization measured at isoglycemia. However, there is a "nonproportional" relationship between glucose uptake and plasma glucose concentration (see 24) that renders the clearance correction inaccurate, and its use also tends to overestimate insulin sensitivity. A third factor that may cause overestimation of insulin sensitivity in NIDDM is the extended time of insulin infusion during clamps (usually 3–4 hours), which exceeds the period of hyperinsulinemia that occurs during normal meals. Thus it is possible that insulin sensitivity measured in NIDDM patients from glucose clamps actually overestimates insulin sensitivity, and that insulin resistance in NIDDM is even greater than the clamp suggests. The minimal model procedure, which may obviate at least some of the problems with the clamp, indicates that insulin sensitivity in NIDDM subjects may be very close to zero in patients with overt disease. Thus it may be concluded that patients with NIDDM in Westernized countries tend to be severely insulin resistant. [This may not, however, be true for all NIDDM patients: for example, Fajans and his colleagues, using the minimal model, have shown that MODY patients are not insulin resistant, and the same is true of nonobese type 2 patients in Japan (25,26).]

In addition, NIDDM patients have severely reduced insulin secretion. In fact, there is often a total absence of first-phase insulin release. In some patients, glucose injection reduces insulin release (27). The degree of insulin secretion in NIDDM is even less, considering that proinsulin accounts for a greater proportion of insulin-like immunoreactivity in plasma in NIDDM patients.

Misleading Results from NIDDM Studies

It is now clear to most investigators that studies of NIDDM patients yield limited information regarding the pathogenesis of the disease. The hyperglycemia itself (that is, glucose toxicity) can be responsible for exacerbating the characteristics of the disease. It has long been known that hyperglycemia will lead to depressed insulin secretion (28), and Kahn and her colleagues, as well as Klip *et al.*, have shown downregulation of insulin-dependent glucose transporter (GLUT4) content in rats under hyperglycemic conditions, reversible by phlorizin-induced normalization of the blood glucose concentration (29,30). Such downregulation will be reflected as insulin resistance. Given these profound effects of hyperglycemia *per se* on insulin secretion and action, and given that hyperglycemia is the hallmark of NIDDM, it is clear that observation of the overt disease state may be quite misleading and may not reveal the primary causes of NIDDM itself. Given this difficulty, it is imperative to study individuals who are going to develop NIDDM or, if this is not possible, to study those who are at high risk of the disease, to identify any preexisting primary metabolic defects.

Longitudinal Studies

Few longitudinal studies of the development of NIDDM exist. Thus it is difficult to establish a precise sequence of events in the development of this condition. However, studies at the Joslin Clinic in Boston, Mass., initiated by Soeldner, Warram, and their colleagues, analyzed in collaboration with our group (31,32), and studies of the natural history of NIDDM in the Pima Native Americans carried out by Bennett, Bogardus and Saad and their colleagues (33,34) suggest the following events.

The Joslin group studied 155 normal offspring of two parents with NIDDM (31,32). The offspring were studied with intravenous glucose tolerance tests (IVGTTs) while glucose tolerance was normal. Over the 25 years of follow-up, 25 of the subjects (16%) developed NIDDM. We analyzed the 3-hour IVGTT, which had been performed on entry to the study, in all the subjects, using the minimal model approach (15). It was clear (Fig. 4) that the individuals who went on to develop NIDDM were the most resistant ones. This resistance could not be accounted for by adiposity alone (estimated as body-mass index, BMI), although BMI is at best a gross indicator of adiposity (35). An additional defect discovered was glucose resistance, that is, reduced glucose effectiveness. In the Joslin study, clear evidence of reduced β-cell function, as reflected by suppressed first-phase insulin release, was not revealed. Thus, the Joslin study strongly implicated insulin resistance, possibly independent of adiposity, as a predictor of future NIDDM.

Studies in the Pima Native Americans have been most revealing in elucidating the progression of NIDDM. It is well documented that this is a very insulin-resistant population (35). Bogardus and his colleagues have produced compelling evidence that insulin resistance in the Pimas is related to family origin, suggesting that this is an inherited characteristic (34) (Fig. 5).

Epidemiological evidence therefore suggests that, in most of the populations studied, insulin resistance is an inherited characteristic, probably exacerbated by obesity, which strongly predicts the development of NIDDM.

Mechanism

The precise cause of inherited insulin resistance in at-risk individuals remains an enigma (Fig. 6). Given the normality of the insulin receptor and the insulin-dependent glucose transporter in subjects with NIDDM (36,37) it has been suggested that a component of the complex insulin signaling pathway may not be expressed normally in at-risk individuals (38). This result would be consistent with reduced mobilization of glucose transporters on stimulation by insulin. Alternatively, a pathway defect, possibly at the level of glycogen synthesis in muscle (39), could, due to a negative feedback phenomenon, suppress glucose transport. It has been suggested that the glucosamine pathway mediates this negative feedback in adipocytes, and this may also be involved in skeletal muscles.

Our group has been examining the delivery of insulin from the blood to insulin

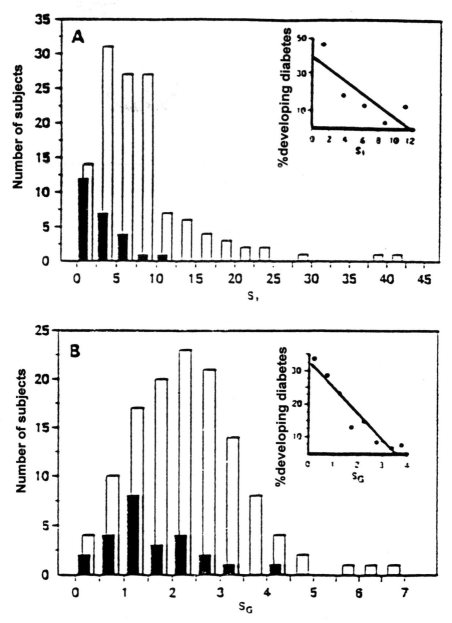

FIG. 4. Distribution of minimal model parameters of insulin sensitivity (S_1; *top*) and glucose effectiveness (S_G; *bottom*) in subjects with normal glucose tolerance at entry into 25-year follow-up study. Insets indicate data as proportion of subjects who subsequently developed diabetes. Reproduced from Martin BC, Warram JH, Krolewski AS, Bergman RN, Soeldner JS, Kahn CR. Role of glucose and insulin resistance in development of type 2 diabetes mellitus: results of a 25-year follow-up study. *Lancet* 1992; 340:925–9.

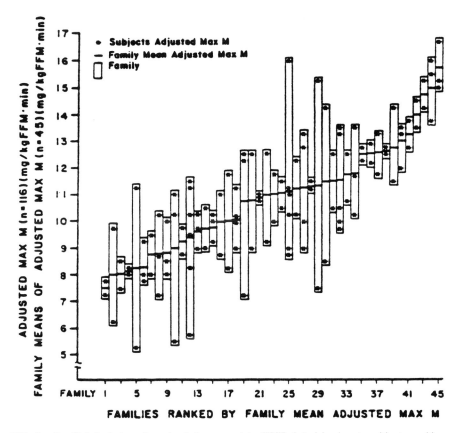

FIG. 5. Familial clustering of maximal glucose uptake ("M"). Asterisks denote subjects, and bars represent families. Reproduced from Lilliojas *et al.* (34).

sensitive cells (40–42). We have reported that insulin moves slowly across the endothelial barrier, and this movement determines the rate of insulin action *in vivo* (Fig. 7). However, whether this transendothelial transport of insulin is impeded in NIDDM and whether there is alteration in such transport in at-risk individuals, has not been investigated. Also, Baron and his colleagues have shown that insulin increases blood flow through insulin-sensitive tissues (43). He has argued that reduction in this action might also result in insulin resistance.

Of course it is impossible here to review the vast amount of information related to the mechanism of insulin resistance. Suffice it to say that severe insulin resistance is a dominant feature in most forms of NIDDM, and that the exact intracellular or transcellular mechanism accounting for it, despite years of research, remains unclear. In fact, as the complexity of the insulin signaling pathways becomes increasingly evident, it appears more likely that the site of insulin resistance will be delineated by the genetic approach (that is, by identifying the gene(s) for NIDDM) than by direct study of the insulin action mechanism in cells.

	yes	probably	no	maybe
Alterations in Blood Flow				●
Transendothelial Insulin Transport				●
Insulin Receptor Structure			●	
Insulin Signalling Pathway		●		
Glucose Transporter Structure			●	
Transporter Shuttle Mechanism				●
Glycogen Synthase		●		
Other Metabolic Pathways				●

FIG. 6. Potential mechanisms of peripheral insulin resistance.

Progression to NIDDM

Will insulin resistance *per se* result in NIDDM? As predicted by the hyperbolic law (Fig. 2), insulin resistance will require increased insulin secretion to maintain glucose tolerance. Kahn *et al.* have shown that experimental induction of insulin resistance with nicotinic acid will, in normal individuals, produce the necessary insulin secretion to maintain glucose tolerance in the normal range (44). Also, insulin resistance is profound in pregnancy, but the great majority of women, even after multiple pregnancies, do not develop diabetes. Finally, theoretical studies have demonstrated that insulin resistance *alone* should not lead to NIDDM (15).

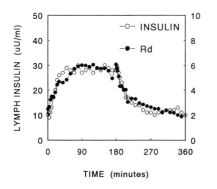

FIG. 7. Dynamics of lymph insulin concentration (reflective of interstitial insulin) and glucose uptake (R_d) during hyperinsulinemic glucose clamp. That dynamics are superimposable indicates that lymph insulin is the signal to which insulin-sensitive tissues respond to utilize glucose, and that transendothelial insulin transport is rate-limiting for insulin action to increase R_d. Adapted from Yang YJ *et al.* (40).

Thus it can be suggested that multiple defects will be necessary to account for the development of NIDDM. How may additional defects be identified? It is reasonable that a combination of insulin resistance *plus* a β-cell defect should result in the diabetic state. Such subtle defects are difficult to identify. One approach that has been useful has been that of Polonsky and his colleagues who have reported that an early sign of developing NIDDM is an alteration in the cyclic characteristics of insulin secretion in response to profound insulin resistance (45). Recently, Lillioja *et al.* have reported a subtle β-cell defect in Pima Indians *before* the onset of NIDDM (46).

Because of the normal compensatory characteristics of the glucose regulating system, it is difficult to pinpoint a β-cell defect, since the pancreatic gain increases to compensate for insulin resistance. However, as we suggested, an early β-cell defect will be reflected in *a failure of β-cell gain to increase appropriately for a given degree of insulin resistance.* Thus, better than simply measuring β-cell secretion, it is important to relate β-cell secretion to insulin sensitivity using the hyperbolic curve. When this was done for Pima Indians, it was clear that those individuals who later went on to develop NIDDM were below the curve (Fig. 8), that is, there was a reduced ability of the β-cell to respond to the insulin-resistance challenge. In addition, examination of subjects with impaired glucose tolerance, who are at higher risk for NIDDM than those with normal glucose tolerance, shows that a significant proportion have reduced β-cell function when considered in relation to the degree of insulin resistance.

Results demonstrating a subtle defect in β-cell gain have likewise been reported for subjects with gestational diabetes. Although this condition can certainly be differentiated from NIDDM, it is similar during the pregnant state when insulin sensitivity is greatly reduced (47). Buchanan has demonstrated that insulin response, although increasing as pregnancy progresses, is significantly suppressed when compared with that in pregnant women without gestational diabetes.

Taken together, the data appear to support the existence of a latent β-cell defect that exists *before* the onset of NIDDM. Thus it is possible to hypothesize that there is insulin resistance and a latent β-cell defect in existence before the onset of the disease; whether *both* these defects are present from birth remains unclear. It seems reasonable to propose that if the degree of insulin resistance is severe, then a moder-

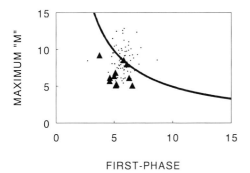

FIG. 8. Reciprocal relationship between glucose uptake at maximal insulin ("M") and first-phase insulin release from longitudinal study in Pima Indians. Of 90 subjects studied (*dots*), 11 eventually developed diabetes (*triangles*). All of the subjects who were to develop diabetes lie on or below the hyperbolic curve described in Eq. 1 (see text), indicating inadequate metabolic compensation. Data kindly provided by C. Bogardus for publication in Bergman RN (15).

ate β-cell defect will culminate in type 2 diabetes; in states of more modest resistance, a more substantial β-cell defect will lead to the disorder. Either way, the hyperbolic law will be violated overall, and diabetes may well ensue.

Catastrophe

The question remains: If predisposition to diabetes is defined as some combination of resistance and reduced β-cell gain, at what point, and for what reason, does homeostasis of glucose fail and hyperglycemia ensue?

The answer to this question may well reside in the concept of glucose toxicity (Fig. 9). It is reasonable to imagine that, with advancing age, there will be a modest reduction in insulin sensitivity, even in at-risk individuals. Such a reduction will represent an increasing stimulus to the β-cell, the gain of which will continue to increase to compensate. Assuming that what is characteristic of NIDDM is a limited

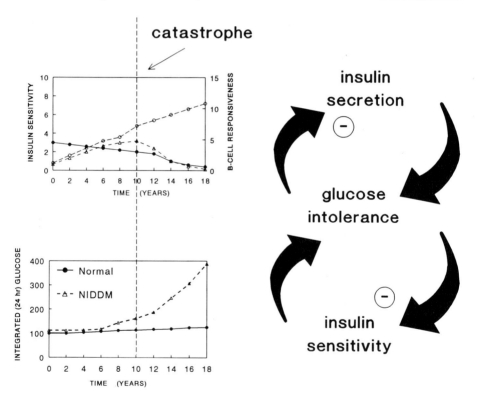

FIG. 9. Proposed scenario (*top panel*) for the pathogenesis of fasting hyperglycemia. Insulin sensitivity decreases with advancing age (*closed circles*), which in healthy individuals, is compensated by increased β-cell responsiveness (*open circles*). In subjects at risk for diabetes, β cells may be unable to adequately increase their gain despite prevailing resistance (*triangles*), and hyperglycemia ensues (*bottom panel*).

ability of the β cell to increase gain in the face of increased resistance, a modest re-regulation of the system regulating glucose will result. In the face of reduced insulin action, insulin will begin to lose its ability to restrain hepatic glucose output, resulting in a slight increment in the fasting glucose level. At a certain point, in those at-risk individuals unable to increase β-cell gain sufficiently to compensate for insulin resistance, glycemia will reach a point where it will *both* exacerbate insulin resistance *and* downregulate insulin secretion. Thus a vicious cycle will emerge in which hyperglycemia downregulates the β cell and limits the ability of insulin to restrain glucose output; the latter will result in increased glycemia, and so on. One may hypothesize that it is this vicious cycle that is responsible for the glucose catastrophe, leading to failure of glucose homeostasis and fasting hyperglycemia.

OTHER MECHANISMS

The insulin resistance/β-cell scenario outlined above may not be the only factor that plays a role in challenging the β cell and hastening the onset of hyperglycemia. In fact, significant amounts of glucose are taken up by tissues independently of insulin, and as insulin resistance (and secretion) worsens, glucose effectiveness becomes an increasingly important player in determining glucose levels and glucose tolerance. Thus it may well be that a reduced glucose effectiveness (that is, glucose resistance) may be a confounding factor contributing to the downfall of the β cell in at least some individuals at risk for NIDDM. Indeed, we found that reduced glucose effectiveness was an independent predictor of NIDDM in the Joslin study (31). In addition, the mechanism by which insulin restrains hepatic glucose production appears to be rather complex (48), and when this interaction is better understood it could well be that other, yet-unidentified factors may contribute to the onset of fasting hyperglycemia as NIDDM develops.

CONCLUSION

Type 2 diabetes is a prevalent disease, and very costly in Westernized countries. Most insidious are the complications of the disease, contributing substantially to the morbidity and mortality of Western populations. Thus it is critical to understand the causes of the disease, so that interventions may become possible. However, as discussed here, type 2 diabetes is a *systemic* disease, involving altered relationships among the liver, muscle, adipose tissue, brain, kidneys, and most other tissues of the body. The intense intercommunication among the various tissues has made it difficult to pinpoint the primary cause of the disease, since the functions of different tissue beds decline in parallel. It can now be said that insulin resistance is a usual contributor, but not the only cause of diabetes. Strong evidence exists for an additional pancreatic β-cell defect, which is difficult to detect because of overall system compensations. Also, the disease is presumably heterogeneous, and different causes may well contribute to single symptomology.

Advances in human genetic research hold the possibility of finding the primary genetic cause in at least some NIDDM cases. If this can be done, by relating phenotypic defects in insulin secretion and/or action to alterations in the human genome, defective genes (and individual proteins) may be identified. Such elucidation may then allow the development of specific pharmaceutical or even genetic therapies to re-control the blood glucose level and thus mitigate the egregious parallel complications of type 2 diabetes mellitus. In the absence of such information, it seems prudent to assume that, for type 2 diabetes as has recently been demonstrated for type 1 (49), control of the blood glucose concentration is a reasonable, prudent approach to minimizing complications.

REFERENCES

1. Riordan JR, Rommens JM, Kerem B, *et al*. Identification of the cystic fibrosis gene: cloning and characterization of complementary DNA. *Science* 1989; 245: 1066–73.
2. Froguel P, Vaxillaire M, Sun F, *et al*. Close linkage of glucokinase locus on chromosome 7p to early-onset non-insulin-dependent diabetes mellitus. *Nature* 1992; 356: 162–4.
3. Stoffel M, Froguel P, Takeda J, *et al*. Human glucokinase gene: isolation, characterization, and identification of two missense mutations linked to early-onset non-insulin-dependent (type II) diabetes mellitus. *Proc Natl Acad Sci USA* 1992; 89: 7698–702.
4. Raben N, Barbetti F, Cama A, *et al*. Normal coding sequence of insulin gene in Pima Indians and Nauruans, two groups with highest prevalence of type II diabetes. *Diabetes* 1991; 40: 118–22.
5. Kusari J, Verma US, Buse JB, Henry RR, Olefsky JM. Analysis of the gene sequences of the insulin receptor and the insulin sensitive glucose transporter (Glut-4) in patients with common-type non-insulin dependent diabetes mellitus. *J Clin Invest* 1991; 88: 1323–30.
6. O'Rahilly S, Choi WH, Patel P, Turner RC, Flier JS, Moller DE. Detection of mutations in insulin-receptor gene in NIDDM patients by analysis of single-stranded conformation polymorphisms. *Diabetes* 1991; 40: 777–82.
7. Cook JTE, Hattersley AT, Christopher P, *et al*. Linkage analysis of glucokinase gene with NIDDM in Caucasian pedigrees. *Diabetes* 1992; 41: 1496–500.
8. National Diabetes Data Group. Classification and diagnosis of diabetes mellitus and other categories of glucose intolerance. *Diabetes* 1979; 28: 1039–57.
9. Bergman RN, Ider YZ, Bowden CR, Cobelli C. Quantitative estimation of insulin sensitivity. *Am J Physiol* 1979; 236: E667–77.
10. Reaven GM. Role of insulin resistance in human disease. (Banting Lecture.) *Diabetes* 1988; 37: 1595–607.
11. Bergman RN, Prager R, Volund A, Olefsky JM. Equivalence of the insulin sensitivity index in man derived by the minimal model method and the euglycemic glucose clamp. *J Clin Invest* 1987; 79: 790–800.
12. Zinman B, Vranic M. Diabetes and exercise. *Med Clin North Am* 1985; 69: 145–57.
13. Swinburn BA, Boyce VL, Bergman RN, Howard BV, Bogardus C. Deterioration in carbohydrate metabolism and lipoprotein changes induced by modern, high fat diet in Pima Indians and Caucasians. *J Clin Endocrinol Metab* 1991; 73: 156–65.
14. Bergman RN, Phillips LS, Cobelli C. Physiologic evaluation of factors controlling glucose tolerance in man: measurement of insulin sensitivity and B-cell glucose sensitivity from the response to intravenous glucose. *J Clin Invest* 1981; 68: 1456–67.
15. Bergman RN. Toward physiological understanding of glucose tolerance: minimal-model approach. (Lilly Lecture.) *Diabetes* 1989; 38: 1512–27.
16. Kahn SE, Prigeon RL, McCulloch DK, *et al*. Quantification of the relationship between insulin sensitivity and B-cell function in human subjects: evidence for a hyperbolic function. *Diabetes* 1993; 42: 1663–72.
17. Porte D Jr. B-cells in type II diabetes mellitus. (Banting Lecture.) *Diabetes* 1991; 40: 166–80.

18. Golay A, Chen YDI, Reaven GM. Effect of differences in glucose tolerance on insulin's ability to regulate carbohydrate and free fatty acid metabolism in obese subjects. *J Clin Endocrinol Metab* 1986; 62: 1081–8.

19. Skor DA, White NH, Thomas L, Santiago JV. Relative roles of insulin clearance and insulin sensitivity in the prebreakfast increase in insulin requirements in insulin-dependent diabetic patients. *Diabetes* 1984; 33: 60–3.

20. Staten M, Worchester B, Szekeres A, *et al*. Comparison of porcine and semisynthetic human insulins using euglycemic clamp-derived glucose-insulin dose-response curves in insulin-dependent diabetes. *Metabolism* 1984; 33: 132–5.

21. Hidaka H, Nagulesparan M, Klimes I, *et al*. Improvement of insulin secretion but not insulin resistance after short term control of plasma glucose in obese Type II diabetics. *J Clin Endocrinol Metab* 1982; 54: 217–22.

22. Rizza RA, Mandarino LJ, Gerich JE. Mechanism and significance of insulin resistance in non-insulin-dependent diabetes mellitus. *Diabetes* 1981; 30: 990–5.

23. Ward GM, Walters JM, Aitken PM, Best JD, Alford FP. Effects of prolonged pulsatile hyperinsulinemia in humans: enhancement of insulin sensitivity. *Diabetes* 1990; 39: 501–7.

24. Best JD, Taborsky GJ, Halter JB, Porte D Jr. Glucose disposal is not proportional to plasma glucose level in man. *Diabetes* 1981; 30: 847–50.

25. Herman WH, Fajans SS, Ortiz FJ, *et al*. Abnormal insulin secretion, not insulin resistance, is the genetic or primary defect of MODY in the RW pedigree. *Diabetes* 1994; 43: 40–6.

26. Taniguchi A, Nakai Y, Fukushima M, *et al*. Pathogenic factors responsible for glucose intolerance in patients with NIDDM. *Diabetes* 1992; 41: 1540–6.

27. Metz SA, Halter JB, Robertson RP. Paradoxical inhibition of insulin secretion by glucose in human diabetes mellitus. *J Clin Endocrinol Metab* 1979; 48: 827–35.

28. Leahy JL, Cooper HE, Deal DA, Weir GC. Chronic hyperglycemia is associated with impaired glucose influence on insulin secretion: a study in normal rats using chronic in vivo glucose infusions. *J Clin Invest* 1986; 77: 908–15.

29. Kahn BB, Shulman GI, DeFronzo RA, Cushman SW, Rossetti L. Normalization of blood glucose in diabetic rats with phlorizin treatment reverses insulin resistant glucose transport in adipose cells without restoring glucose transporter gene expression. *J Clin Invest* 1991; 87: 561–70.

30. Klip A, Marette A, Dimitrakoudis D, *et al*. Effect of diabetes on glucoregulation: from glucose transporters to glucose metabolism in vivo. *Diabetes Care* 1992; 15: 1747–66.

31. Martin BC, Warram JH, Krolewski AS, Bergman RN, Soeldner JS, Kahn CR. Role of glucose and insulin resistance in development of type 2 diabetes mellitus: results of a 25-year follow-up study. *Lancet* 1992; 340: 925–9.

32. Warram JH, Martin BC, Krolewski AS, Soeldner JS, Kahn CR. Slow glucose removal rate and hyperinsulinemia precede the development of Type II diabetes in the offspring of diabetic parents. *Ann Intern Med* 1990; 113: 909–15.

33. Saad MF, Knowler WC, Pettitt DJ, Nelson RG, Mott DM, Bennett PH. The natural history of impaired glucose tolerance in the Pima Indians. *N Engl J Med* 1988; 319: 1500–6.

34. Lillioja S, Mott DM, Zawadzki JK, *et al*. In vivo insulin action is familial characteristic in nondiabetic Pima Indians. *Diabetes* 1987; 36: 1329–35.

35. Lillioja S, Bogardus C. Obesity and insulin resistance: lessons learned from the Pima Indians. *Diabetes Metab Rev* 1988; 5: 517–40.

36. Eriksson J, Koranyi L, Bourey R, *et al*. Insulin resistance in Type 2 (non-insulin-dependent) diabetic patients and their relatives is not associated with a defect in the expression of the insulin-responsive glucose transporter (GLUT-4) gene in human skeletal muscle. *Diabetologia* 1992; 35: 143–7.

37. Taylor SI. Molecular mechanisms of insulin resistance: lessons from patients with mutations in the insulin-receptor gene. (Lilly Lecture.) *Diabetes* 1992; 41: 1473–90.

38. Shoelson SE, Kahn CR. Phosphorylation, the insulin receptor, and insulin action. In: Draznin B, Melmed S, LeRoith D, eds. *Molecular and cellular biology of diabetes mellitus*. Vol II. *Insulin action*. New York: Alan R Liss, 1989: 23–33.

39. Kida Y, Esposito-del Puente A, Bogardus C, Mott DM. Insulin resistance is associated with reduced fasting and insulin-stimulated glycogen synthase phosphatase activity in human skeletal muscle. *J Clin Invest* 1990; 85: 476–81.

40. Yang YJ, Hope ID, Ader M, Bergman RN. Insulin transport across capillaries is rate limiting for insulin action in dogs. *J Clin Invest* 1989; 84: 1620–8.

41. Ader M, Poulin RA, Yang Y, Bergman RN. Dose response relationship between lymph insulin and glucose uptake reveals enhanced insulin sensitivity of peripheral tissues. *Diabetes* 1992; 41: 241–52.
42. Poulin RA, Steil GM, Moore DM, Ader M, Bergman RN. Dynamics of glucose production and uptake are more closely related to insulin in hindlimb lymph than in thoracic duct lymph. *Diabetes* 1994; 43: 180–90.
43. Laakso M, Edelman SV, Brechtel G, Baron AD. Decreased effect of insulin to stimulate skeletal muscle blood flow in obese man. *J Clin Invest* 1990; 85: 1844–52.
44. Kahn SE, Beard JC, Schwartz MW, *et al.* Increased B-cell secretory capacity as mechanism for islet adaptation to nicotinic-acid-induced insulin resistance. *Diabetes* 1989; 38: 562–8.
45. Polonsky KS, Given BD, Hirsch LJ, Tillil H, Shapiro ET, Beebe C, Frank BH, Galloway JA, van Cauter E. Abnormal patterns of insulin secretion in non-insulin-dependent diabetes mellitus. *N Engl J Med* 1988; 318: 1231–9.
46. Lillioja S, Mott DM, Spraul M, *et al.* Insulin resistance and insulin secretory dysfunction as precursors of non-insulin-dependent diabetes mellitus: prospective studies of Pima Indians. *N Engl J Med* 1993; 329: 1988–92.
47. Buchanan TA, Metzger BE, Freinkel N, Bergman RN. Insulin sensitivity and B-cell responsiveness to glucose during late pregnancy in lean and moderately obese women with normal glucose tolerance or mild gestational diabetes. *Am J Obstet Gynecol* 1990; 162: 1008–14.
48. Ader M, Bergman RN. Peripheral effects of insulin dominate suppression of fasting hepatic glucose production. *Am J Physiol* 1990; 258: E1020–32.
49. Hoogwerf BJ, Brouhard BH. Glycemic control and complications of diabetes mellitus: practical implications of the Diabetes Control and Complications Trial (DCCT). *Cleve Clin J Med* 1994; 61: 34–7.

DISCUSSION

Dr. Phenekos: Could you comment on another possible factor in the development of insulin resistance, which is the loss of regular pulsatility of insulin, thus downregulating the insulin receptor? We have, of course, similar examples from other biological systems, such as the LHR antagonist downregulating the receptors in the pituitary.

Dr. Bergman: I think Polonsky has shown very beautifully that loss of pulsatility is one of the earliest changes in the onset of type 2 diabetes and may be the earliest indicator of a β-cell defect. This is certainly true in those individuals who have a specific genetic defect that we can relate to a β-cell defect, the MODY (Maturity Onset Diabetes in the Young) for example. However, my view of this is that pulsatility itself is an indicator of, but not a cause of, the pathogenesis of type 2 diabetes. I think it is an early indicator of a β-cell defect. I had the opportunity of talking to Polonsky about this recently. He has been comparing pulsatility with first-phase insulin secretion, corrected for the hyperbolic relationship that I showed, and it turns out that there is a relative decrease in first-phase insulin secretion when compared with a normal hyperbolic curve; in other words the first phase corrected for insulin resistance and the pulsatility factor both seem to disappear at the same time. So my view is that the pulsatility factor is an indicator of an early β-cell defect, but I don't believe it is the cause of insulin resistance in type 2 diabetes. On the whole, workers in the field do not believe that receptor downregulation is the cause of insulin resistance; it may occur as a result of hyperinsulinemia, which itself is a result of the impaired glucose tolerance state.

Dr. Marliss: The concept of glucose effectiveness is not one that is easy to understand. Perhaps you would amplify it somewhat and tell us where the glucose is going that is not necessarily insulin-dependent, and in what way you think that it might be a source of the primary defect.

Dr. Bergman: Girard discussed the same concept in different language. When the blood sugar goes up it has a choice of destination, particularly under normal meal conditions. It can go into the insulin-sensitive tissues, that is, the muscle or the adipose tissue, or it can go into the non-insulin-sensitive tissues, that is, the liver (which is very sensitive to hypoglycemia), the gut, and the brain. Under normal meal conditions, there is a relatively even distribution of glucose between the insulin-dependent and the insulin-independent tissues. As insulin resistance develops, the insulin-sensitive tissues, which are now less insulin-sensitive, have a reduced capacity to take up glucose. Our concept is that under those conditions the insulin-independent tissues, particularly liver, brain and gut, will then take up a greater and greater proportion of the blood sugar. This accounts for the reduced glucose tolerance—the blood sugar is raised for a longer period of time and it will be taken up increasingly by the non-insulin-dependent tissues.

In the true NIDDM state, you have a condition in which there is little insulin secretion because the β cell is very dysfunctional, and you have a highly insulin-resistant state, so even if you did secrete insulin it wouldn't do anything. The NIDDM patient therefore has to exist essentially independently of any dynamic insulin function. Insulin does very little for the type 2 diabetic except possibly to help maintain the fasting blood sugar. Therefore most of the glucose uptake in that case will be by the insulin-independent tissues, and this will result in a decreased glucose tolerance. What then becomes important are the other glucose transporters, which will determine the way in which glucose is taken up by the non-insulin-dependent tissues, in other words the non-GLUT4 transporters. The concept then is that your glucose effect under such conditions will be determined by whether you have an adequate or an inadequate provision of non-insulin-dependent transporters; this could have a lot to do with the progression to type 2 diabetes because, if you have a large abundance of such transporters, you can deal better with insulin resistance, and the need for insulin secretion is reduced. If you have a deficiency of that transporter the reverse is true.

Dr. Swift: As pediatricians we see very little NIDDM, but the one group we do see occasionally is the MODY group. I was very interested to hear your reference to a genetic abnormality there. Would you expand upon the results of those investigations regarding chromosome 20 and β-cell abnormalities?

Dr. Bergman: Several families have been identified in France as well as in Michigan in the USA in which MODY has been very carefully studied. I am most familiar with the studies done by Fajans. He has been following maturity-onset diabetes of the young for many years. He has measured β-cell function and insulin sensitivity in the MODY families and found a high prevalence of β-cell defect, defined by a reduced pulsatility and reduced insulin secretion. A study of the genetics of those families showed that in some of them there was a variety of deletions in the gene for glucokinase, which supports the concept that glucokinase is the β-cell glucose receptor. In addition, they recently found a defect in chromosome 20 in at least one of these families, although they have yet to identify the metabolic result of this chromosomal defect.

Dr. Cowett: I am fascinated by your comment on the direct *versus* the indirect effect of insulin. Is it fair to summarize this by suggesting that what you are really talking about is glucose autoregulation?

Dr. Bergman: I think that autoregulation usually refers to glucose control of glucose uptake by the liver. This is the effect of raised glucose, not raised insulin, acting either by suppressing glucose output by the liver or increasing glucose uptake by the liver. The concept of insulin's indirect effect incorporates two ideas: first, that it is an effect of insulin per se, not glucose, on liver glucose output or glucose uptake, and second, that the effect of insulin per se is mediated through an extra-hepatic effect of the hormone.

Dr. Nattrass: Can you tell us what you specifically mean by insulin sensitivity and insulin resistance?

Dr. Bergman: Insulin resistance is the failure of insulin to stimulate adequate glucose uptake. This is a very narrow definition, and I am following a tradition in the field that was a result of the development of the glucose clamp, in which the effect of insulin in stimulating glucose uptake under euglycemic conditions is the main target of interest. Of course it is true that insulin action has many different targets and insulin resistance or sensitivity can be defined in many different ways. Clearly the inhibition of lipolysis by insulin is a very important factor in insulin sensitivity and there is evidence that this is controlled independently of the effect of insulin on glucose uptake. So I don't believe that the effect of insulin on glucose uptake *per se* is the only type of insulin resistance. Let me call it a subclass of insulin resistance, one that is very important if you are talking about diseases in which hyperglycemia is involved.

Dr. Nattrass: You are saying that you think that insulin resistance in, say, glucose uptake into tissues can be divorced from insulin resistance relating to its ability to inhibit lipolysis, or do they always go hand in hand?

Dr. Bergman: I am quite certain that they can be divorced. I am also certain that the effect of insulin on the liver and its effect on the periphery can be divorced. That is quite clear because there are insulin-resistant individuals who have diabetes and there are insulin-resistant individuals who do not have diabetes. People with insulin resistance but without hyperglycemia can be shown to have a substantial degree of insulin resistance; in fact it may be almost impossible to show any effect of insulin on glucose uptake by the periphery and yet the liver produces glucose at an appropriate rate because the fasting blood sugar is not elevated. Other individuals may have an elevated hepatic glucose production, but insulin stimulation of glucose uptake in the periphery may not be much reduced. So I agree with you, these things are controlled independently and it is quite clear that hepatic insulin resistance probably comes later in the pathogenesis of type 2 than peripheral insulin resistance, because it seems to be responsible for the hyperglycemia.

Dr. Girard: I would like to make a comment on glucokinase and MODY. The glucokinase gene is expressed both in pancreatic β cells and in the liver, and the main difference between the liver and β cells is that in the β cells a promotor region and the first exon of glucokinase are different from in the liver, although the other exons are exactly the same. In the deletions and mutations that have been described for glucokinase, most of the deletions are in exons 2 to 7, so they probably affect both the liver and the pancreatic β cells. Unfortunately the effect of these deletions on hepatic glucose uptake has not been tested properly. It is likely that there is no defect in the β cell in these cases, but the liver is unable to take up glucose in an appropriate manner.

Dr. Crofford: Did I understand correctly that you are attributing the entire effect of insulin in reducing hepatic glucose output to an indirect mechanism rather than accepting that there may be both direct and indirect effects?

Dr. Bergman: No you didn't, and let me try to support my position. If you increase glucagon you can easily show a direct effect of insulin on glucose output by the liver, so under hyperglucagonemic conditions, I agree, and I believe that the effect of insulin is direct. However the great proportion of the basal glucose output by the liver is independent of glucagon and what we are focusing on in our laboratory is that part of the glucose production. What is the evidence that this effect is indirect? We have done experiments in which we increased portal insulin, which of course also increased systemic insulin, and we then did additional experiments in which the systemic insulin was raised to the same extent but the portal insulin was much lower. The suppression of glucose output was exactly the same in the two situations. We believe that most of the suppression of fasting glucose output in normal dogs is mediated by a peripheral mechanism, not a direct one. We maintain that most of the suppression of glucose output in these conditions is not mediated directly via the hepatic insulin receptor. We have recently repeated all these experiments under conditions in which the glucagon was completely suppressed, because we wanted to make sure that this mechanism was not due to insulin-mediated glucagon suppression, and we got exactly the same result.

Diabetes, edited by Richard M. Cowett,
Nestlé Nutrition Workshop Series,
Vol. 35. Nestec Ltd.,
Vevey/Raven Press, Ltd., New York © 1995.

Diabetes in Pregnancy

Patrick M. Catalano

Department of Reproductive Biology, Case Western Reserve University
at MetroHealth Medical Center, 2500 MetroHealth Medical Center,
Cleveland, Ohio 44109-1998, USA

Diabetes mellitus is the most common endocrine disorder that occurs during human gestation. In the United States, diabetes (including gestational diabetes) affects approximately 3–5% of all pregnant women (1) or about 70,000–100,000 women per year. Before the discovery of insulin, there was significant maternal and fetal mortality associated with diabetes during pregnancy. Since the discovery of insulin in the 1920s and the implementation of rigorous glucose control in the last decade, the incidence of maternal and fetal mortality has been reduced to that observed in the general obstetrical population with normal glucose tolerance. However, increased maternal and fetal morbidity, however subtle, persists.

The main aim of this chapter will be to review the alterations in carbohydrate metabolism that occur during normal gestation and the effect these changes have on women with diabetes mellitus. Although the issue of fetal malformations associated with poor glucose control during embryogenesis is a significant and important problem in women with type 1 diabetes mellitus, the focus of this review will be on the more prevalent alterations in carbohydrate metabolism in women developing glucose intolerance during pregnancy, or gestational diabetes. The alterations in carbohydrate metabolism that develop over the course of 9 months in women developing gestational diabetes may serve as a model for the development of type 2 diabetes over a period of decades in nonpregnant individuals.

LONGITUDINAL CHANGES IN CARBOHYDRATE METABOLISM DURING NORMAL GESTATION

The longitudinal changes in carbohydrate metabolism provide for both maternal and fetal growth and energy requirements. Previously, estimates of the alterations in basal and postprandial glucose metabolism relied upon interpretation of plasma glucose and insulin concentrations. However, with the advent of newer techniques such as stable isotopes of glucose to estimate basal endogenous (primarily hepatic) glucose production (2), glucose clamps (3) and minimal modeling (4) to estimate insulin sensitivity, we are now better able to characterize the normal alterations in glucose metabolism during pregnancy.

Basal Endogenous Glucose Production

There is evidence for a progressive decrease in plasma glucose and increase in plasma insulin concentrations with advancing gestation (5). Taken together, these data support the concept that there is either no change or an increase in hepatic insulin sensitivity during pregnancy. However, Kalhan *et al.* (6) and Cowett *et al.* (7) in separate studies using stable isotope methodologies have previously shown that there were no significant differences in basal endogenous glucose turnover or production in normal pregnant women at term when the data were expressed per kg of body weight. However, when the data were expressed in relationship to pregravid weight, basal endogenous glucose production was increased in late gestation. In our own longitudinal studies (8) in nonobese women with normal glucose tolerance using 6-6 ^{2}H$_2$ glucose evaluated prior to conception, in early gestation (12–14 weeks), and in late gestation (34–36 weeks), there were no significant changes in basal endogenous glucose production in early gestation but a significant ($p = 0.0005$) 30% increase in total basal glucose production by late gestation (Fig. 1). The significant increase in basal endogenous glucose production persisted when corrected for fat-free mass ($p = 0.05$). The decrease in plasma glucose concentration was most probably the

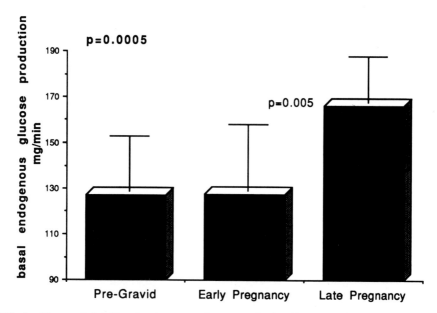

FIG. 1.   Changes in total basal endogenous glucose production. Error bars, SD. Reproduced with permission of *Am J Obstet Gynecol* 1992; 167: 913–9.

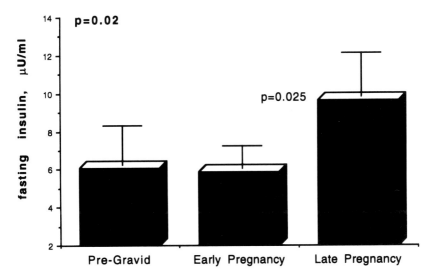

FIG. 2. Changes in fasting insulin. Error bars, SD. Reproduced with permission of *Am J Obstet Gynecol* 1992; 167: 913–9.

result of an increased maternal volume of distribution as well as of increased feto-placental glucose utilization in late gestation. These data in addition to the significant increases in basal insulin concentration during pregnancy (Fig. 2) are evidence for decreased basal hepatic insulin sensitivity to glucose in late gestation.

Beta Cell Response to Glucose Infusion

Insulin response to a glucose stimulus increases with advancing gestation. Various investigators have described increased insulin response to either an oral (5) or intravenous glucose challenge (9) in late pregnancy compared with either a nonpregnant control group or the same subjects examined after delivery. In early pregnancy, however, the changes in insulin response to a glucose challenge are less clear. In studies by Spellacy *et al.* (10), there was no significant difference in insulin response to an intravenous glucose challenge at 13–15 weeks gestation when compared with the same subjects evaluated after delivery. In our own studies in nonobese women evaluated prior their conceiving and in early and late gestation (11), there was a significant 120% increase in first-phase insulin response and a 50% increase in second-phase insulin response by 12–14 weeks gestation. The mean increase in insulin response by late pregnancy was 350% for the first-phase response and 300% for the second-phase response, as compared with the pregravid response (Fig. 3). Whether the differences in reported insulin response in early gestation are a result of different amounts of glucose used for the intravenous glucose challenges or persistent increases in postpartum insulin response remains unknown.

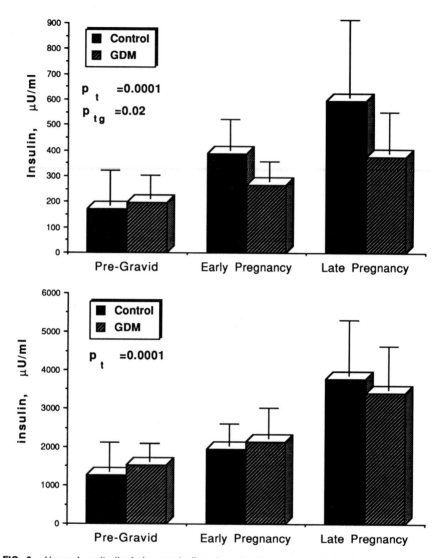

FIG. 3. *Upper:* Longitudinal changes in first-phase insulin response during intravenous glucose tolerance test. Error bars, SD. *Lower:* Longitudinal changes in second-phase insulin response during intravenous glucose tolerance test. Error bars, SD. P_t, change over time; P_{tg}, time-group interaction; GDM, gestational diabetes mellitus. Reproduced with permission of *Am J Physiol* 1993; 264 (*Endocrinol Metab* 27): E60–67.

Peripheral Insulin Sensitivity

On the basis of an increase in plasma insulin and glucose concentrations after a glucose challenge, particularly in late gestation, most investigators agree that there is decreased insulin sensitivity to glucose in late pregnancy (12). Employing more sophisticated methodologies, Fisher *et al.* (13), using a high-dose glucose infusion test, Buchanan *et al.* (14), using the minimal model technique, and in separate studies Ryan (15) and Catalano (11), using the hyperinsulinemic-euglycemic clamp, have all found significant decreases in maternal insulin sensitivity of between 33% and 78% in late pregnancy. In our own longitudinal studies using the hyperinsulinemic-euglycemic clamp (11), there was a 39% decrease in insulin sensitivity in early pregnancy ($p < 0.04$) and a 56% decrease by late pregnancy ($p = 0.005$), compared with pregravid measurements (Fig. 4). In addition, there was essentially complete ($\geq 90\%$) suppression of endogenous glucose production during insulin infusion in women with normal glucose tolerance, both pregravid and during early and late gestation.

Most of these estimates of insulin sensitivity in late pregnancy, however, are probably overestimates of true maternal insulin sensitivity. This is because even using the clamp methodology there is significant noninsulin-mediated glucose utilization by the placenta and fetus. Glucose utilization by the placenta and fetus in the human has not been quantified. However, estimates in maternal and feto-placental tissues have been obtained by Hay *et al.* (16) using the pregnant ewe model. From their studies, approximately one-third of the maternal glucose utilization is accounted for by uter-

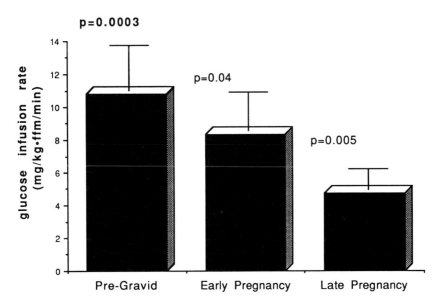

FIG. 4. Changes in glucose infusion rate during hyperinsulinemic-euglycemic clamp. Error bars, SD. Reproduced with permission of *Am J Obstet Gynecol* 1991; 165: 1667–1672.

ine, placental, and fetal tissues. Hence the decrease in peripheral insulin sensitivity observed in late gestation is equivalent, if not greater than, that described in many patients with type 2 diabetes mellitus.

Reproductive Hormones Associated with Alterations in Glucose Metabolism

The mechanisms associated with decreased insulin sensitivity during pregnancy have not been well characterized. Various reproductive hormones have been implicated in the alterations in insulin sensitivity during gestation. For example, estrogen has been associated with both an increase and a decrease in insulin sensitivity. Estrogen has previously been shown to improve glucose tolerance in partially pancreatectomized animal models (17). In contrast, Kojima et al. (18), using an intravenous insulin tolerance test, found decreased insulin sensitivity with the doses of ethinyl estradiol found in oral contraceptives. Progesterone, unlike estrogen, may not affect glucose tolerance but may increase glucose-stimulated insulin response (19), alter insulin clearance (18), and modify the route of glucose metabolism (20).

Decreased insulin sensitivity in late gestation has been ascribed to a variety of reproductive hormones. In late pregnancy, there are increased concentrations of both free and bound cortisol (21). In nonpregnant subjects, Rizza et al. (22) have described increases in endogenous glucose production and decreased insulin sensitivity using multidose hyperinsulinemic-euglycemic clamps. Since there was normal insulin binding to erythrocytes and monocytes, with a shift to the right, but near maximal glucose utilization during high-dose insulin infusion, the authors concluded that the decrease in insulin sensitivity was best explained by a postreceptor defect. Moreover, from data obtained using multidose insulin clamps in late pregnancy, Ryan et al. (15) postulated that postreceptor defects in insulin action were a potential mechanism to explain the decreases in insulin sensitivity in late gestation.

Human placental lactogen (or human chorionic somatomammotropin), which accounts for approximately 10% of all placental protein production, is a polypeptide hormone secreted by the syncytiotrophoblast and shares many of the biological properties of human growth hormone (23). Twelve-hour overnight infusions of human placental lactogen result in impaired glucose tolerance in response to an oral glucose challenge (24). Kalkhoff et al. (25) have also shown that in women with normal glucose tolerance, postpartum infusions of human placental lactogen result in increases in plasma glucose in response to an oral glucose challenge, but no change in insulin concentrations. In contrast, in subjects with subclinical diabetes mellitus, infusions of human placental lactogen result in frankly abnormal glucose tolerance, with increases in both glucose and insulin response. The mechanisms responsible for these alterations in glucose metabolism are, however, not yet well defined.

Lastly, prolactin has been implicated in decreased insulin sensitivity. Plasma concentrations of prolactin increase 5–10-fold with advancing gestation. Gustafson et al. (26) measured the plasma insulin and glucose response to an oral glucose challenge in women with hyperprolactinemia in comparison with an age 1 and weight-matched control group. They described increases in both basal and postglucose challenge insulin and glucose concentrations in women with elevated plasma prolactin. The results of these studies were supported by experiments by the same investigators using an animal model (27). Short-term prolactin administration in adult female rats resulted in increased insulin responses to an intravenous glucose challenge. Whether these alterations in insulin and glucose response resulted from a decrease in insulin sensitivity or an enhanced β-cell response remains unknown. However, in our own longitudinal studies of the changes in insulin sensitivity with advancing gestation, using the hyperinsulinemic-euglycemic clamp model (28), we were unable to correlate decreases in insulin sensitivity with the changes in any reproductive hormone, including estrogen, progesterone, human chorionic gonadotropin, prolactin, cortisol, and human placental lactogen.

LONGITUDINAL CHANGES IN CARBOHYDRATE METABOLISM DURING GESTATION IN WOMEN WITH GESTATIONAL DIABETES

O'Sullivan has shown that women developing gestational diabetes are at increased risk of diabetes mellitus in later life (29). Over the years, these results have been confirmed in various ethnic groups by multiple investigators (30,31). Although, women with gestational diabetes were believed initially to be at risk for both type 1 and type 2 diabetes mellitus in later life, the available evidence now suggests these women are primarily at increased risk for type 2 diabetes (32). As such, the development of gestational diabetes in women with normal glucose tolerance may serve as a paradigm for the pathogenesis of type 2 diabetes mellitus in later life in this at-risk population.

Basal Endogenous Glucose Production

Although basal insulin concentrations increase with advancing gestation in women with gestational diabetes, there is a great deal of overlap in women with gestational diabetes and those with normal glucose tolerance (33). Similarly, although the basal or fasting plasma glucose concentrations may be increased in late gestation in women with gestational diabetes as compared with women with normal glucose tolerance, most often it is the postprandial glucose values that are significantly increased. Moreover, a raised fasting glucose concentration in women with gestational diabetes may be the single best predictor of an abnormal glucose tolerance test soon after delivery (34) and may be useful in the identification of the women whose glucose intolerance existed before conception but was unrecognized as such (35).

Basal endogenous glucose production has been reported to be similar in women with normal glucose tolerance and gestational diabetes. Separate studies by Kalhan *et al.* (6), Cowett *et al.* (7), and Catalano *et al.* (33) using stable isotope methods have shown similar significant increases in endogenous glucose production in late pregnancy in women with normal glucose tolerance and gestational diabetes, even

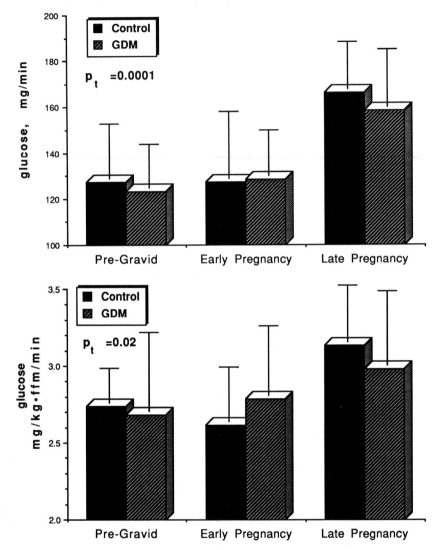

FIG. 5. *Upper:* Longitudinal changes in total basal endogenous glucose production. Error bars, SD. *Lower:* Longitudinal changes in total basal endogenous glucose production expressed in mg/ kg fat-free mass/min. Error bars, SD; P_t change over time; GDM, gestational diabetes mellitus. (Reproduced with permission of *Am J Physiol* 1993; 264 (*Endocrinol Metab* 27): E60–67.

when corrected for weight (Fig. 5). However, during insulin infusion with the hyper-insulinemic-euglycemic clamp, we have shown that there is evidence of impaired suppression of endogenous glucose production in late gestation in women with gestational diabetes. Endogenous glucose production was only 80% suppressed in women with gestational diabetes as compared with the 95% suppression in women with normal glucose tolerance. Otherwise, as was found in women with normal glucose tolerance, there was essentially complete suppression of hepatic glucose production in women with gestational diabetes before pregnancy and in early gestation.

Cell Response to Glucose Infusion

Decreased insulin response to a glucose challenge in late pregnancy in women with gestational diabetes has been described by several investigators, although the degree of insulin sensitivity has varied considerably. Yen *et al.* (36) described a decrease in first-phase insulin response and a decrease in glucose disposal using the intravenous glucose tolerance test in women with gestational diabetes in late gestation. Recently, Buchanan *et al.* (14), using the minimal model in late gestation, showed that women with gestational diabetes had a significant decrease in first-phase insulin response, but insulin sensitivity was similar to that of a normal pregnant control group. Lastly, in our own prospective longitudinal study of nonobese women developing gestational diabetes (33), we described a significant decrease in first-phase insulin response using the intravenous glucose tolerance test in late gestation in comparison with a control group (Fig. 3). The decrease in first-phase response, however, developed gradually with advancing gestation and only with a progressive decrease in insulin sensitivity to glucose. Although there was an increase in second-phase insulin response in women with gestational diabetes ($p<0.001$), there were no significant differences between the groups.

Peripheral Insulin Sensitivity

Increased, decreased, and no change in peripheral insulin sensitivity to glucose have all also been suggested as potential factors in the development of gestational diabetes. Ryan *et al.* (15) showed that there was a 40% decrease in insulin sensitivity in women with gestational diabetes in late pregnancy in comparison with a control group, using the hyperinsulinemic-euglycemic clamp. Although there was an increase in insulin response to a test meal in women with gestational diabetes as compared with a pregnant control group, the first-phase insulin response was not examined. In contrast, Fisher *et al.* (37), using a glucose infusion test in nonobese women with gestational diabetes, described increased insulin sensitivity in late pregnancy. These investigators suggested that the increased insulin sensitivity was compensating for the low insulin response found in these women. As noted previously, Buchanan *et al.* (14), using the minimal model technique, showed that in late gestation women with gestational diabetes had a significant decrease in first-phase insulin response, but insulin sensitivity was not different from that found in a pregnant control group. Lastly, we described the longitudinal changes in insulin sensitivity using the hyperinsulinemic-euglycemic clamp in nonobese women who developed abnormal glucose intolerance, in comparison with a matched control group (33). Although women with

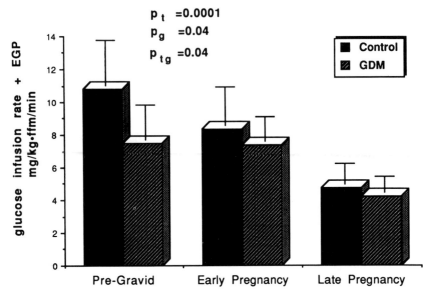

FIG. 6. Longitudinal changes in peripheral insulin sensitivity as indicated by infusion of glucose required to maintain euglycemia (90 mg/dl) + endogenous glucose production during insulin infusion. Error bars, SD; P_t, change over time; P_g, difference between groups; P_{tg}, time-group interaction; GDM, gestational diabetes mellitus. (Reproduced with permission of *Am J Physiol* 1993; 264 (*Endocrinol Metab* 27): E60–67.

gestational diabetes had decreased insulin-stimulated glucose uptake or insulin sensitivity in comparison with the control group. These differences were greatest before conception and in early pregnancy, and by the late third trimester the differences in insulin sensitivity were much smaller in rate as compared with pregravid measurements (Fig. 6). In women with gestational diabetes or decreased insulin sensitivity before conception, there was very little change in insulin sensitivity from the time prior to conception through early gestation as compared with the 40% decrease in insulin sensitivity in the control group. Furthermore, in some very insulin-resistant individuals, there was actually an increase in insulin sensitivity in early gestation as compared with pregravid measurements. An increase in insulin sensitivity in early gestation in individuals with a high degree of insulin resistance may help to explain the decrease in insulin requirements observed in some women with type 1 diabetes in early pregnancy.

CONCLUSION

In summary, in nonobese women with normal glucose tolerance there is a progressive decrease in insulin sensitivity with advancing gestation. There is a significant 30% increase in basal endogenous glucose production despite an increase in basal insulin concentration and a progressive 60% decrease in peripheral insulin sensitivity, as estimated by the hyperinsulinemic-euglycemic clamp. Endogenous glucose production, however, decreases appropriately during insulin infusion. Accordingly, the decrease in insulin sensitivity is associated with a 3.0–3.5-fold increase in insulin respond by late pregnancy.

In contrast, we have observed that decreased insulin sensitivity is the only abnormality of carbohydrate metabolism found before conception in nonobese women developing abnormal glucose tolerance during pregnancy. In these women, there is essentially no change in insulin sensitivity in early gestation but a significant decrease in sensitivity by late pregnancy. A relative decrease in first phase insulin response is observed only in comparison with a control group and in association with a progressive decrease in insulin sensitivity. Likewise, impaired suppression of endogenous glucose production with insulin infusion develops only in late gestation. The progression of abnormalities of carbohydrate metabolism in women developing gestational diabetes (that is, decreased peripheral insulin sensitivity), followed by a relatively diminished increase in insulin response and an impaired suppression of endogenous glucose production during an insulin infusion, is consistent with the models of the pathogenesis of type 2 diabetes mellitus proposed by DeFronzo (38) and Bogardus *et al.* (39) (in the Pima Indians). Further longitudinal studies in various ethnic and weight groups are needed in order to elucidate more fully the abnormalities of glucose metabolism in pregnant women.

REFERENCES

1. Gabbe SG, Mestman JH, Freeman RK, Anderson GV, Lowensohn RI. Management and outcome of Class A diabetes mellitus. *Am J Obstet Gynecol* 1977; 127: 465–9.
2. Wolfe RR. Tracers in metabolic research: radioisotope and stable isotope/mass spectrometry methods. Chapter 9. Specific applications: glucose metabolism. New York: Alan R Liss, 1984: 113–21.
3. DeFronzo RA, Tobin JD, Andres R. Glucose clamp technique: a method for quantifying insulin secretion and resistance. *Am J Physiol* 1979; 237: E214–23.
4. Bergman RN, Ider YZ, Bowden CR, Cobelli C. Quantitative estimation of insulin sensitivity. *Am J Physiol* 1979; 236: E667–77.
5. Lind T, Billewicz WZ, Brown G. A serial study of changes occurring in the oral glucose tolerance test during pregnancy. *J Obstet Gynaecol Br Cwlth* 1973; 80: 1033–9.
6. Kalhan SC, D'Angelo LJ, Savin SM, Adam PAJ. Glucose production in pregnant women at term gestation: sources of glucose for human fetus. *J Clin Invest* 1979; 63:388–94.
7. Cowett RA, Susa JB, Kahn CB, Gilotti B, Oh W, Schwartz R. Glucose kinetics in nondiabetic and diabetic women during the third trimester of pregnancy. *Am J Obstet Gynecol* 1983; 146: 773–80.
8. Catalano PM, Tyzbir ED, Wolfe RR, Roman NM, Amini SB, Sims EAH. Longitudinal changes in basal hepatic glucose production and suppression during insulin infusion in normal pregnant women. *Am J Obstet Gynecol* 1992; 167: 913–19.
9. Spellacy WN, Goetz FC. Plasma insulin in normal late pregnancy. *N Engl J Med* 1963; 268: 988–91.
10. Spellacy WN, Goetz FC, Greenburg BZ, Ellis J. Plasma insulin in normal "early" pregnancy. *Obstet Gynecol* 1965; 25: 862–5.
11. Catalano PM, Tyzbir ED, Roman NM, Amini SB, Sims EAH. Longitudinal changes in insulin release and insulin resistance in non-obese pregnant women. *Am J Obstet Gynecol* 1991; 165: 1667–72.
12. Freinkel N. Banting Lecture 1980: Of pregnancy and progeny. *Diabetes* 1980; 29: 1023–35.
13. Fisher PM, Sutherland HW, Bewsher PD. The insulin response to glucose infusion in normal human pregnancy. *Diabetologia* 1980; 19: 15–20.
14. Buchanan TZ, Metzger BE, Freinkel N, Bergman RN. Insulin sensitivity and β-cell responsiveness

to glucose during late pregnancy in lean and moderately obese women with normal glucose tolerance or mild gestational diabetes. *Am J Obstet Gynecol* 1990; 162: 1008–14.

15. Ryan EA, O'Sullivan MJ, Skyler JS. Insulin action during pregnancy: studies with the euglycemic clamp technique. *Diabetes* 1985; 34: 380–9.

16. Hay WW, Sparks JW, Wilkening RB, Battalgia FC, Meschia G. Partition of maternal glucose production between conceptus and maternal tissues in sheep. *Am J Physiol* 1983; 245: E347–50.

17. Houssay BA, Foglia VG, Rodriguez RR. Production or prevention of some types of experimental diabetes by oestrogens or corticosteroids. *Acta Endocrinologica* 1954; 17: 146–64.

18. Kojima T, Lindheim SR, Duffy DM, Vijod MA, Stanczyk FZ, Lobo RA. Insulin sensitivity is decreased in normal women by doses of ethinyl estradiol used in oral contraceptives. *Am J Obstet Gynecol* 1993; 169: 1540–4.

19. Kalkhoff RK, Jacobson M, Lemper D. Progesterone, pregnancy and the augmented plasma insulin response. *J Clin Endocrinol* 1970; 31: 24–8.

20. Sutter-Dub MT, Dazey B, Vergnaad MT, Madec AM. Progesterone and insulin resistance in the pregnant rat. *Diabete Metab* 1981; 7: 97–104.

21. Gibson M, Tulchinsky D. The maternal adrenal. In: Tulchinsky D, Ryan KJ, eds. *Maternal-fetal endocrinology*. Philadelphia: WB Saunders, 1980: 129–43.

22. Rizza RA, Mandarino LJ, Gerich JE. Cortisol-induced insulin resistance in man: impaired suppression of glucose production and stimulation of glucose utilization due to a postreceptor defect of insulin action. *Clin Endocrinol Metab* 1982; 54: 131–8.

23. Osathanondh R, Tulchinsky D. Placental polypeptide hormones. In: Tulchinsky D, Ryan KJ, eds. *Maternal-fetal endocrinology*. Philadelphia: WB Saunders, 1980: 17–42.

24. Beck P, Daughaday WH. Human placental lactogen:studies of its acute metabolic effects and disposition in normal man. *J Clin Invest* 1967; 46: 103–10.

25. Kalkhoff RK, Richardson BL, Beck P. Relative effects of pregnancy, human placental lactogen and prednisolone on carbohydrate tolerance in normal and subclinical diabetic subjects. *Diabetes* 1969; 18: 153–75.

26. Gustafson AB, Banasiak MF, Kalkhoff RK, Hagen TC, Kim H-J. Correlation of hyperprolactinemia with altered plasma insulin and glucagon: similarity to effects of late human pregnancy. *J Clin Endocrinol Metab* 1980; 51: 242–6.

27. Gustafson A, Banasiak M, Kalkhoff R, Hagen T, Kim H. Prolactin induced hyperinsulinemia. *Clin Res* 1978; 26: 720A (abstract).

28. Catalano PM, Tyzbir ED, Nakajima ST, Chapitis J, McAuliffe T, Sims EAH. Longitudinal changes in insulin sensitivity: relationship to pregravid insulin sensitivity and alterations in hormone concentrations during gestation. In: *Proceedings of the 37th Annual Meeting of the Society for Gynecologic Investigation,* St Louis, Missouri, March 21–24, 1990. St Louis, Society for Gynecology Investigation, 1990, Abstract 177.

29. O'Sullivan JB. Body weight and subsequent diabetes mellitus. *JAMA* 1982; 248: 949–52.

30. Kjos SL, Buchanan TA, Greenspoon JS, Montoro M, Bernstein GS, Mestman JH. Gestational diabetes mellitus: the prevalence of glucose intolerance and diabetes mellitus in the first two months post partum. *Am J Obstet Gynecol* 1990; 163: 93–8.

31. Damm P, Kühl C, Bertelsen A, Mølsted-Pedersen L. Predictive factors for the development of diabetes in women with previous gestational diabetes mellitus. *Am J Obstet Gynecol* 1992; 167: 607–16.

32. Metzger BE, Roston SM, Cho NH, Radvany R. Prepregnancy weight and antepartum insulin secretion predict glucose intolerance five years after gestational diabetes mellitus. *Diabetes Care* 1993; 16: 1598–605.

33. Catalano PM, Tyzbir ED, Wolfe RR, *et al.* Carbohydrate metabolism during pregnancy in control subjects and women with gestational diabetes. *Am J Physiol* 1993;264 (*Endocrinol Metab* 27): E60–7.

34. Catalano PM, Vargo KM, Bernstein IM, Amini SB. Incidence and risk factors associated with abnormal postpartum glucose tolerance in women with gestational diabetes. *Am J Obstet Gynecol* 1991; 165: 914–9.

35. Metzger BE, Bybee DE, Freinkel N, Phelps RL, Radvany RM, Vaisrub N. Gestational diabetes mellitus: correlations between the phenotypic and genotypic characteristic of the mother and abnormal glucose tolerance during the first year postpartum. *Diabetes* 1985; 34(Suppl. 2): 111–5.

36. Yen SCC, Tsai CC, Vela P. Gestational diabetogenesis: quantitative analysis of glucose-insulin interrelationship between normal pregnancy and pregnancy with gestational diabetes. *Am J Obstet Gynecol* 1971;111: 792–800.

37. Fisher PM, Sutherland HW, Bewsher PD. The insulin response to glucose infusion in gestational diabetes. *Diabetologia* 1980; 19: 10–4.
38. DeFronzo RA. Lilly Lecture, 1987. The triumvirate: cell, muscle, liver: a collusion responsible for NIDDM. *Diabetes* 1988; 37: 667–87.
39. Bogardus C, Lillioja S, Bennett PH. Pathogenesis of NIDDM in Pima Indians. *Diabetes Care* 1991; 14(suppl 3): 685–90.

DISCUSSION

Dr. Schwartz: I have trouble in understanding your use of fat-free mass as a reference for your glucose data. I thought that adipose tissue was an insulin-sensitive tissue and therefore would be metabolized to glucose.

Dr. Catalano: The reason why we use fat-free mass for both the basal measurements and the clamp measurements is that basal endogenous glucose production is not dependent upon insulin-sensitive tissue. You are looking at brain tissue and in pregnancy you are looking at non-insulin-mediated disposal to the fetus. The reason why we use the fat-free mass during the clamp studies is that about 80–90% of glucose disposal during a clamp is related to muscle tissue, which is primarily lean tissue. We have analyzed the data in relation to body weight per kg and there is no significant difference in any of the values.

Dr. Cowett: Were any of the normal or gestational diabetes (GDM) babies specifically large for gestational age?

Dr. Catalano: Some babies were large for gestational age. I think the heaviest baby in the group weighed 4.5 kg but I can't tell you the exact proportion; my guess is probably 15–20%.

Dr. Zoppi: Were the mothers obese before pregnancy or did they become obese during pregnancy?

Dr. Catalano: These studies were specifically looking at nonobese women, so I can't answer the question. What we are trying to do now, using the same study design, is to look at women with more than 25% body fat. The data are too preliminary to give you an answer except to say that, as you might anticipate, they were more insulin-resistant before pregnancy.

Dr. Bergman: I would be careful about drawing conclusions about suppression of hepatic glucose output between 80% and 90% when you are using any isotope dilution method. With such a small group, it is really very difficult to interpret an 80% *versus* a 90% suppression during a clamp as being different. My own view is that one should be quite conservative about these kinds of numbers because of the many potential errors in measuring hepatic glucose output.

Dr. Catalano: We looked at it statistically and made the assumption based on a statistical analysis. We also added label to the 20% glucose infusion during the clamp, so it was the type of study in which you could decrease the likelihood of getting negative numbers for hepatic glucose production. Finally, we have repeated the study with additional women, and it appears that we are finding the same result. I agree that it is reasonable to be conservative but there is certainly a trend in the direction shown.

Dr. Zoupas: Can you give us an explanation why most GDM patients need more and more insulin in late pregnancy, while some need less.

Dr. Catalano: My own simplistic answer is that if you look at the people who need less insulin in late pregnancy you will see that they tend to be the women who have the biggest babies. With a big baby and a big placenta, you have increased non-insulin-mediated glucose disposal and as a result you may not need as much insulin. I admit that this is speculation.

Dr. Zoupas: I have noticed that the earlier you start insulin treatment in GDM the better the end result. When you start insulin late in pregnancy your result is really very poor. Do you agree?

Dr. Catalano: Yes I do. The one thing that has been most disappointing to obstetricians is that glucose control in late pregnancy correlates very poorly with growth. You can prevent problems such as fetal death, but the relationship to fetal growth is poor. Our own speculation is that whatever controls fetal growth probably also controls placental growth, and we think that in early pregnancy there are abnormalities of carbohydrate metabolism that affect placental growth in women who later develop gestational diabetes.

Dr. Nattrass: I would like to criticize the use of the term *insulin sensitivity* when you are really just talking about glucose disposal into tissues. This seems to me to be particularly apposite in pregnancy. If, for example, as Bergman suggested, you can divorce changes in insulin sensitivity in the glucose-consuming tissues from lipolytic insulin sensitivity, you could see changes in pregnancy in lipolytic insulin sensitivity that would allow a greater delivery of substrates such as fatty acids and ketone bodies to tissues that would normally consume glucose. In that case you might interpret the changes you see as a difference in insulin sensitivity when in practice the tissues are thinking that they don't need to take up so much glucose because they are quite happy utilizing fatty acids or ketone bodies.

Dr. Catalano: We have done indirect calorimetric studies but I did not present the data because of time constraints. If you believe indirect calorimetry, the results show there is an increase in carbohydrate oxidation in early pregnancy, so while indeed there may be more lipolysis going on at this time, the evidence from indirect calorimetry is that carbohydrate oxidation increases proportionally more than lipolysis.

Dr. Bergman: Has anyone tried to normalize insulin sensitivity in an animal model by normalizing the known contra-insulin hormones of pregnancy? I think that there may well be a neural component to this.

Dr. Catalano: The only thing we found that correlated with the change in insulin sensitivity was the initial insulin sensitivity. If you are very insulin-sensitive that tends to indicate that you would have a large decrease in sensitivity. On the other hand if you are very insulin-resistant, it would tend to indicate that the changes would be relatively small. I am not aware of any animal data that have related insulin sensitivity to either hormonal or neural input. The data that I have reviewed were primarily human.

Dr. Bergman: I think neural mechanisms are more rapidly turned on and off than hormonal ones. A possible analogue to this is the diurnal rhythm in insulin sensitivity. There is a tremendous insulin resistance in the afternoon and insulin sensitivity goes up and down every day by large amounts. Nobody has explained that either, and it could be that there is a common mechanism between the normal diurnal rhythm of insulin sensitivity and the insulin resistance in pregnancy.

Dr. Catalano: The only comment I have is anecdotal. If you look at insulin requirements in pregnancy, you find that, unlike the nonpregnant state, insulin requirements during pregnancy seem to be relatively uniformly spread out over the day. So, based on clinical data, I would think that some of the normal variation is lost in pregnancy, whatever the overriding changes in insulin sensitivity. As another example, the diurnal variation in cortisol is less pronounced in pregnancy.

Dr. Hoet: Did you choose your study women? Did you select them according to their own birth weight?

Dr. Catalano: No. We selected them only in relation to whether they had a normal previous pregnancy *versus* a previous history of gestational diabetes. That was the only selective criterion other than being healthy.

Dr. Hoet: Birthweight of the mother could be very important if, as you and Bergman were saying, thinness at birth is related to insulin resistance later in life. Among your sample you would have had a mix of women who were small for gestational age, normal for gestational age, or even overweight for gestational age, and therefore you would have a very heterogenous group. I feel that your data should be examined in relation to the birthweight of the women themselves because that is very definitely going to influence their insulin sensitivity once they are adult.

Dr. Catalano: We tried to recruit only women in the normal group, who had no history of any diabetes in the family. I would be hesitant to look at birthweight because it is only one variable relating to fetal growth. What does it mean if a baby weighs 3.5 kg unless I also have the length? And I would even argue further that unless I have the percent of body fat I am only getting a one-dimensional view of a three-dimensional person.

Dr. Hoet: But the fact is that there is a relationship between thinness at birth and insulin resistance later on, so the weight alone at a particular length of gestation is an important variable in glucose metabolism in later life. I believe this is a concept that we must introduce into our ways of looking at this subject.

Dr. Girard: If we accept that insulin sensitivity during the euglycemic clamp is related to an insulin effect on skeletal muscle, one component that is very important is skeletal muscle triglyceride concentration. That could be a crucial factor in the insulin resistance during pregnancy, and it has not been very thoroughly investigated.

Dr. Catalano: I agree.

Dr. Marliss: As diabetologists, we tend to define diabetes and glucose in terms of insulin. I am pleased that Nattrass continues to want to have them defined in terms of lipid, and I was even more pleased that you indicated that amino acids may have some relevance in the setting you describe. I would like to propose a hypothesis: the reason why the people you study become insulin-resistant is a *physiological* one related to corresponding alterations in amino acid turnover and protein kinetics. As you pointed out, and especially in late gestation, one of the main tasks of the fetus is to lay down a great deal of protein. If the mother has insulin resistance with regard to protein kinetics there will be a higher turnover of amino acids and therefore greater amino acid availability to the fetus. Studies on the turnover of labeled glycine have shown an increased turnover in pregestational diabetes, even in well-controlled cases, and there was a very direct correlation between this and fetal size in terms of outcome. So on the one hand it is probably a very physiological thing for the individual to do and desirable, but on the other hand, if exaggerated, it may contribute to the macrosomia.

Diabetes, edited by Richard M. Cowett,
Nestlé Nutrition Workshop Series,
Vol. 35. Nestec Ltd.,
Vevey/Raven Press, Ltd., New York © 1995.

Maternal Diabetes: Consequences for the Offspring

An Experimental Model in the Rat

K. Holemans, L. Aerts, J. Verhaeghe, and F.A. Van Assche

U.Z. Gasthuisberg, Dept Obstet Gynecol, Herestraat 49, 3000 Leuven, Belgium

The physiological changes of pregnancy tend to reset glucose homeostasis in the direction of diabetes. About 2–3% of all pregnant women develop abnormal glucose tolerance in pregnancy. Pregnancy complicated by diabetes leads to increased perinatal mortality and morbidity. Functional and morphological changes are present at cellular and tissue level. Furthermore, there are implications for the long-term effects of maternal diabetes on the offspring.

Progress in understanding the fetal consequences in diabetic pregnancy and its long-term effects has been made possible by the use of rats in experimental models. Hyperglycemia during pregnancy (first generation), induced by streptozotocin (1,2) or during a glucose infusion (3–6), has a profound influence on fetal development and metabolism, and disturbances in glucose handling persist into the second and third generation offspring of these rats.

FETAL AND LONG-TERM RESULTS OF EXPERIMENTAL DIABETES

Granulated β cells can be recognized in the fetal pancreas of the rat from day 17 or 18 of gestation. From day 20 on, the endocrine cells accumulate in clusters; the contribution of β cells to the islet population remains low, but ultrastructurally the β cells appear mature, replete with secretory granules, and comparable to those of adult rats. During the last two days before birth, the islets show a dramatic expansion and the typical organization in mantle islets with a central core of β cells becomes apparent (1).

In fetuses of streptozotocin-diabetic rats, a similar evolution to control fetuses is observed, but the development of the endocrine pancreas is enhanced by the increased blood glucose concentrations, which results in hypertrophy and hyperplasia of the islets from day 20 of gestation until birth. When maternal hyperglycemia is severe, the β cells of these fetuses become degranulated, due to overstimulation by the excessive glucose concentrations. At day 20 of gestation, decreased pancreatic and plasma insulin concentrations characterize the fetuses of severely streptozotocin-diabetic rats. These data have been confirmed in fetuses of spontaneously diabetic BB rats (7). Similar findings have also been reported in very poorly controlled human diabetes (8). With the appearance of small islets of Langerhans (day 20 of gestation), glucose-stimulated insulin release can be triggered *in vivo*. The transition from a fetal-to an adult-type of insulin release in response to glucose occurs during the last days of gestation and parallels quantitative rather than qualitative changes within the β cell (9). In contrast, glucose-stimulated insulin release was absent from pancreases of severely hyperglycemic (15.1 mM) fetuses (9). Incubation of fetal islets with other secretagogues also results in the absence of an insulin response in the fetuses of highly hyperglycemic rats. Only arginine induced a sustained monophasic insulin release, suggesting that the defect may be related to stimulus-secretion coupling (3,4).

Diabetes in the maternal rat not only affects pancreatic development and function; it also involves other important aspects of fetal metabolism. Because of accentuated catabolism in the maternal rat, the fuel supply to the fetus is abundant. Fetal glucose concentrations are a reflection of maternal glucose concentrations (1,10). Hepatic glycogen accumulation has been reported to be decreased in hypoinsulinemic fetuses of streptozotocin-diabetic rats (1). The influx of amino acids from the maternal side is significantly reduced in microsomic fetuses of diabetic rats, while amino acid transport to their overweight littermates is greatly increased (11). Amino acid levels are therefore markedly decreased in fetuses of severely diabetic rats (1,10). Plasma triglyceride and non-esterified fatty acid (NEFA) concentrations and liver triglyceride content are highly increased in fetuses of severely diabetic rats (1,10).

Severe diabetes in rats is associated with fetal growth retardation as a result of fetal malnutrition. Fetal hypoinsulinemia and a reduced number of insulin receptors on target cells (12) in fetuses of severely diabetic rats may lead to a reduction in fetal glucose uptake; a reduced fetal glucose uptake has been demonstrated in hypoinsu-linemic streptozotocin-injected fetal lambs (13).

After birth, the glucose diet of the fetus changes into the high-fat diet of the suckling rat. The amount of endocrine tissue does not increase further, while the pancreatic insulin content exceeds adult values. Plasma insulin concentrations decrease and remain low till weaning (14). At weaning, the high-fat diet of the suckling rat is changed into a high-carbohydrate diet. The mass of endocrine tissue and plasma insulin concentrations increase, while pancreatic insulin content decreases (14). The suckling-weaning transition in rats is associated with an increase in insulin sensitivity of the peripheral tissues (15), which may be conferred by an enhanced expression of the GLUT4 glucose transporter (16).

Newborns of severely diabetic rats have a decreased body weight. As in the control group, the lactation period represents a steady-state period in the development of the endocrine pancreas. Severely diabetic rats are too ill to feed their offspring properly. The pups, already small at birth, remain smaller than normal, with a lower growth rate and reduced β-cell mass. Malnutrition results in hypoglycemia and subsequent hypo-activity of the β cells (14).

TABLE 1. *Body weight, plasma glucose and plasma insulin concentrations of first- and second-generation control and diabetic rats and of their third generation fetuses*

	Control			Diabetic		
	Body weight (g)	Glucose (mmol/liter)	Insulin (nmol/liter)	Body weight (g)	Glucose (mmol/liter)	Insulin (nmol/liter)
First generation						
Pregnant	290 ± 3 (16)	4.1 ± 0.1 (16)	0.38 ± 0.03 (13)	285 ± 4 (22)	22.6 ± 0.5*** (23)	0.11 ± 0.01** (22)
Second generation						
Nonpregnant	213 ± 2 (39)	5.4 ± 0.1 (38)	0.17 ± 0.01 (34)	179 ± 2*** (49)	5.3 ± 0.1 (46)	0.26 ± 0.01*** (44)
Pregnant	293 ± 3‡ (35)	4.3 ± 0.1‡ (49)	0.40 ± 0.02‡ (34)	270 ± 3***,‡ (37)	4.7 ± 0.1**,† (45)	0.34 ± 0.01*,† (40)
Third generation						
Fetuses	2.10 ± 0.03 (65)	2.3 ± 0.1 (21)	0.72 ± 0.05 (10)	2.12 ± 0.02 (112)	2.7 ± 0.1** (48)	0.96 ± 0.05** (44)

The measurements were made at 100 days of age in nonpregnant animals, on day 20 of gestation in pregnant animals, and in third generation fetuses. Values are means ± SEM for the number of rats in parentheses.
* $p < 0.05$, ** $p < 0.01$, *** $p < 0.001$, diabetic *versus* control.
† $p < 0.01$, ‡ $p < 0.001$, pregnant *versus* nonpregnant.

At adult age (3 months), the offspring of diabetic rats appear to have recovered from the influences of a perinatal diabetic environment. They have a morphologically normal endocrine pancreas and normal plasma glucose concentrations (17). Plasma insulin concentrations are normal (18) or increased (19) (Table 1).

Body weight in the offspring of severely diabetic rats remains below normal. Plasma glucagon and triglyceride levels are decreased, but plasma amino acid levels can be regarded as normal (1).

When these offspring, reared by their own diabetic mothers, are submitted to a 3-hour glucose infusion, they manage to maintain glucose levels within the control range, but in the presence of high insulin levels, resulting in an increased insulin-to-glucose ratio (20). In *in vivo* insulin-captation experiments, an increased renal clearance was found (18). These data suggest that there was insulin resistance in the offspring of diabetic rats.

In order to quantitate and characterize the insulin resistance in the female offspring of streptozotocin-diabetic pregnant rats (SDF rats), we applied the euglycemic hyperinsulinemic clamp at various insulin infusion rates in order to obtain an insulin dose-response curve. The exogenous glucose infusion rate required to maintain euglycemia at steady-state plasma insulin concentrations is generally considered to be a measure of the effect of insulin on total body glucose metabolism. In SDF rats, the dose-response curve was shifted to the right with a decreased maximum effect. This finding indicates that total body glucose metabolism is both less sensitive and less responsive to insulin in SDF rats compared with control rats (21). The use of [3-³H]-glucose allowed us to determine the effect of insulin on hepatic glucose production and peripheral glucose utilization (22). The insulin resistance involves the peripheral tissues as well as the liver (21). The peripheral tissues of SDF rats are less sensitive to insulin

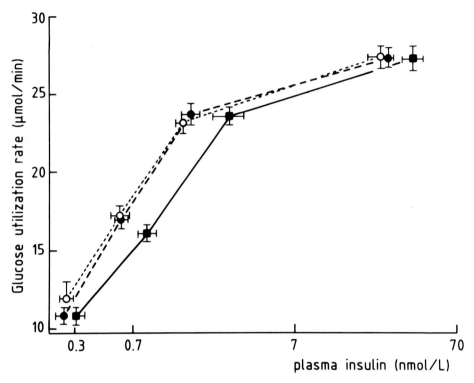

FIG. 1. Insulin dose-response curves for stimulation of glucose utilization in age-matched (●---●) and weight-matched (○---○) control rats and adult offspring of streptozotocin-diabetic rats (■---■). Data are means, error bars, SEM of 5–11 experiments.

(half-maximal effect), but they display a normal responsivity to insulin (maximum effect; Fig. 1), confirming previous results of the ^{123}I-insulin captation experiments (18). In this study, the authors suggested that the increased uptake of radioactive insulin by the kidney might be attributed to a decreased uptake of insulin by the peripheral extrahepatic tissues (18). Since in the clamp studies all rats were in the postabsorptive state, the glucose production rate in these studies equals the actual glucose production rate. The insulin dose-response curve for inhibition of hepatic glucose production (Fig. 2) in SDF rats obviously shows that the liver in these animals is both less sensitive and less responsive to insulin (21).

With the exception of the liver, the hyperinsulinemic clamp does not allow identification of the tissues contributing to the peripheral insulin resistance. To determine which peripheral tissues contribute to the decreased glucose disposal we used the 2-deoxy-[1-³H]-D-glucose technique in basal conditions and during a clamp at physiological hyperinsulinemia. We thus determined the glucose metabolic index, which is a measure for glucose utilization, in five skeletal muscles, the diaphragm muscle, white adipose tissue, and two control tissues (brain and duodenum). As could be

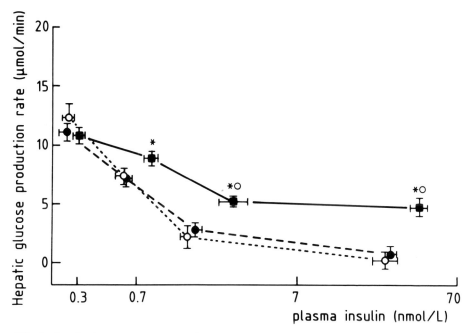

FIG. 2. Insulin dose-response curves for inhibition of endogenous glucose production in age-matched (●---●) and weight-matched (○---○) control rats and adult offspring of streptozotocin-diabetic rats (■---■). Data are means, error bars, SEM of 5–11 experiments. *$p < 0.05$ versus age-matched control rats; °$p < 0.05$ versus weight-matched control rats.

expected, skeletal muscles are primarily responsible for the peripheral insulin resistance that characterizes SDF rats (Fig. 3) (2). Indeed, the glucose metabolic index in the skeletal muscles of SDF rats was 9–29% and 25–70% lower than in control rats under basal conditions and at physiological hyperinsulinemia, respectively. Muscles are the main reservoir of insulin-sensitive tissues within the mammalian body, representing 36–40% of the body weight. Their contribution to the whole glucose turnover is about 36% in postabsorptive control rats and 50% during euglycemic hyperinsulinemia (23).

Offspring of streptozotocin-diabetic rats are resistant to the action of insulin at the hepatic and peripheral level. The tissues contributing to the peripheral insulin resistance are mainly skeletal muscle, as determined with the 2-deoxy-D-glucose technique.

The offspring of diabetic rats develop signs of glucose intolerance when they become pregnant; they have a greater degree of glycemia than do normal pregnant rats, and the number of granulated β cells in the endocrine pancreas does not increase as in normal rat gestation (1). These data would suggest that a defect is present in SDF rats in the pregnancy-induced response of the β cells to glucose. Because normal pregnancy is a state of severe physiological insulin resistance, we wanted to investigate whether the insulin resistance present in SDF rats is further aggravated during

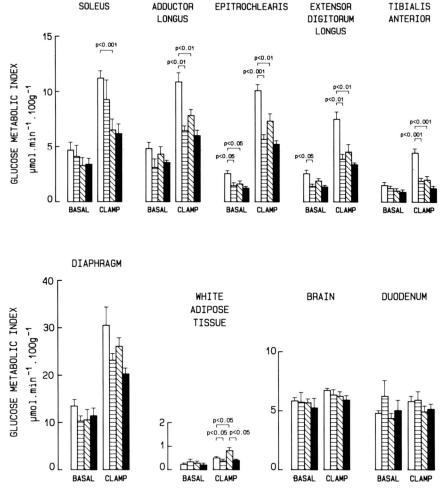

FIG. 3. *In vivo* glucose metabolic index in soleus, adductor longus, epitrochlearis, extensor digitorum longus and tibialis anterior muscles; and of diaphragm, white adipose tissue, brain, and duodenum in nonpregnant (□) and pregnant (■) control rats and in nonpregnant (⊠) and pregnant (■) offspring of rats made diabetic with streptozotocin under basal conditions and at physiological hyperinsulinemia. Data are means, error bars, SEM of 5–10 experiments.

gestation. For this purpose, we again used the euglycemic hyperinsulinemic clamp technique (19). The insulin dose-response curves for the increase of glucose metabolic clearance rate over basal values (Fig. 4) (19) and inhibition of endogenous glucose production (Fig. 5) (19) obviously show that the insulin resistance of pregnancy is not mirrored in SDF rats: there is no further decrease in the peripheral tissue sensitivity to insulin, while there is only a small decrease in the hepatic insulin sensitivity. Overall

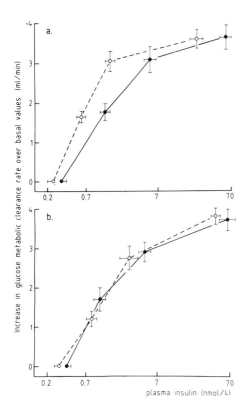

FIG. 4. Insulin dose-response curves for the increase in glucose metabolic clearance rate over basal values in **(a)** nonpregnant (O---O) and pregnant (●---●) control rats and **(b)** nonpregnant (O---O) and pregnant (●---●) offspring of streptozotocin-diabetic rats. Data are means, error bars, SEM of 5–8 experiments.

there are no differences in insulin sensitivity between pregnant control rats and pregnant SDF rats (19). This is also apparent from the glucose metabolic indices determined in various peripheral tissues of both pregnant control rats and pregnant SDF rats (Fig. 2) (2). Although the insulin resistance was not markedly aggravated during pregnancy in SDF rats, a syndrome of gestational diabetes ensued in these rats. The increase in circulating insulin concentrations, as seen in normal pregnancy, was blunted; as a result, pregnant SDF rats had lower insulin concentrations than pregnant control rats. In addition, nonfasting glucose levels were increased (Table 1), and NEFA levels were markedly elevated (21).

The exact cause of the hepatic and peripheral insulin resistance in adult offspring of diabetic rats is unknown at present. Insulin action on target tissues might be altered by a decreased receptor number and/or affinity, or by a postreceptor defect (24). Changes in the levels of counterregulatory hormones could also be involved, for example glucagon stimulates insulin-inhibited hepatic glucose production (24). In the basal state and during hyperinsulinemia, glucagon levels are not significantly different in SDF rats and control rats. This suggests that glucagon is probably not involved in the hepatic insulin resistance observed in SDF rats (21). Raised NEFA levels

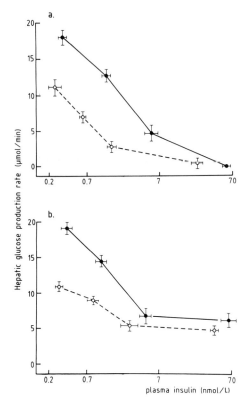

FIG. 5. Insulin dose-response curves for inhibition of endogenous glucose production in **(a)** nonpregnant (O---O) and pregnant (●---●) control rats and **(b)** nonpregnant (O---O) and pregnant (●---●) offspring of streptozotocin-diabetic rats. Data are means, error bars, SEM of 5–8 experiments.

are known to reduce insulin-stimulated glucose disposal, especially in muscle (25). Although NEFA levels are lower in basal conditions in SDF rats, hyperinsulinemia decreased NEFA to a lesser extent in SDF rats than in control rats. However, plasma NEFA levels do not reach significantly higher levels during extreme hyperinsulinemia in SDF rats. This suggests that NEFA do not inhibit glucose utilization in SDF rats (21).

When the second generation offspring of streptozotocin-diabetic rats become pregnant, they develop gestational diabetes. This means that their fetuses (third generation) also develop in an abnormal intrauterine milieu. Indeed these fetuses display islet hyperplasia, β-cell degranulation (1), hyperinsulinemia, hyperglycemia (Table 1) (19), and they are macrosomic (1).

At adult age, the third generation offspring of streptozotocin-diabetic pregnant rats have impaired glucose tolerance with high glucose levels (20). Similar results were also obtained in the third generation offspring of glucose-infused hyperglycemic pregnant rats (5).

These data clearly show that a diabetogenic tendency is transmitted from the pregnant streptozotocin-diabetic rat to her fetuses, with consequences persisting into adulthood and into the next generation (20). The transmission of diabetes via the maternal line has been confirmed in the adult offspring of rats made hyperglycemic by a continuous glucose infusion during the last week of pregnancy (5,26). Very recently, Gauguier *et al.* (27) found, besides a genetic inheritance, a higher maternal than paternal transmission of diabetes in the GK rat, a model of spontaneous non-insulin-dependent diabetes mellitus (NIDDM) without obesity. This finding, however, was not confirmed by Abdel-Halim *et al.* (28).

The inducing factor of the insulin resistance, which characterizes the adult offspring of severely streptozotocin-diabetic rats, must be the abnormal perinatal milieu of the diabetic maternal rat to which the developing fetus has to adapt. Indeed, normalization of maternal glycemia from day 15 of gestation by islet transplantation prevents the occurrence of a disturbed glucose tolerance in the offspring (29). The studies of Grill *et al.* (30) and of Ktorza *et al.* (26) strongly suggest that the diabetic or hyperglycemic intrauterine milieu must be responsible for the metabolic alterations observed in the offspring, since in both studies the offspring were reared by nondiabetic or normoglycemic foster mothers. Ryan *et al.* (31) also found the existence of an insulin resistance in offspring of streptozotocin-diabetic rats, which appears to be related to the degree of hyperglycemia they were exposed to during fetal life.

COMPARISON WITH THE HUMAN

Although hyperglycemia of such severity is rarely encountered in humans, our data suggest that poorly controlled diabetes during pregnancy may affect the glucose-insulin homeostasis in the offspring from diabetic women. It remains difficult, however, to compare the metabolic impact of severe streptozotocin-diabetes in the rat with (treated) insulin-dependent and non-insulin-dependent diabetes in women.

Tight metabolic control before pregnancy and throughout pregnancy has reduced perinatal morbidity and mortality over the last decades. Neonatal problems are predominantly related to overfeeding the fetus, associated with fetal hyperinsulinemia, since the other well-known neonatal complications (hypoglycemia, hypocalcemia, polycythemia, and respiratory distress) can be reduced by intensive management. However, maternal diabetes still compromises fetal development and behavior. An important fetal target organ is the endocrine pancreas.

The human fetal endocrine pancreas comprises about 5% of the total pancreatic volume. The pancreas is derived from two buds of the primitive gut, a dorsal and a ventral primordium; these two buds fuse to form the pancreas. The dorsal primordium develops into the tail and the superior part of the head of the pancreas; the ventral primordium develops into the lower part of the pancreatic head (32). The endocrine pancreatic system is derived from the ductuli. The first stage is the formation of knots, which then become independent from the ductuli to endocrine islets. In these primitive islets the different cell types are intermingled. From about 16 weeks of fetal life typical mantle islets are seen, with a central core of β cells (insulin-producing) and a mantle of non-β cells. Identification of the different cell types is possible with electron-optical and immunocytochemical methods or by a combination of both (33).

The β cells have large granules, their core can be electron dense (dark granules), sometimes even crystalline, or more electron lucent (light granules). These β granules contain insulin. The α cells have smaller granules than the β cells, and the core is electron dense with a closely fitting membrane. Some α cells have larger granules than others. The α granules contain glucagon. D cells have granules heterogeneous in size and electron density; they contain somatostatin. Pancreatic polypeptide (PP) cells have small and electron-dense granules containing pancreatic polypeptide. The lower part of the pancreatic head, which originates from the ventral primordium, contains a high proportion of PP cells and is called the *PP-rich zone*. A fifth cell type (D_1 cell) has been described by Van Assche et al. (33), which has very small granules. This cell type occurs in close relationship with nerve fibres. The hormonal content of the granules is still unknown.

The islets of Langerhans in fetuses of diabetic mothers are more numerous and larger than those in normal fetuses. Innumerable small islets composed of only a few cells can be demonstrated. The islet capillaries are congested. The β cells have an enlarged and hyperchromatic nucleus. In about 30% of the cases, an infiltration by eosinophilic polymorphs is present in and around the islets. These immunological changes, as shown by eosinophilic infiltration in the fetal pancreatic islets, are present only in type 1 diabetes and not in infants born to gestational diabetic mothers. It is possible that these immunological changes protect against the development of diabetes in later life (34). Increased volume density of the endocrine tissue and an increased percentage of insulin producing β cells are present in fetuses of insulin-dependent diabetic mothers and of mothers with gestational diabetes. This β-cell hyperplasia is responsible for the fetal hyperinsulinism (34,35). Furthermore, in poorly controlled diabetes, degranulation of the fetal islets can also be observed (8).

It can be concluded that the diabetic intrauterine milieu induces changes in the fetal endocrine pancreas and in fetal metabolism, which can have consequences throughout later adult life. However, there are conflicting data about the incidence of diabetes in the offspring of insulin-dependent diabetic women. Although Farquhar (36) has shown that the incidence of insulin-dependent diabetes is 20 times higher in children of diabetic mothers than in the control population, Warram et al. (37) have shown that children of diabetic fathers have a greater risk of subsequent insulin-dependent diabetes than do children of diabetic mothers. The epidemiological data in gestational diabetes are more consistent. The risk of NIDDM is significantly higher when the mother rather than the father had this disorder (38). Furthermore, 35% of women with gestational diabetes are the daughters of diabetic mothers, compared with only 5% of normoglycemic pregnant women, and gestational diabetes occurs more frequently in the offspring of diabetic mothers (35%) than in the offspring of diabetic fathers (7%) (39). Most convincing are the studies carried out in Pima Indians, in whom there is an extraordinarily high incidence of NIDDM. These studies have clearly shown that, in addition to a genetic transmission of diabetes, diabetes during pregnancy increases the incidence of impaired glucose tolerance in their children. At the age of 15–19 years, the incidence was 33%, *versus* 1.4% in the offspring of mothers who developed diabetes after pregnancy (40). An extensive study over several generations showed a significant predominance of NIDDM in great-grandmothers of insulin-dependent diabetics on the maternal side when compared with the paternal side. In addition, a significant predominance of familial diabetes aggregation in first- and second-degree relatives was found on the maternal side when compared with the paternal side. Systematic prevention of hyperglycemia and impaired glucose tolerance in pregnant women has significantly decreased the prevalence of diabetes mellitus in their children (41).

The existence of maternal component in the transmission of NIDDM is widely accepted. Both genetic and environmental factors might contribute to the maternal transmission of diabetes. Besides an intrauterine effect in the transmission of NIDDM, there is transmission of an X-linked susceptibility locus or inheritance of mitochondrial DNA that is transmitted exclusively from mother to offspring (42).

Strict metabolic control is necessary for all pregnant women with diabetes, because the deleterious effects for the offspring, engendered by maternal diabetes, are not confined to the fetal and neonatal period, but extend into adulthood and the next generation.

REFERENCES

1. Aerts L, Holemans K, Van Assche FA. Maternal diabetes during pregnancy: consequences for the offspring. *Diabetes Metab Rev* 1990; 6: 147–67.
2. Holemans K, Van Bree R, Verhaeghe J, Aerts L, Van Assche FA. In vivo glucose utilization by individual tissues in virgin and pregnant offspring of severely diabetic rats. *Diabetes* 1993; 42: 530–6.
3. Bihoreau MT, Ktorza A, Kervran A, Picon L. Effect of gestational hyperglycemia on insulin secretion in vivo and in vitro by fetal rat pancreas. *Am J Physiol* 1986; 251: E86–91.
4. Bihoreau MT, Ktorza A, Picon L. Gestational hyperglycemia and insulin release by the fetal rat pancreas in vitro. *Diabetologia* 1986; 29: 434–9.
5. Gauguier D, Bihoreau MT, Ktorza A, Berthault MF, Picon L. Inheritance of diabetes mellitus as a consequence of gestational hyperglycemia in rats. *Diabetes* 1990; 49: 734–9.
6. Ktorza A, Girard J, Kinebanyan MF, Picon L. Hyperglycemia induced by glucose infusion in the unrestrained pregnant rat during the last three days of gestation. Metabolic and hormonal changes in the mother and the fetus. *Diabetologia* 1981; 21: 569–74.
7. Verhaeghe J, Peeters TL, Vandeputte M, Rombauts W, Bouillon R, Van Assche FA. Maternal and fetal endocrine pancreas in the spontaneously diabetic BB rat. *Biol Neonate* 1989; 55: 298–308.
8. Van Assche FA, Aerts L and De Prins FA. Degranulation of the insulin producing B cells in an infant of a diabetic mother. Case Report. *Br J Obstet Gynaecol* 1983; 90: 182–185.
9. Kervran A, Randan J, Girard JR. Dynamics of glucose-induced plasma insulin increase in the rat fetus at different stages of gestation. Effects of maternal hypothermia and fetal decapitation. *Biol Neonate* 1979; 35: 242–8.
10. Herrera E, Palacin M, Martin A, Lasuncion MA. Relationship between maternal and fetal fuels and placental glucose transport in rats with maternal diabetes of varying severity. *Diabetes* 1985; 34: 42–46.
11. Kim JS, Yoon Y, Kim Y. New model for infants of diabetic mothers. In: Shafrir E, Renold AE, eds. *Lessons from animal diabetes*. London: John Libbey, 1984: 676–84.
12. Mulay S, Philip A, Salomon S. Influence of maternal diabetes on fetal rat development. Alterations of insulin receptors in fetal liver and lung. *J Endocrinol* 1983; 98: 401–10.
13. Phillips AF, Rosenkrantz TS, Clark RM, Knox I, Chafiin DG, Raye JR. Effects of fetal insulin deficiency on growth and development in fetal lambs. *Diabetes* 1991; 40: 20–7.
14. Aerts L, Van Assche FA. Endocrine pancreas in the offspring of rats with experimentally induced diabetes. *J Endocrinol* 1981; 88: 81–8.

15. Issad T, Coupé C, Pastor-Anglada M, Ferré P, Girard J. Development of insulin sensitivity at weaning in the rat. Role of nutritional transition. *Biochem J* 1988; 251: 685–90.
16. Leturque A, Postic C, Ferré P, Girard JR. Nutritional regulation of glucose transporter in muscle and adipose tissue of weaned rats. *Am J Physiol* 1991; 260: E588–93.
17. Aerts L, Van Assche FA, Faure A, Sutter-Dub MT. Effects of treatment with progestrone and oestradiol-17β on the endocrine pancreas in ovariectomized rats: ultrastructural variations in the B cell. *J Endocrinol* 1980; 84: 317–20.
18. Aerts L, Sodoyez-Goffaux F, Sodoyez JC, Malaisse WJ, Van Assche FA. The diabetic intrauterine milieu has a long-lasting effect on insulin secretion by the B cells and on insulin uptake by target tissues. *Am J Obstet Gynecol* 1988; 159: 1287–92.
19. Holemans K, Aerts L, Van Assche FA. Absence of pregnancy-induced alterations in tissue sensitivity in the offspring of diabetic rats. *J Endocrinol* 1991; 131: 387–93.
20. Van Assche FA, Aerts L. Long-term effects of diabetes and pregnancy in the rat. *Diabetes* 1985; 34: 116–8.
21. Holemans K, Aerts L, Van Assche FA. Evidence for an insulin resistance in adult offspring of pregnant streptozotocin-diabetic rats. *Diabetologia* 1991; 34: 81–5.
22. Burnol AF, Leturque A, Ferré P, Girard J. A method for quantifying insulin sensitivity in vivo in the anesthetized rat: the euglycemic clamp technique coupled with isotopic measurement of glucose turnover. *Reprod Nutr Dev* 1983; 23: 429–35.
23. Ferré P, Leturque A, Burnol AF, Pénicaud L, Girard JR. A method to quantify glucose utilization in vivo in skeletal muscle and white adipose tissue of the anaesthetized rat. *Biochem J* 1985; 228: 103–10.
24. Olefsky JM. Insulin resistance and insulin action: an in vitro and in vivo perspective. *Diabetes* 1981; 30: 148–61.
25. Randle P, Garland P, Hales C, Newsholme E, Denton R, Pogson C. Interaction of metabolism and the physiological role of insulin. *Recent Prog Horm Res* 1966; 22: 1–48.
26. Ktorza A, Gauguier D, Bihoreau MT, Berthault MF, Picon L: Adult offspring from mildly hyperglycemic rats show impairment of glucose regulation and insulin secretion which is transmissible to the next generation. In: Shafrir E, ed. *Frontiers in diabetes research. Lessons from animal diabetes III.* London: Smith-Gordon, 1990: 555–60.
27. Gauguier D, Nelson I, Bernard C, *et al.* Higher maternal than paternal inheritance of diabetes in GK rats. *Diabetes* 1994; 43: 220–4.
28. Abdel-Halim SM, Guenfi A, Luthman H, Grill V, Ependic I, Ostenson CG. Impact of diabetic inheritance on glucose tolerance and insulin secretion in spontaneously diabetic GK-Wistar rats. *Diabetes* 1994; 43: 281–8.
29. Aerts L, Van Assche FA. Transplantation in diabetic pregnant rats normalizes glucose homeostasis in their offspring. *J Dev Physiol* 1992; 17: 283–7.
30. Grill V, Johannson B, Jalkanen P, Eriksson UY. Influence of severe diabetes mellitus early in pregnancy in the rat: effects on insulin sensitivity and insulin secretion in the offspring. *Diabetologia* 1991; 34: 373–84.
31. Ryan EA, Liv D, Crawford J, Bell R, Tang J. Insulin resistance in adult offspring of diabetic mothers. *Diabetes* 1993; 42: 86A. (Abstract)
32. Pictet R, Rutter W. Development of the embryonic endocrine pancreas. In: Steiner DF, Freinkel N, eds. *Handbook of physiology.* Baltimore: Williams and Watkins Co. 1972; 7,I: 25–66.
33. Van Assche FA, Aerts L, Gepts W. The different cell types in the endocrine pancreas. *Diabetologia* 1982; 16: 151–2.
34. Van Assche FA. Management problems in the pregnant diabetic. *Fetal Maternal Med Rev* 1993; 5: 29–37.
35. Naeye RL. Infants of diabetic mothers: quantitative morphologic study. *Pediatrics* 1965; 35: 980–9.
36. Farquhar JW. Prognosies of babies born to diabetic mothers in Edinburgh. *Arch Dis Child* 1969; 44: 36–40.
37. Warram JH, Martin BC, Krolewski AJ. Possible mechanisms for the diminished risk of NIDDM in the children of diabetic mothers. In: Andreani D, Bompiani G, Di Mario G, Galluzo A, eds. *Immunobiology of normal and diabetic pregnancy.* New York: John Wiley, 1990: 221–8.
38. Knowler W, Pettitt DJ, Kunzelman CL, Everhart J. Genetic and environmental determinants of non-insulin-dependent diabetes mellitus. *Diabetes Res Clin Pract* 1985; suppl 1: S309.
39. Martin AO, Simpson JL, Ober C, Freinkel N. Frequency of diabetes mellitus in probands with gestational diabetes: possible maternal influence on the predisposition to diabetes. *Am J Obstet Gynecol* 1985; 151: 471–3.

40. Pettitt DJ, Aleck KA, Baird HR, Carraher MJ, Bennett PH, Knowler WC. Congenital susceptibility to NIDDM. Role of the intrauterine environment. *Diabetes* 1988; 37: 622–8.
41. Dörner G, Plagemann A, Reinagel H. Familial diabetes aggregation in type 2 diabetics: gestational diabetes as apparent risk factor for increased diabetes susceptibility in the offspring. *Exp Clin Endocrinol* 1987; 89: 84–90.
42. Cox NJ. Maternal component in NIDDM transmission. How large an effect? *Diabetes* 1994; 43: 166–8.

DISCUSSION

Dr. Schwartz: I have a question concerning your streptozotocin model where you showed that low-dose streptozotocin results in macrosomia with what you call *decreased insulin secretion*. I assume what you mean is *decreased insulin mass* in the β-cell mass. The simplest view that we have had over the years is that hyperglycemia of the mother is transmitted to the fetus who is then stimulated to secrete excess insulin. Your model apparently has macrosomia with decreased insulin.

Dr. Van Assche: No, in mild diabetes there is an increased amount of insulin in the fetus and an increase in β-cell function, so the amount of endocrine tissue is increased. Thus in mild diabetes there is hyperinsulinism in the fetus and macrosomia. In severe diabetes, I agree with you, we have hypoinsulinism and we have intrauterine growth retardation. So from that point of view there is a similarity with the human situation.

Dr. Schwartz: My other question concerns intrauterine growth retardation (IUGR). My simple mind wonders what is the driving force in that situation. If you look at the infant weight, the controls were, as I recall, around 2000 g and the IUGR infants were 1000 g. If you look at the mass of the β cell or the islets it appears to be about 50% of control in the IUGR offspring, so it seems that the islet mass was proportional to the mass of the infant.

Dr. Van Assche: Morphometry means that in a certain area of the pancreas, always in the tail, you measure the proportion of endocrine tissue. This is very difficult to do, and I completely accept your point. To obtain the exact weight of the pancreas is hard because even a tiny bit of fat can change the weight significantly. However, it is a generally accepted morphological principle that "volume density" means the amount of a recognizable part of an organ compared with the total organ mass in a certain area. We have always used an area of 0.5 cm^2 where we measure morphometrically the amount of endocrine tissue, so in this case the overall weight of the pancreas is not important.

Dr. Swift: I would like to emphasize the importance of the length of the baby. I don't know of any data that relate maternal diabetes to the length of the baby at birth. People talk of macrosomia, but what do they mean by macrosomia? In practice they mean obesity, and nobody has ever accurately measured birth length. I would like to hear of any data relating to fetal or infant length.

Dr. Van Assche: When we describe macrosomia in the rat this refers not only to increased weight but also to increased length. Our experimental model of intrauterine growth retardation had not only a reduction in weight, but also a reduction in length. Maybe Catalano has more data on the human situation.

Dr. Catalano: We have data on maybe 300 babies, about 150 normals and 150 from women with mild gestational diabetes. When the data are corrected for gestational age and sex, we find that despite what we consider adequate control the principal difference between an infant of a diabetic mother and of a control mother is the amount of fat. The distribution of the fat is similar to that in a type 2 diabetic, *i.e.*, central rather than peripheral. So in our data at least there was no difference in length or head circumference, etc.

Dr. Dakou: Were the measurements done specifically as part of the study or were they taken from the records? That would introduce a great deal of uncertainty.

Dr. Catalano: They were done prospectively by a specifically trained person.

Dr. Dakou: I was impressed by your data from anencephalic fetuses. It appears that besides nutrient stimulation of the β cell you also need an intact hypothalamic-pituitary axis. Do you need growth hormone related factors to stimulate β-cell growth?

Dr. Van Assche: We developed a model whereby decapitating the fetuses of diabetic mother rats *in utero* we could confirm what we have shown in the anencephalic human. There is some indication that endocrine stimulation from the hypothalamus and the hypophysis is important. It has also been shown that estrogen in the fetus stimulates endocrine growth.

Dr. Guesry: If I followed what you said correctly, your data would suggest that in countries where the rate of intrauterine growth retardation is very high, as in Bangladesh with a 30% incidence, all those undergrown infant girls are at risk of becoming diabetic themselves.

Dr. Van Assche: It is very difficult to speculate on this. I am not an epidemiologist. I think that intrauterine growth retardation is related to diseases in later life, not only diabetes but also lung disorders and other diseases. From the work of David Barker translated to what is now happening in the underdeveloped countries, this indeed is a problem. We must wait for further epidemiological data.

Dr. Zoupas: From your beautiful studies, can you give us an explanation for sudden intrauterine death in the diabetic mother's child?

Dr. Van Assche: The only thing we have seen (and this has been supported by the King's College Hospital group) is severe hypoglycemia in the fetus in cases of fetal distress.

Dr. Hoet: You showed that the β cells in the pancreas of a child born to a mother with very severe diabetes were degranulated. Would you like to comment on the vascularity of the islets?

Dr. Van Assche: The vascularity was decreased.

Dr. Bergman: To follow up on this comment, I think there may well be alterations in perfusion patterns, capillary density, endothelial cell transport potential, and so on, and it would be very interesting to look at capillary density morphometrically in these offspring. If vascular abnormalities are present, the insulin resistance might be continued in further generations.

Dr. Van Assche: I completely agree with you; I believe that diabetes in pregnancy and preeclampsia are both endothelial disorders.

Dr. Siadati: What is the cause of transient neonatal diabetes?

Dr. Van Assche: It is suggested that there is an immaturity of the fetal β cell at birth; these infants need insulin and the majority recover. However, as far as I know about 25–30% of them become diabetic in childhood.

Diabetes, edited by Richard M. Cowett,
Nestlé Nutrition Workshop Series,
Vol. 35. Nestec Ltd.,
Vevey/Raven Press, Ltd., New York © 1995.

The Infant of the Diabetic Mother

Richard M. Cowett

Department of Pediatrics, Women and Infants' Hospital of Rhode Island; Department of Pediatrics, Brown University School of Medicine, Providence, Rhode Island 02905–2401, USA

The infant of the diabetic mother (IDM) is a prime example of the problems that may exist in the neonate secondary to maternal disease (diabetes). From a developmental standpoint, the normal neonate is in a transitional state of glucose homeostasis. The fetus is completely dependent on its mother for glucose delivery, and the adult is considered to have precise control of glucose homeostasis, since plasma glucose concentration is regulated to a fine degree (1). In contrast, maintenance of glucose homeostasis may be a major problem even for the normal neonate (2). The precarious nature of this situation is emphasized by the numerous problems associated with neonatal hypoglycemia and hyperglycemia during this period of life. The IDM can be used to document not only how far we have come in understanding the pathophysiology of glucose disequilibrium, but also how far we need to go (3–5).

Although many infants of diabetic mothers have an uneventful perinatal course, there is still an increased risk of glucose disequilibrium. In this review, I shall enumerate the metabolic abnormalities that the IDM may encounter in relation to glucose metabolism and evaluate the pathophysiologic basis for their occurrence.

PERINATAL MORTALITY AND MORBIDITY

While the IDM may have greater morbidity than the neonate of the nondiabetic woman (Table 1), many infants of insulin-dependent diabetic women may experience an uneventful clinical course, and even more infants of gestational diabetic women do well (3–5). Theoretically, the better the metabolic control of the diabetic pregnant patient, the greater the potential for a normal neonate. Over the last decade or so, perinatal mortality, except for congenital anomalies, has approached that for neonates born to nondiabetic mothers (6,7).

Studies of perinatal morbidity and mortality from diverse centers attest to the increasing success of these principles. In 1974, Pedersen *et al.* published a review of their experiences over a 26-year period with an analysis of 1332 diabetic pregnancies (8). Perinatal mortality varied directly with the severity of maternal diabetes as judged by two commonly used maternal classification schemes: White's original

TABLE 1. *Morbidity in the infant of the diabetic mother*

Asphyxia	Macrosomia
Birth injury	Neurologic instability
Caudal regression	Organomegaly
Congenital anomalies	Polycythemia and hyperviscosity
Double outlet right ventricle	Respiratory distress
Heart failure	Respiratory distress syndrome
Hyperbilirubinemia	Septal hypertrophy
Hypocalcemia	Small left colon syndrome
Hypoglycemia	Transient hematuria
Hypomagnesemia	Truncus arteriosus
Increased blood volume	

classification of diabetes in pregnancy, and Pedersen's Prognostically Bad Signs in Pregnancy (PBSP) classification. White's revised classification (Table 2) is based on duration of diabetes and the presence of late vascular complications (9), while the PBSP classification (Table 3) includes abnormalities of the current pregnancy.

An updated report from the Joslin Clinic service supports the importance of these factors, especially preeclampsia (pretoxemia) as a significant cause of morbidity in the pregnant diabetic. Of 420 patients in the series with insulin-dependent type 1 diabetes, 110, or 26.2%, delivered before 37 weeks, compared with an incidence of

TABLE 2. *White's classification of diabetes in pregnancy (modified)*

Gestational diabetes	Abnormal glucose tolerance test, but euglycemia maintained by diet alone or, if diet alone insufficient, insulin required
Class A	Diet alone, any duration or onset age
Class B	Onset age 20 years or older and duration less than 10 years
Class C	Onset age 10–19 years or duration 10–19 years
Class D	Onset age under 10 years, duration over 20 years, background retinopathy, or hypertension (not preeclampsia)
Class R	Proliferative retinopathy or vitreous hemorrhage
Class F	Nephropathy with over 500 mg/day proteinuria
Class RF	Criteria for both R and F coexist
Class H	Arteriosclerotic heart disease clinically evident
Class T	Previous renal transplantation

TABLE 3. *Prognostically Bad Signs of Pregnancy (PBSP)*

Chemical pyelonephritis
Precoma or severe acidosis
Toxemia
"Neglectors"

9.7% in the nondiabetic population. One-third of the premature deliveries related to preeclampsia. They concluded that a major problem of the diabetic pregnancy was related to preeclampsia and its association with prematurity (10). The risk to the fetus was increased when the PBSP classification was added to the White classification.

The relationship between the two was emphasized by Diamond *et al.* (11) who studied 199 pregnancies from 1977 to 1983. They noted that the presence of PBSP increased the perinatal mortality rate from 7.3% to 17.1% and was predictive of pulmonary morbidity in general (31.6% *versus* 16.3%). The authors concluded that the combination of the two is still as predictive as had been found by Pedersen. While these investigators noted an improvement in nondiabetic pregnancy outcome during this same period, they emphasized that the improved classification scheme combined with increased experience were the major reasons for the improved results in the diabetic pregnancy. This improved perinatal mortality has been confirmed at many centers in the United States and Europe. While the frequency of macrosomia has decreased, the rate is still usually higher than that in neonates born to nondiabetic women. In a survey of macrosomic neonates (large for gestational age; >95 percentile weight for gestational age), most have been born to obese mothers, not all of whom have glucose intolerance as judged by postpartum glycohemoglobin studies (12,13). Nevertheless, the gestational diabetic with glucose intolerance during late pregnancy often remains undiagnosed and may have a neonate with a greater risk of perinatal complications.

Glycosylated hemoglobin (HbA_1C) has been widely touted as a measure of long-term control of diabetic persons. However, recent reports reflect increasing disenchantment with its reliability. While higher HbA_1 levels were noted in women diagnosed as having gestational diabetes, a relatively low sensitivity in detecting gestational diabetes was confirmed. HbA_1 levels and oral glucose tolerance test (OGTT) indices did not correlate well, and delivery of large for gestation neonates was not associated with higher HbA_1 levels (14).

In this same regard, Cano *et al.* studied the relationship of maternal glycosylated hemoglobin and fetal β cell activity with birth weight (15). A population of 40 maternal-neonatal pairs was studied, of whom 17 were diabetic pregnancies. Insulin and C-peptide were measured in cord blood and were compared with maternal HbA_1 levels. HbA_1 did not correlate with weight for gestational age at birth, while insulin and C-peptide concentrations did. The investigators suggested that, in populations with good diabetes control, blood glucose concentration, as monitored by HbA_1 levels, is not the major determinant of fetal growth.

In contrast, Pollak *et al.* studied glucitollysine concentrations in umbilical cord extracts as a spin-off of the measurement of glycation processes in biologic samples (16). The results of 12 samples from the infants of diabetic mothers were compared with 14 control samples from infants with normal mothers. Using ion exchange chromatography followed by reverse-phase high-pressure liquid chromatography, these investigators noted higher glucitollysine levels in the IDM compared with controls.

The levels were even higher in the IDM with congenital malformations. The investigators suggested that nonenzymatic glycation of fetal tissue does occur as a result of *in utero* exposure to cumulative glycemia.

Teramo *et al.* have published data from Helsinki, Finland, relating to perinatal mortality (17). Their study focused on two time periods: 1970–1971 and 1975–1977. In 1974, the principles of obstetric monitoring and the treatment of pregnant diabetic women and their neonates were updated. The review focused on the differences resulting from those changes in management. Specifically, this involved increased monitoring and more frequent hospital admissions for metabolic control, especially in the third trimester. In 1975–1977, all diabetic patients were admitted to hospital from the 32nd week of pregnancy until delivery. Strict maintenance of normoglycemia (blood glucose <120 mg/dl) was the goal of management and, in the latter years, a permanent interdisciplinary team was in charge of the treatment of these patients. Gestational age of the neonates was increased significantly; however, mean birth weights were unchanged. The perinatal mortality rate fell markedly, as did neonatal morbidity. The authors concluded that, while advances were obvious, the final answers were far from apparent because of the significant neonatal morbidity still present.

Similar conclusions about strict metabolic control were mentioned by Jerwell *et al.*, who evaluated their experience in Norway between 1967 and 1976 (18). A total of 1035 births to diabetic mothers were registered during the 10-year period. Not only did perinatal mortality fall by 30%, but the duration of gestation increased from 35.5 to 37 weeks over the same period. The number of neonates with appropriate weight for gestational age (AGA) increased from 53.3%–70.0%. The care of these pregnant diabetic women was more commonly carried out in university clinics and regional hospitals (from 38.7% in 1967–1968 to 77.1% in 1975–1976). The impact of these interventions did not affect malformation rates, which were still more common by a factor of 50% in infants born to these women compared with the general population.

More recently, maternal glucose variability was studied in 154 pregnant diabetic patients who were admitted to hospital for a month prior to delivery. It was found that reduced within-day plasma glucose variability was significantly correlated with enhanced neonatal outcome (that is, there was a decreased incidence of complications), but that there was no correlation between maternal glucose variability and the birth weight of the neonate. The investigators acknowledged that absence of glucose variability would not ensure prevention of neonatal complications (19).

Roberts and Patterson (20) reported on a 20-year experience involving 1528 pregnancies of diabetic women. Of these, 571 had type 1 diabetes and 957 had gestational diabetes. The perinatal mortality rate fell from 15.2%–2% in those with type 1 diabetes and from 6.7%–0.5% for those with gestational diabetes. The authors related the improvement in mortality to better glucose control. They reported, as have others, that the major outstanding problem related to the persistently high incidence of congenital malformations.

Another evaluation was performed in which normoglycemia was maintained in diabetic women with evidence of vascular disease (21). While improvement was noted in many of the side effects of vascular compromise (proteinuria, retinopathy, etc.), a wide range in the birthweight of the infants (including macrosomia) was noted, in spite of normal hemoglobin A_1 determinations.

Coustan and Imarah attempted to use prophylactic insulin treatment in women with gestational diabetes to reduce the incidence of macrosomia, operative delivery, and birth trauma. The results showed a partial decline in complications with tightened maternal metabolic control (22). Subsequently, the same group evaluated a randomized clinical trial of insulin pump or intensive conventional therapy. Twenty-two pregnant diabetic women were randomized to conventional therapy or insulin pump therapy. No significant differences were found with either regimen. Excellent therapy was achieved with both (23).

A more recent review of the use of insulin therapy was reported by Thompson *et al.* (24). One-hundred-eight gestational diabetic women were randomized to receive diet plus insulin or diet alone to maintain glycemic control. The investigators reported that if the patients were treated for at least 6 weeks with diet plus insulin, the mean birth weight, incidence of macrosomia, and ponderal index were reduced. No patient who weighed less than 90 kg and maintained euglycemic control delivered a neonate who weighed more than 4000 g. The authors concluded that maternal obesity or failure to achieve glycemic control should alert the clinician to an increased risk of macrosomia.

The same conclusion was reached by Larsen *et al.*, who found that maternal obesity (>95%) was associated with an odds ratio of 2.2 of macrosomia (BW >4000 g) compared with 1.0 for women who weighed between the 25th and the 75th percentile (25).

An extension of the above was reported by Nordlander *et al.*, who evaluated factors that influence neonatal morbidity in gestational diabetes (26). Perinatal morbidity was significantly more frequent in women with gestational diabetes (23%) than in a control group (13%). The occurrence of large for gestational age neonates was not different between the groups. Of infants born to gestational diabetic women, those who presented with morbidity were of shorter gestational age at delivery, were delivered more frequently by cesarean section, and had mothers who had a higher prepregnancy weight and a greater area under the glucose tolerance curve. Gestational age at delivery and maternal prepregnancy weight were the most significant factors. The investigators concluded that factors besides blood glucose control during pregnancy were critical in determining neonatal outcome in gestational diabetic pregnancies.

Hanson *et al.* (27) evaluated factors influencing neonatal morbidity in diabetic pregnancies. They evaluated maternal duration of diabetes, third-trimester blood glucose control, gestational age at delivery, mode of delivery, and hypertension in 92 consecutive pregnancies of White's classes B through F. Morbidity was classified as none, minor, or severe, and no differences were noted in the former two groups. Those with severe morbidity had longer duration of maternal diabetes, shorter gestational age at birth, higher rates of cesarean section, and higher frequency of toxemia.

The most significant single factor was the gestational age of the pregnancy. Glucose control between 70 and 153 mg/dl did not influence morbidity.

Hunter *et al.* (28) compared neonatal mortality rates among infants of women with insulin-dependent diabetes and infants of women without diabetes using an historical cohort analysis between 1980 and 1989. There were 230 infants in the former group and 460 infants in the latter group. The infants born to diabetic mothers had higher incidences of glucose infusions, birth weight $\geq$90th percentile, and neonatal jaundice, but no differences in the incidence of respiratory distress, polycythemia, or hypocalcemia. Glycosylated hemoglobin levels were not related to birth weight. Nearly 25% of the infants were delivered before 37 weeks' gestation, nearly half because of maternal hypertension. The investigators suggested that neonatal morbidity is more likely to be determined by the gestational age at delivery than by the maternal diabetes.

In contrast, Persson and Hanson evaluated the outcome in a population with strictly individualized glucose control from their own institution and from a multicenter network (29). They noted a normal premature delivery rate of 8.9% and a low rate of maternal hypoglycemia and concluded that strictly individualized management programs offer the optimum neonatal outcome.

Finally, a recent evaluation known as the Diabetes in Early Pregnancy Study considered maternal postprandial glucose levels and infant birth weight. Recruited before conceiving, 323 diabetic and 361 control women were evaluated for fasting and non-fasting venous plasma glucose concentrations measured on alternate weeks during the first trimester and monthly thereafter. A greater percentage of infants of diabetic mothers were $\geq$90th percentile for birthweight compared with the control group (28.5% *versus* 13.1%, $p < 0.0001$). After adjusting for specific maternal indications, monitoring of nonfasting glucose concentrations was thought to be necessary to prevent macrosomia (30).

A conclusion from many of the studies that have been cited might be that the maintenance of a normal metabolic state, including euglycemia, should diminish, but will not completely eradicate, the increased perinatal and neonatal mortality and morbidity noted in the diabetic pregnancy.

PATHOGENESIS OF THE EFFECTS OF MATERNAL DIABETES ON THE FETUS

As yet, no single pathogenic mechanism has been clearly defined to explain the diverse problems observed in infants of diabetic mothers. Nevertheless, many of the effects can be attributed to maternal metabolic (glucose) control. Pedersen and his colleagues originally emphasized the relationship between maternal glucose concentration and neonatal hypoglycemia (31) (Table 4). His simplified hypothesis recognized that maternal hyperglycemia was paralleled by fetal hyperglycemia, which stimulated the fetal pancreas, resulting in islet cell hypertrophy and β-cell hyperplasia with increased insulin content. Following separation of the fetus from the mother,

TABLE 4. *Components for the hypothesis of hyperinsulinism in the infant of the diabetic mother*

1. Islet hyperplasia and β cell hypertrophy
2. Obesity and macrosomia
3. Hypoglycemia with low free fatty acids concentration
4. Rapid glucose disappearance rate
5. (a) Higher plasma insulin-like activity after glucose infusion
   (b) Umbilical vein reactive immunoinsulin increase
6. C-peptide and proinsulin concentrations increased

the former was no longer supported by placental glucose transfer, with the result that neonatal hypoglycemia occurred.

Hyperinsulinemia *in utero* affects diverse organ systems, including the placenta. Insulin acts as the primary anabolic hormone of fetal growth and development, resulting in visceromegaly (especially of the heart and liver) and macrosomia. In the presence of excess substrate (glucose), increased fat synthesis and deposition occur during the third trimester. Fetal macrosomia is reflected by increased body fat, muscle mass, and organomegaly but not by an increased size of the brain or kidneys (32,33). After delivery there is a rapid fall in plasma glucose with persistently low concentrations of plasma free fatty acids (FFA), glycerol, and β-hydroxybutyrate. In response to an intravenous glucose stimulus, plasma insulin-like activity is increased, as is plasma immunoreactive insulin (determined in the absence of maternal insulin antibodies) and plasma C-peptide (34). The insulin response to intravenous arginine is also exaggerated in infants of gestationally diabetic mothers (35).

In a follow-up study using the chronic hyperinsulinemic fetal rhesus monkey, Susa and coworkers studied neonatal insulin secretion following delivery (36). They gave 300 μg/kg of glucagon to stimulate insulin secretion. Compared with controls, the experimental group had a blunted insulin and C-peptide response to the glucagon infusion. The investigators suggested that fetal hyperinsulinemia resulted in inhibition of insulin synthesis and secretion in extrauterine life.

MacFarlane and Tsakalakos suggested that the initial increase in fetal size due to fetal hyperinsulinemia was implicated in the development of hypoxemia. The limitation in fetal oxygen availability altered differential utilization of glucose and increased α-glycerophosphate synthesis in the fetal adipocyte, which resulted in fetal adiposity (37).

The response to an oral glucose load results in an earlier plasma insulin rise than in normal neonates, although the area under the insulin curve is similar (38). During the initial hours after birth, the response to an acute intravenous bolus of glucose in infants of diabetic mothers compared with normal controls is a rapid rate of glucose disappearance from the plasma (39). In contrast, the rise in plasma glucose concentration following stepwise hourly increases in the rate of infused glucose, occurs even at normal rates of infusion, that is, 4–6 mg/kg/min (40,41). The latter may be attributed to a persistence of hepatic glucose output, which is similar to that of the normal infant.

Alterations of plasma glucocorticoids and growth hormone have not been significant in infants of diabetic mothers. Definitive studies of the somatomedins (IGF-1, IGF-2) are currently being reported. As an example, Hill *et al.* studied insulin-like growth factors in fetal macrosomia in neonates whose mothers did or did not have diabetes (42). Cord blood concentrations of IGF-I, total IGF, and IGF binding protein were determined in 15 term infants of diabetic mothers and 29 term neonates of nondiabetic mothers. Although there was a relationship between cord IGF and total IGF concentration in large for gestational age *versus* appropriate for gestational age neonates of nondiabetic mothers, there was no such relationship in infants of diabetic mothers. IGF binding proteins were not different in any group. The authors concluded that the absence of increased IGF concentration in infants of diabetic mothers suggested that these growth factors are not involved in the development of macrosomia in such infants. In contrast, urinary excretion of catecholamines was diminished, especially in neonates with low plasma glucose concentrations (43). In addition, plasma glucagon levels were less raised after delivery than in normal neonates (44).

Recent studies of insulin receptors on fetal monocytes isolated from placental blood of infants of gestationally diabetic mothers (IGDM) at delivery indicated that these infants had more receptor sites per monocyte than normal adults or normal neonates (45). Monocytes from both normal neonates and IGDM showed greater affinity for insulin than did those from adults. Furthermore, in the presence of increased ambient levels of plasma insulin, monocytes from the IGDM seemed to develop increased (not decreased) concentrations of insulin receptors, as well as an increased affinity for the hormone. The significance of these observations in relation to the physiologic effects of insulin are unclear. However, there are implications for competition of insulin and its antibodies for receptor sites and for the resulting insulin-sensitive tissues.

In a more recent evaluation, the role of insulin receptors in macrosomia and the tendency to hypoglycemia was studied in infants of diabetic mothers and control infants at between 3 and 14 days of age. The infants of diabetic mothers were macrosomic. Plasma-free insulin concentrations in cord blood were 15-fold higher in these infants compared with controls, and threefold higher in peripheral venous blood. Hypoglycemia was noted in 12 of 17 IDMs but in none of the control neonates. In umbilical blood, insulin binding to erythrocytes was not different between groups but decreased during the first weeks at a more rapid rate in IDM, because of decreased receptor affinity and receptor concentration in these infants. Thus insulin binding was similar in spite of gross hyperinsulinemia in the IDM, the latter resulting in macrosomia and hypoglycemia that decreased early on in the neonatal period (46).

KINETIC ANALYSIS OF THE IDM

Application of *in vivo* kinetic analysis has been used by numerous investigators to evaluate the infant of the diabetic mother metabolically. An early study using stable nonradioactive isotopes was reported by Kalhan *et al.* (using [1-^{13}C]glucose and the prime constant infusion technique) (47). These investigators measured systemic glucose production rates in five normal (nondiabetic) and five infants of insulin-dependent diabetics at 2 hours of age. As expected, the infant of the diabetic mother had a lower glucose concentration during the study compared with the infant of the nondiabetic mother. For the first time, the authors reported that the IDM had a lower systemic glucose production rate. They suggested that decreased glucose output was related to inhibited glycogenolysis. They speculated that increased insulin and decreased glucagon and catecholamine responses resulted in decreased systemic output. What was fascinating about this report was that for the time studied (the late 1970s) the diabetic women were considered to be in excellent control, having been admitted to hospital during the last four weeks of the pregnancy to achieve strict metabolic control (maternal blood glucose between 50 and 150 mg/dl). Yet the systemic glucose production rates of these neonates were lower than those of the control neonates.

A further evaluation of the infant of the diabetic mother was reported by the same group five years later in 1982 (48). Again focusing on neonates of mothers in "strict control" the authors evaluated systemic glucose production in five infants of insulin-dependent mothers, one infant of a gestational diabetic mother, and five infants born to normal mothers. The blood glucose measurements were in a more restricted range (36–104 mg/dl) than in the previous series, and the mothers were controlled in a hospital setting for 3–4 weeks before delivery. In this series, systemic glucose production rates were similar in the diabetic women and the controls. However, the investigators, like other groups (49), carried their analyses a significant step further. They infused exogenous glucose, which can diminish endogenous glucose production because of the precise control known to be the hallmark of the adult. The infants of diabetic mothers did not show as great a suppression of endogenous glucose production as the adults. The investigators concluded that altered regulation of glucose production may be secondary to intermittent maternal hyperglycemia, even in women whose diabetes was strictly controlled.

These studies parallel the work of the Brown University group that studied glucose kinetics in the neonate. Using 78% enriched D[U-^{13}C] glucose, 16 infants of diabetic women (10 insulin-dependent and six chemical dependent) were compared with five infants of normal nondiabetic women. Four insulin-dependent mothers and five infants of chemical diabetic mothers received 0.45% saline as the stable isotopic tracer diluent to determine basal endogenous glucose production (Fig. 1). All of the mothers were evaluated relative to control mothers by hemoglobin A$_1$C and maternal plasma glucose and/or cord vein glucose determinations at delivery. None of the women was maintained in the hospital before study. There was a similarity between basal glucose production rates in the neonates studied with no exogenous glucose infused. The investigators concluded that good metabolic control of the maternal diabetic state would help maintain euglycemia (50). However, in a subsequent analysis in which neonates of nondiabetic mothers received glucose exogenously to maintain euglycemia, a heterogeneity continued to exist in the ability of the neonates to depress endogenous glucose production (51). These latter data parallel other work from the

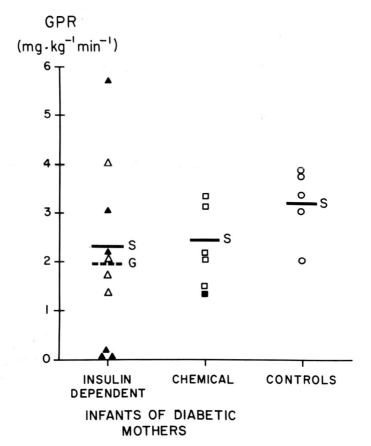

FIG. 1. Glucose production rate (GPR) for the infants of diabetic mothers and controls. The solid bar indicates the mean rate of production within each group. The filled symbols denote neonates who received exogenous glucose as the isotopic tracer diluent, and the empty symbols denote neonates who received 0.45% saline as the isotopic tracer diluent. From Cowett RM, Susa JB, Giletti B, et al. Variability of endogenous glucose production in infants of insulin dependent diabetic mothers. *Pediatr Res* 1980; 14: 570A. (Abstract); Cowett RM, Susa JB, Giletti B, Oh W, Schwartz R. Glucose kinetics in infants of diabetic mothers. *Am J Obstet Gynecol* 1983; 146: 781–6, with permission.

same group that reflects the transitional nature of glucose metabolism in the term and preterm infant, born both to diabetic and to nondiabetic mothers (47,52).

Another recent evaluation of postnatal glucose kinetics in neonates born to tightly controlled, insulin-dependent diabetic mothers was reported from Groningen, The Netherlands, by Baarsma *et al.* (53). These investigators studied 15 mother-infant pairs from the beginning of pregnancy until birth and then measured glucose kinetics on the first day. Alternate substrates, free fatty acids, and ketone bodies were also measured. There was no relationship between diabetic control in the mothers and glucose kinetics in the neonates. Glucose production was significantly lower in neonates studied at the end of the first day (Fig. 2) and the lower rate of production

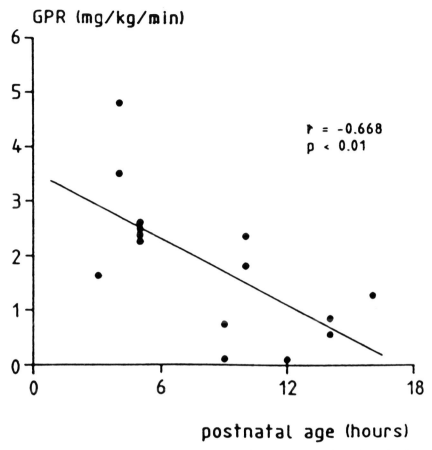

FIG. 2. Relationship between glucose production rate (GPR) and postnatal age, determined cross-sectionally in 15 infants of diabetic mothers. From Baarsma R, Reijngoud D-J, van Asselt WA, van Doormaas JJ, Berger R, Okken A. Postnatal glucose kinetics in newborns of tightly controlled insulin dependent diabetic mothers. *Pediatr Res* 1993; 34: 443–7, with permission.

was associated with increased concentrations of ketone bodies. The high glucose production rate early in the first day was probably secondary to glycogenolysis. The investigators concluded that glucose kinetics in infants of tightly controlled diabetic mothers appear to be normal.

The realization that neonatal glucose homeostasis is in a transitional state is further supported by studies in which maternal control was evaluated in a group of gestationally diabetic women in relation to the birthweights of their infants (54). If the Pedersen hypothesis were correct, birthweights of the neonates should correlate with the degree of control of the mother during the pregnancy. There was a lack of correlation between birthweight and mean maternal plasma glucose concentration during the third trimester of pregnancy in this group of gestational diabetics (Fig. 3). This lack of correlation further supports the heterogeneity of the diabetic state and suggests

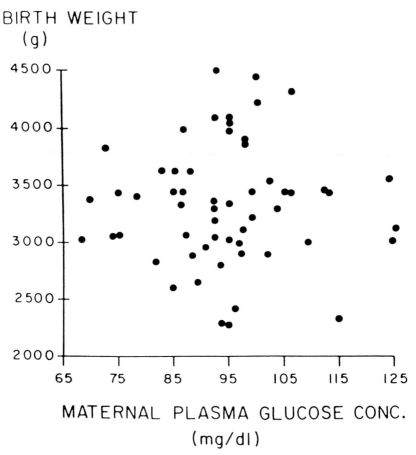

FIG. 3. Lack of correlation between birth weight of the neonate and mean maternal plasma glucose concentration (mg/dl) during the last trimester of pregnancy in women with gestational diabetes. From Widness JA, Cowett RM, Coustan DR, Carpenter MW, Oh W. Neonatal morbidities in infants of mothers with glucose intolerance in pregnancy. *Diabetes* 1985; 34(suppl 2): 61–5, with permission.

that, as control of glucose is multifactorial, control of fetal growth is likewise multifactorial. Similar conclusions led Freinkel and others to conclude that mixed nutrients (amino acids, free fatty acids, etc.) other than glucose are important in fetal-neonatal metabolic control (55,56), as shown schematically in Fig. 4. This concept is an important one for ongoing research.

Support for the concept has recently been provided by Kalkhoff *et al.* (57), who studied the relationship between neonatal birthweight and maternal plasma amino acid profiles in lean and obese, nondiabetic women and in type 1 diabetic pregnant women. HbA$_1$, plasma glucose, and total amino acid profiles were increased in diabetic subjects compared with controls. No differences were present between obese

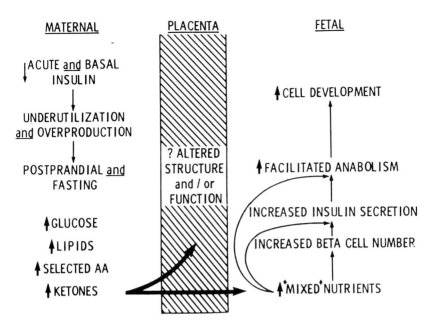

FIG. 4. Fetal growth in insulinogenic diabetic pregnancy secondary to maternal mixed nutrients. Reproduced from Freinkel N. Of pregnancy and progeny. The Banting Lecture. *Diabetes* 1980; 29: 1023–35, with permission.

and lean control groups. Plasma glucose concentrations and profiles of HbA₁ did not correlate with relative weights of the neonates, while average total plasma amino acid concentrations did. The authors concluded that maternal plasma amino acid profiles may influence fetal weight generally and affect the development of neonatal macrosomia.

Patel and Kalhan have evaluated glycerol kinetics in infants of diabetic mothers (58). They noted the possibility of intermittent hyperglycemia and hyperinsulinemia *in utero* and suggested that lower concentrations of plasma FFA concomitant with lower plasma glucose concentrations were secondary to decreased mobilization of fatty acids from adipose tissue. Since glycerol is released in a 1:3 molar ratio with fatty acids, they measured glycerol turnover using [2-¹³C]glycerol. Unexpectedly in the macrosomic infants that were studied, a normal adaptive response to fasting was noted that could assist in maintaining euglycemia.

A recent study has focused on the concept of alternate substrates in relation to the morbidity of macrosomia (59). The investigators measured plasma glucose, glycosylated hemoglobin, glycosylated protein, insulin, and triglyceride concentrations in gestational diabetes to determine their relationship to glucose intolerance and macrosomia. Plasma triglyceride concentration was the only estimation that was significantly associated with birth weight corrected for gestational age (birthweight ratio) ($p < 0.05-< 0.01$). Using multivariate analysis, triglyceride concentration was associated with birthweight ratio even when maternal prepregnancy weight gain and the

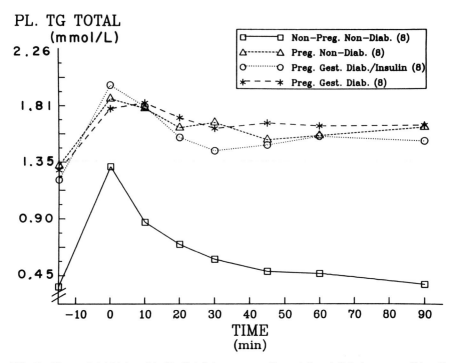

FIG. 5. Plasma total triglyceride (Tg Total) in women with gestational diabetes on or off insulin compared with pregnant nondiabetic women and nonpregnant nondiabetic women. From Cowett RM, Carr SR, Ogburn PL. Lipid tolerance testing in pregnancy. *Diabetes Care* 1993; 16: 51–56, with permission.

correlations between prepregnancy weight gain and triglyceride and birthweight ratio were controlled ($p < 0.019$). The investigators concluded that triglyceride concentration may be a physiological contributor to infant birthweight.

In contrast, we performed a lipid tolerance test in women with gestational diabetes, both on and off insulin, and compared the results to control groups who were pregnant nondiabetic or not pregnant. Figure 5 shows the plasma total triglyceride concentration over time in these groups. Although pregnancy appeared to be associated with a decreased rate of triglyceride lipolysis compared with the nonpregnant state, no differences were noted in lipid metabolism among normal pregnant and relatively well-controlled gestational diabetic patients (60).

Further work is necessary to understand the glucose kinetics and the relationships between glucose and lipid kinetics in neonates, especially infants born to well-controlled as well as poorly controlled diabetic women.

HYPOGLYCEMIA

A rapid fall in plasma glucose concentration following delivery is characteristic of the infant of the diabetic mother. Values less than 35 mg/dl in term neonates and less than 25 mg/dl in preterm neonates are abnormal and may occur within 30 minutes of clamping the umbilical vessels. Factors that are known to influence the degree of hypoglycemia include prior maternal glucose homeostasis and maternal glycemia during delivery (2). In inadequately controlled pregnancy diabetes, the fetal pancreas will have been stimulated to synthesize excessive insulin, which may readily be released. Administration of intravenous dextrose during the intrapartum period, which results in maternal hyperglycemia (>125 mg/dl) will be reflected in the fetus and will exaggerate the infant's normal postdelivery fall in plasma glucose concentration. In addition, hypoglycemia may persist for 48 hours or may develop after 24 hours.

As noted previously, fetal hyperinsulinemia is associated with suppressed concentrations of plasma free fatty acids and/or with variably diminished hepatic glucose production in the neonate. Other factors that may contribute to the development of hypoglycemia include defective counterregulation by catecholamines and/or glucagon.

The neonate shows transitional control of glucose metabolism, which suggests that a multiplicity of factors affect homeostasis. Many of the factors are similar to those that influence homeostasis in the adult. What is different in the neonate is that various stages of maturation exist for each factor. Prior work, in conjunction with glucose infusion studies, can be summarized to suggest that there is blunted splanchnic (hepatic) responsiveness to insulin in the neonate, both in infants of diabetic mothers and in preterm and term infants of nondiabetic mothers, compared with the adult (51). What have not been studied, but are of particular interest, are the many counter-insulin hormones that influence metabolism. If insulin is the primary glucoregulatory hormone, then counter-insulin hormones assist in balancing the effect of insulin and other factors.

One should probably evaluate all of the counter-insulin hormones but those that have been studied and are of particular interest in the infant of the diabetic mother have been of the sympatho-adrenal neural axis. There are many studies that have looked at epinephrine and norepinephrine concentrations in infants of diabetic mothers. The results are quite variable. An early study involved 11 infants of diabetic mothers, only two of whom were gestational. Urinary excretion of catecholamines was measured and compared with 10 infants of normal mothers. Urinary norepinephrine and epinephrine levels did not increase in the infants of diabetic women who were severely hypoglycemic but did rise in infants whose mothers were mildly hypoglycemic (43).

These results parallel investigations of Stern *et al.* who suggested that hypoglycemia may be secondary to an adrenal medullary exhaustion phenomenon (61). This would itself be secondary to longstanding hypoglycemia in the infant of the diabetic mother (presumably from the fetal period and related to poor control of maternal diabetes). In further studies, however, Keenan *et al.* noted normal increases in plasma glucose and free fatty acids and normal falls in plasma insulin in response to exogenous administration of epinephrine (62). This confirmed the exhaustion theory. A

parallel explanation was given by Young *et al.* to explain the high plasma norepinephrine concentrations in the infant of the diabetic mother, whose degree of euglycemic
control was not reported except that some of the neonates were borderline large for
gestational age (63). These investigators speculated that the infant of the diabetic
mother exposed to excessive quantities of glucose may be subject to chronic sympathoadrenal stimulation.

In another series, Artel *et al.* measured plasma epinephrine and norepinephrine
concentrations in infants of diabetic mothers (64). Increased levels of both hormones
were found, although the variation was markedly increased in the IDM. The investigators speculated that hypoglycemia after birth may be secondary to adrenal exhaustion
producing temporary depletion later in the neonatal period. This temporary depletion
might account for the appearance of hypoglycemia noted clinically by others. In a
follow-up to evaluate whether the neonatal changes were related to maternal metabolic control, plasma glucose, catecholamines, and glucagon were measured in the
neonatal period in 10 neonates of well-controlled class B diabetic women. Good
control resulted in appropriate counterregulatory hormone responses comparable
with those neonates of normal mothers. The investigators concluded that epinephrine
and glucagon levels, which paralleled the development of euglycemia, were significant factors in perinatal glucose homeostasis (65).

A series by Broberger *et al.* (66) evaluated sympathoadrenal activity in the first
12 hours after birth in infants of diabetic mothers (nine from women with type 1
diabetes and 13 from women with insulin-treated gestational diabetes). Failure to
observe differences in plasma epinephrine and norepinephrine levels between the
IDM and control neonates was believed to be secondary to good metabolic control
of the diabetic mother.

However, other factors related to sympathoadrenal activity in the neonate may be
of importance. In a continuing evaluation of the transitional nature of neonatal glucose
metabolism, relating both to insulin and to counter-insulin factors, we infused epinephrine in two doses (50 or 500 mg/kg/min) in a newborn lamb model and glucose
kinetics (turnover) were measured with [6-^{3}H]glucose. The newborn lamb showed a
blunted response to the lower dose of epinephrine infused. We speculated that the
neonate has blunted responsiveness to this important counter-insulin stimulus. If this
occurs in the diabetic state, it could partially account for the hypoglycemia that is
found clinically (67,68).

Thus the infant of the diabetic mother is a prime example of the potential for
glucose disequilibrium in the neonate. Because of the transitional state of glucose
homeostasis in the neonatal period, accentuation of disequilibrium may be enhanced
in such infants secondary to metabolic alterations present in the diabetic mother. A
great deal of work is necessary to fully appreciate the pathophysiology.

CONCLUSION

Although there has been continuing improvement in the outcome of neonates born
to diabetic mothers, they remain a high-risk population. Optimal results are obtained

when meticulous, medical-obstetric care throughout pregnancy is combined with expert neonatal supervision following delivery. Many of the risks previously identified now occur less often, however, further investigations are necessary to clarify the specific pathology of the metabolic abnormalities.

ACKNOWLEDGMENTS

We wish to express our appreciation to Ms. Patricia Knight for her expert secretarial assistance.

REFERENCES

1. Wolfe RR, Allsop J, Burke JF. Glucose metabolism in man: responses to intravenous glucose. *Metabolism* 1979; 28: 210–20.
2. Cowett RM. Pathophysiology, diagnosis and management of glucose homeostasis in the neonate. In: Lockhart J, ed. *Clinical problems in pediatrics*. Chicago: Yearbook, 1985; 15: 1–43.
3. Cowett RM. The metabolic sequelae in the infant of the diabetic mother. In: Jovanovic L, ed. *Controversies in diabetes and pregnancy*. New York: Springer-Verlag, 1988: 149–71.
4. Cowett RM. The infant of the diabetic mother. In: Hay WW, ed. *Neonatal nutrition and metabolism*. St Louis: Mosby Yearbook 1991; 419–31.
5. Cowett RM. The infant of the diabetic mother. In: Sweet AY, Brown E, eds. *Medical and surgical complications of pregnancy: effects on the fetus and newborn*. Chicago: Yearbook, 1991; 302–17.
6. Jovanovic L, Druzin M, Peterson CM. Effects of euglycemia on the outcome of pregnancy in insulin-dependent diabetic women as compared with normal control subjects. *Am J Med* 1980; 68: 105–12.
7. Kitzmiller JL, Cloherty JP, Younger MD, *et al*. Diabetic pregnancy and perinatal morbidity. *Am J Obstet Gynecol* 1978; 131: 560–8.
8. Pedersen J, Molsted-Pedersen L, Andersen B. Assessors of fetal perinatal mortality in diabetic pregnancy. Analyses of 1332 pregnancies in the Copenhagen series 1946–1972. *Diabetes* 1974; 23: 302–5.
9. Hare JW, White P. Gestational diabetes and the White classification. *Diabetes Care* 1980; 3: 394.
10. Greene MF, Hare JW, Krache M, *et al*. Prematurity among insulin requiring diabetic gravid women. *Am J Obstet Gynecol* 1989; 161: 106–11.
11. Diamond MD, Salyer SL, Vaughn WK, *et al*. Reassessment of White's clarification and Pedersen's prognostically bad signs of diabetic pregnancies in insulin dependent diabetic pregnancies. *Am J Obstet Gynecol* 1987; 156: 599–604.
12. Pollak A, Brehm R, Havelec L, *et al*. Total glycosylated hemoglobin in mothers of large for gestational age infants: a postpartum test for undetected maternal diabetes? *Biol Neonate* 1983; 40: 129–35.
13. Widness JA, Schwartz HC, Zeller WP, *et al*. Glycohemoglobin in postpartum women. *Obstet Gynecol* 1983; 57: 414–21.
14. Cocilovo G, Guerra S, Colla F, *et al*. Glycosylated hemoglobin (HbA$_1$) assay as a test for detection and surveillance of gestational diabetes. A reappraisal. *Diabetes Metab* 1987; 13: 426–30.
15. Cano A, Barcelo F, Fuentet T, *et al*. Relationship of maternal glycosylated hemoglobin and fetal beta cell activity with birthweight. *Gynecol Obstet Invest* 1986; 22: 91–6.
16. Pollak A, Salzer HR, Lischka A, *et al*. Nonenzymatic glycation of fetal tissue in diabetic pregnancy. Estimation of the glucitollysine content of umbilical cord extracts. *Acta Paediatr Scand* 1988; 77: 481–4.
17. Teramo K, Kuusisto AN, Raivio KO. Perinatal outcome of insulin-dependent diabetic pregnancies. *Ann Clin Res* 1979; 11: 146–55.
18. Jerwell J, Bjerkedal T, Moe N. Outcome of pregnancies in diabetic mothers in Norway 1967–1976. *Diabetologia* 1980; 18: 131–4.
19. Artal R, Golde SH, Dorey F, *et al*. The effect of plasma glucose variability on neonatal outcome in the pregnant diabetic patient. *Am J Obstet Gynecol* 1983; 147: 537–41.
20. Roberts AB, Patterson NS. Pregnancy in women with diabetes mellitus, twenty-years experience: 1968–1987. *N Z Med J* 1990; 103: 211–3.

21. Jovanovic R, Jovanovic L. Obstetric management when normoglycemia is maintained in diabetic women with vascular compromise. *Am J Obstet Gynecol* 1984; 149: 617–23.
22. Coustan DR, Imarah J. Prophylactic insulin treatment of gestational diabetes reduces the incidence of macrosomia, operative delivery, and birth trauma. *Am J Obstet Gynecol* 1984; 150: 836–42.
23. Coustan DR, Reece EA, Sherwin RS, *et al*. A randomized clinical trial of the insulin pump vs intensive conventional therapy in diabetic pregnancies. *JAMA* 1986; 108: 329–30.
24. Thompson DJ, Porter KB, Gunnells DJ, *et al*. Prophylactic insulin in the management of gestational diabetes. *Obstet Gynecol* 1990; 75: 960–4.
25. Larsen CE, Serdula MK, Sullivan KM. Macrosomia: influence of maternal overweight among a low income population. *Am J Obstet Gynecol* 1990; 162: 490–4.
26. Norlander E, Hanson U, Persson B. Factors influencing neonatal morbidity in gestational diabetic pregnancy. *Br J Obstet Gynecol* 1989; 96: 671–8.
27. Hanson U, Persson B, Stangenberg M. Factors influencing neonatal morbidity in diabetic pregnancy. *Diabetes Res* 1986; 3: 71–6.
28. Hunter DJ, Burrows RF, Mohilde PT, Whyte RK. Influence of maternal insulin dependent diabetes mellitus on neonatal morbidity. *Can Med Assoc J* 1993; 149: 47–52.
29. Persson B, Hanson U. Insulin dependent diabetes in pregnancy: impact of maternal blood glucose control on the offspring. *J Paediatr Child Health* 1993; 29: 20–3.
30. Peterson LJ, Peterson CM, Reed CF, *et al*., and the National Institute of Child Health and Human Development. The maternal post prandial glucose levels and infant birth weight: diabetes in early pregnancy study. *Am J Obstet Gynecol* 1991; 164: 103–11.
31. Pedersen J. The pregnant diabetic and her newborn. 2nd ed. Baltimore: Williams and Wilkins, 1977.
32. Naeye RL. Infants of diabetic mothers: a quantitative morphologic study. *Pediatrics* 1964; 35: 980–8.
33. Susa JB, McCormick KL, Widness JA, *et al*. Chronic hyperinsulinemia in the fetal rhesus monkey. Effects on fetal growth and composition. *Diabetes* 1979; 28: 1058–63.
34. Block MD, Pildes RS, Mossabhou NA, *et al*. C-peptide immunoreactivity (CRP): a new method for studying infants of insulin-treated diabetic mothers. *Pediatrics* 1974; 53: 923–8.
35. King KC, Adam PAJ, Yamaguchi K, *et al*. Insulin response to arginine in normal newborn infants and infants of diabetic mothers. *Diabetes* 1974; 23: 816–20.
36. Susa JB, Boylan JM, Sehgal P, *et al*. Impaired insulin secretion in the neonatal rhesus monkey after chronic hyperinsulinemia in utero. *Proc Soc Exp Biol Med* 1990; 194: 209–15.
37. MacFarlane CM, Tsakalakos N. The extended Pedersen hypothesis. *Clin Physiol Biochem* 1988; 6: 68–73.
38. Pildes RS, Hart RJ, Warner R, Cornblath M. Plasma insulin response during oral glucose tolerance tests in newborns of normal and gestational diabetic mothers. *Pediatrics* 1969; 44: 76–82.
39. Isles PE, Dickson M, Farquhar JW. Glucose intolerance and plasma insulin in newborn infants of normal and diabetic mothers. *Pediatr Res* 1966; 2: 198–208.
40. Adam PAJ, King KC, Schwartz R. Model for investigation of intractable hypoglycemia. Insulin-glucose interrelationships during steady state infusion. *Pediatrics* 1968; 41: 91–105.
41. King KC, Adam PAJ, Clements GA, Schwartz R. Infants of diabetic mothers: attenuated glucose uptake without hyperinsulinemia during continuous glucose infusions. *Pediatrics* 1969; 44: 381–92.
42. Hill WC, Pelle-Day G, Kitzmiller JL, *et al*. Insulin like growth factors in fetal macrosomia with and without maternal diabetes. *Hormone Res* 1989; 32: 178–82.
43. Light IJ, Sutherland JM, Loggie JM, *et al*. Impaired epinephrine release in hypoglycemic infants of diabetic mothers. *N Eng J Med* 1967; 277: 394–8.
44. Bloom SR, Johnston DT. Failure of glucagon release in infants of diabetic mothers. *BMJ* 1972; 4: 453–4.
45. Kaplan SA, Neufeld ND, Lippe BM, *et al*. Maternal diabetes and the development of the insulin receptor. In: Merkatz IR, Adam PAJ, eds. *The diabetic pregnancy. A perinatal perspective*. New York: Grune & Stratton, 1979: 169–73.
46. Lautala P, Puukka R, Knip M, *et al*. Postnatal decrease in insulin binding to erythrocytes in infants of diabetic mothers. *J Clin Endocrinol Metab* 1988; 66: 696–701.
47. Kalhan SC, Savin SM, Adam PAJ. Attenuated glucose production rate in newborn infants of insulin-dependent diabetic mothers. *N Eng J Med* 1977; 296: 375–6.
48. King KC, Tserng KY, Kalhan SC. Regulation of glucose production in newborn infants of diabetic mothers. *Pediatr Res* 1982; 16: 608–12.
49. Cowett RM, Susa JB, Giletti B, *et al*. Variability of endogenous glucose production in infants of insulin dependent diabetic mothers. *Pediatr Res* 1980; 14: 570A. (Abstract)

50. Cowett RM, Susa JB, Giletti B, Oh W, Schwartz R. Glucose kinetics in infants of diabetic mothers. *Am J Obstet Gynecol* 1983; 146: 781–6.
51. Cowett RM, Oh W, Schwartz R. Persistent glucose production during glucose infusion in the neonate. *J Clin Invest* 1983; 71: 467–73.
52. Cowett RM, Andersen GE, Maguire CA, Oh W. Ontogeny of glucose kinetics in low birth weight infants. *J Pediatr* 1988; 112: 462–5.
53. Baarsma R, Reijngoud D-J, van Asselt WA, van Doormaas JJ, Berger R, Okken A. Postnatal glucose kinetics in newborns of tightly controlled insulin dependent diabetic mothers. *Pediatr Res* 1993; 34: 443–7.
54. Widness JA, Cowett RM, Coustan DR, Carpenter MW, Oh W. Neonatal morbidities in infants of mothers with glucose intolerance in pregnancy. *Diabetes* 1985; 34(suppl 2): 61–5.
55. Freinkel N. Of pregnancy and progeny. The Banting Lecture. *Diabetes* 1980; 29: 1023–35.
56. Milner RDG. Amino acids and beta cell growth in structure and function. In: Merkatz IR, Adam PAJ, eds. *The diabetic pregnancy. A perinatal perspective.* New York: Grune & Stratton 1979; 37: 145–53.
57. Kalkhoff RK, Kandaraki E, Morrow PG, *et al.* Relationship between neonatal birth weight and maternal plasma amino acid profiles in lean and obese nondiabetic women and in type 1 diabetic pregnant women. *Metabolism* 1988; 37: 234–9.
58. Patel D, Kalhan S. Glycerol metabolism and triglyceride-fatty acid cycling in the human newborn: effect of maternal diabetes and intrauterine growth retardation. *Pediatr Res* 1992; 31: 52–8.
59. Knoop RH, Magee MS, Walden CE, Bonet B, Benedetto TJ. Prediction of infant birth weight by GDM screening tests. Importance of plasma triglycerides. *Diabetes Care* 1992; 11: 1605–13.
60. Cowett RM, Carr SR, Ogburn PL. Lipid tolerance testing in pregnancy. *Diabetes Care* 1993; 16: 51–56.
61. Stern L, Ramos A, Leduc J. Urinary catecholamine excretion in infants of diabetic mothers. *Pediatrics* 1968; 42: 598–605.
62. Keenan WJ, Light IJ, Sutherland JM. Effects of exogenous epinephrine on glucose and insulin levels in infants of diabetic mothers. *Biol Neonate* 1972; 21: 44–53.
63. Young BJ, Cohen WR, Rappaport EB, *et al.* High plasma norepinephrine concentrations at birth in infants of diabetic mothers. *Diabetes* 1979; 28: 697–9.
64. Artel R, Platt LD, Kummula RK, *et al.* Sympatho-adrenal activity in infants of diabetic mothers. *Am J Obstet Gynecol* 1982; 42: 436–9.
65. Artal R, Doug N, Wu P, *et al.* Circulating catecholamines and glucagon in infants of strictly controlled diabetic mothers. *Biol Neonate* 1988; 53: 121–5.
66. Broberger U, Hansson U, Lagercrantz H, *et al.* Sympatho-adrenal activity and metabolic adjustment during the first 12 hours after birth in infants of diabetic mothers. *Acta Paediatr Scand* 1984; 73: 620–5.
67. Cowett RM. Decreased response to catecholamines in the newborn: effect on glucose kinetics in the lamb. *Metabolism* 1988; 37: 736–40.
68. Cowett RM. Alpha adrenergic agonists stimulate neonatal glucose production less than beta adrenergic agonists in the lamb. *Metabolism* 1988; 37: 831–6.

DISCUSSION

Dr. Bartsokas: Although you did not touch on the subject, would you speculate on the cause of the cardiomyopathy in infants of diabetic mothers?

Dr. Cowett: It has been shown that there is increased glycogen in the heart in cases of cardiomyopathy but I do not know the origin of the congenital cardiac malformations that occur.

Dr. Nattrass: What changes do you find in the catecholamines? What effect would such changes have upon the delivery of substrates, for example fatty acids and also gluconeogenic substrates, in view of the changes that you find in glucose production?

Dr. Cowett: We know there are increases in catecholamine production but the stresses responsible for this are not well understood. The fact is that the pregnancies that are considered to be under stress produce the biggest infants, so there seems to be a positive correlation between increased catecholamines and the size of the infant.

Dr. Catalano: I have a question regarding the timing of your kinetic studies in the newborn. How important is it to time when you do the measurements and to ensure that the timing is equal between groups? Is there a delay of enzyme maturation in the liver that may affect the time when you study an infant of a diabetic mother as compared with an infant of a woman who has normal glucose metabolism?

Dr. Cowett: Kalhan's studies were done at 2 hours, ours tended to be done between 24 and 72 hours. Until now we have not studied newborns before 24 hours of age, and we have no studies after 72 hours. Early on, in the first hours, glycogenolysis is likely to be predominant. From alanine studies, Bier and colleagues have suggested that gluconeogenesis probably begins at around 6 hours of age, but it has not been looked at earlier than that. The response that Kalhan showed was not only a response of glucagon but also of catecholamines, and it has been suggested that this occurs in the infant of the diabetic mother as well.

Dr. Schwartz: Many years ago, Drash and I independently studied glucagon responses in babies. When we gave glucagon to a normal newborn infant, the hyperglycemic response was slow and delayed and very different from what one sees in an older infant or an adult, where you get a prompt response with a rise of glucose in 30 minutes. In the newborn, the rise occurs over 120 minutes. I believe that the insulin response that you showed was initially low and also delayed, in contrast to the adult, and I wonder whether you can reconcile that with your hypothesis about catecholamines and glucose and insulin effectiveness.

Dr. Cowett: The concern in the infant of the diabetic mother has always been that there is a blunted catecholamine response. Paul Wu showed that the response was blunted compared with normal when glucagon was given to the infant of the diabetic mother.

Dr. Bergman: I don't know whether Dr. Schwartz is going to cover this, but I was interested in his insulin-infused rhesus monkey model. I was very curious about the blood sugar, for example, and what effect this may have on the developing brain. I assume that blood sugar would have been very low in the fetus. This could also have an impact on the metabolism of the mother, who has to deliver large amounts of glucose to the fetus.

Dr. Schwartz: May I answer this? Our first study was of *in utero* hyperinsulinemia that had no effect on maternal glucose or any other variable that we could measure and that caused a slight decrease in umbilical artery glucose in the fetus, but no decrease in umbilical vein glucose because of maternal-fetal transfer. The other study was to take this model and to produce neonatal hypoglycemia deliberately. We delivered the fetuses with the insulin infusion pump intact, put a catheter in the umbilical vein, and followed blood glucose serially for 12–14 hours while inducing severe hypoglycemia. We also had a control group. These two groups were then put in the monkey baby nursery and reared. When the monkeys were growing and stabilized they were transferred to the university and went through an elaborate 2-year blinded analysis. This analysis could not discriminate between the two groups of monkeys. So severe neonatal hypoglycemia in the monkey apparently has no consequences as far as development is considered. These results have been published (1).

Dr. Girard: The fetal and neonatal brain is relatively well protected against hypoglycemia since the brain can take up lactate to a very large extent and this is capable of covering its energy needs. This has been very well demonstrated (2).

Dr. Bergman: What is the enzymatic mechanism of this, compared with the normal adult brain?

Dr. Girard: It is probably the capacity of the blood-brain barrier to transfer dicarboxylic acid very efficiently. There is also glucose transporter expression that allows the brain to take up glucose even in the presence of hypoglycemia.

Dr. Cowett: Does that persist, or when does it diminish?

Dr. Girard: It seems to decrease with development, but it is very particularly efficient during the neonatal period. It has been demonstrated recently (3) in the adult that lactate is capable of replacing glucose as a fuel for the brain during hypoglycemia.

Dr. Schwartz: The classical example of that is type 1 glycogen storage disease where you get severe hypoglycemia, blood sugars at zero for example, and lactate that are 12–15 mM, extraordinarily high. Lactate uptake by the brain has been shown in older children (2).

Dr. Drash: Are you willing to extrapolate to the human situation? Should we have no concern about the effect of maternal hypoglycemia on the fetus?

Dr. Schwartz: No, I would not say that at all.

Dr. Swift: This is a very worrying discussion for pediatricians involved in neonatal care. Infants of diabetic mothers who have in the past became hypoglycemic seem to be normal mentally on long-term follow up, but Alan Lucas's data from Cambridge published in recent years suggests that the one identifiable variable relating to poor outcome in children who were preterm is hypoglycemia in the preterm nursery. Of course that might relate to overall nutrition rather than just to hypoglycemia, but perhaps you would like to comment.

Dr. Cowett: We are familiar with Lucas' data. It does not really equate with work in the monkey, and I am concerned that their data have not been confirmed by others. Many different components are usually operative when the infant becomes hypoglycemic, so it is hard to tease out one variable. However, we should be cautious in suggesting that this model shows that hypoglycemia does not have any effect on the human; it simply says that in this model the monkeys grew up seemingly normal.

Dr. Marliss: Along the same lines, I was very impressed by the rates of endogenous glucose production in the small-for-gestational age subjects you showed. If I remember correctly, it was in the neighborhood of 6 or even more mg per kg per minute. Is that because those individuals have disproportionately large brains and if you were to look at glucose production with some other denominator it might be somewhat less impressive?

Dr. Cowett: The infants were all appropriate for gestational age and their head circumferences were over the 10th and under the 90th percentile. We would agree, however, that there is an increased glucose production based on an increased brain size relative to body size in small-for-dates infants. It has been shown by others that there is a correlation between glucose turnover and brain size indirectly measured by head circumference in a heterogeneous age group of infants.

Dr. Drash: I would like to ask Girard about the time course of lactate adaptation. Type 1 glycogen storage disease is a very interesting model in this regard. Years ago we treated some of these children with diazoxide and they ran around the house with blood sugars of 5 or 10 mg/dl (0.3–0.6 mM) and were absolutely asymptomatic. However, when we put them on diazoxide and maintained their blood sugars around 50 or 60 mg/dl (2.7–3.3 mM) they then developed severe hypoglycemic symptoms with very mild falls in blood sugar so we had to abandon diazoxide therapy. I did not think in terms of lactate at the time. I thought we were probably dealing with ketone bodies. But I felt that what we had done was to remove a very important metabolic adaptation, and once they had lost it they could not regain it quickly. I wonder if there are any data on the time course of this adaptation?

Dr. Girard: From the data obtained in the rat, the adaptation seems to be rapid, but in order for lactate to replace glucose as a fuel you must have a high plasma-lactate concentration. So in a situation in which you have an infusion of insulin, you probably stimulate glucose metabolism in peripheral tissue and provide more lactate. In a situation in which you have a very low lactate concentration in the blood the brain is not protected at all.

REFERENCES

1. Schrier AM, Brady PW, Church RM *et al.* Neonatal hypoglycemia in the rhesus monkey: effect on development and behavior. *Infant Behavior and Development* 1990; 13: 189–207.
2. Fernandez J, Berger R, Smit GPA. Lactate as a cerebral metabolic fuel for glucose-6-phosphatase deficient children. *Pediat Res* 1984; 18: 335–9.
3. Maran A, Cranston I, Lomas J, MacDonald I, Amiel SA. Protection by lactate of cerebral function during hypoglycaemia. *Lancet* 1994; 343: 16–20.

Diabetes, edited by Richard M. Cowett,
Nestlé Nutrition Workshop Series,
Vol. 35. Nestec Ltd.,
Vevey/Raven Press, Ltd., New York © 1995.

Clinical Presentation of Type 1 Diabetes in Childhood

Robert Schwartz and Patricia A. Walsh

Division of Pediatric Endocrinology and Metabolism, Department of Pediatrics, Rhode Island Hospital, and Brown University School of Medicine, Providence, Rhode Island 02903, USA

HISTORY (1)

The Papyrus Ebers contained reference to a condition that may have been diabetes mellitus dating back to before 1500 BC. A good clinical description was given by Celsus (30 BC–50 AD). He described the cardinal symptoms in detail: polyuria, polydipsia, polyphagia, and weight loss. Aretaeus of Cappadocia (81–138 AD) (Roman Asia Minor) named the disorder *diabetes* from the Greek word for siphon or to pass through. Chinese writings in 200–600 AD contained similar observations. The ancients noted that ants were attracted by a "sweetness of the urine" and that carbuncles frequently plagued victims of this disease. Paracelsus (1493–1541 AD) thought the white deposit left by the urine was salt and therefore added salt to the diet as therapy. Initially it was thought to be a disease of the kidneys. Indian physicians made diagnostic use not only of inspection, palpation, and auscultation, but also of smelling and tasting. Note was made of the sweet taste of diabetic urine (*madhumeha*) (2). The Japanese made similar observations. Avicenna, a well-known Arab physician, gave a very complete description of the disorder around 1000 AD. Thomas Willis (1621–1675) also noted the urine to be "wondrous sweet as if imbued with honey." Dobson realized that the serum was sweet, while Cullen (1710–1790) added the word *mellitus* in Edinburgh.

The next major phase was concerned with chemical analysis of blood and urine, recognizing reducing substances with iron or copper reagents. It was not until the 1950s that practical enzymatic analysis of glucose *per se* was developed.

In 1869, Paul Langerhans, a medical student, first identified clusters of cells later identified as the pancreatic islets. In 1889, Joseph von Mering and Oskar Minkowski successfully performed a total pancreatectomy in the dog, producing hyperglycemia and glycosuria, and finally death with ketosis and coma. Minkowski recognized the significance of these findings and tested the urine for sugar, thus finally associating the pancreas with diabetes.

TABLE 1. *Status of 750 diabetic children in 1931*

	Total number of cases	Number living Oct. 1931	% Living
Period First Seen			
Naunyn (1898–1914)	61	1	2
Allen (1914–1922)	170	49	28
Banting (1922–1931)	519	483	93

From White P (3).

The next 30 years were devoted in large measure to identifying the elusive agent produced by the pancreas. While many investigators had near success, it was the team of Banting, Best, Collip, and Macleod in Toronto, Ontario, that produced the first major product. Their description of correction of hyperglycemia in a depancreatectomized dog was a remarkable achievement.

Before 1921, therapy was primarily dietary, as presented in Strasbourg by Naunyn and in the USA by Frederick Allen. Both were convinced that semistarvation was important and that carbohydrate was not the key to management. Sodium bicarbonate was added to stabilize acidosis.

In addition to the symptoms noted above, management of diabetes was associated with profound weight loss. This was not due to dehydration but rather to loss of tissue mass resulting in marasmus. The administration of insulin produced a dramatic reversal in body composition, as noted in 1922 in an early patient, a 3-year-old boy who weighed 6.8 kg (15 lb). In just 2 months of insulin therapy, he weighed 13 kg (29 lb) and looked cherubic. Thus was opened the insulin era and the consequences of long-term survival with diabetes. Priscilla White summarized survival from diabetes in 1931 (3) (Table 1).

CRITERIA FOR DIAGNOSIS (4)

Diabetes Mellitus in Children

Either of the following are considered diagnostic for diabetes: 1. the presence of the classic symptoms of diabetes, such as polyuria, polydipsia, ketonuria, and rapid weight loss, together with a random plasma glucose >200 mg/dl (11.1 mM); 2. in an asymptomatic individual, both a raised fasting glucose concentration and a sustained increase in glucose concentration during an oral glucose tolerance test (OGTT) on more than one occasion. Both the 2-hour blood sample and some other sample taken between administration of the glucose dose (1.75 g/kg ideal body weight, up to a maximum of 75 g) and 2 hours later must meet the following criteria:

Fasting value: Venous plasma >140 mg/dl (7.8 mmol/liter); venous whole blood >120 mg/dl (6.7 mmol/liter); capillary whole blood >120 mg/dl (6.7 mmol/liter)

2-hour OGTT value and an intervening value: Venous plasma >11.1 mmol/liter (200 mg/dl); venous whole blood >10.0 mmol/liter (180 mg/dl); whole capillary blood ≥11.1 mmol/liter (200 mg/dl).

Normal Glucose Levels in Children

Fasting value: Venous plasma <7.2 mmol/liter (130 mg/dl); venous whole blood <6.4 mmol/liter (115 mg/dl); capillary whole blood <6.4 mmol/liter (115 mg/dl)
2-hour OGTT value: Venous plasma <7.8 mmol/liter (140 mg/dl); venous whole blood <6.7 mmol/liter (120 mg/dl); whole capillary blood <7.8 mmol/liter (140 mg/dl).

Urine glucose (enzyme methods) or reducing substances are nonspecific and provide a basis for suspicion of the need to analyze blood or plasma for glucose.

INCIDENCE AND SYMPTOMS

In 1932, Priscilla White reported on 750 children with insulin-dependent diabetes, with an equal distribution between the sexes. She later summarized her experience with 4054 cases. In the earlier series, she described peaks of incidence at 3, 5, 8, and 12 years. In the later series (Fig. 1) she noted the peak in girls to be 10 years while that in boys was at 13 years (5). She attributed these differences to the onset of puberty. Our series is too small to draw any inferences. A complete discussion of the epidemiology of diabetes is presented in the chapter by Drash.

Danowski (6) reported that 89.5% of his patients had polyuria or polydipsia or both (Table 2). This is similar to our own recent experience of 93%. The exceptions are equally important. One 10-year-old girl was asymptomatic and was seen by her pediatrician for an annual examination in May. A routine urine test indicated 55.5 mM glucose (1000 mg/dl), but it was negative for ketones. A random blood glucose concentration was 21.7 mM (390 mg/dl), while a fasting blood glucose concentration was 13 mM (235 mg/dl). In October, another youngster, a 14-year-old male who was asymptomatic, fractured a fibula. Routine blood investigation indicated hyperglycemia. His orthopedist performed an oral glucose tolerance test that was abnormal. His admission blood glucose was 17.9 mM (322 mg/dl) while his HbAlc was 8.8% (normal less than 6.6%).

Of the other major manifestations, weight loss is no different from adults in frequency, occurring in about 60% of newly diabetic children. Appetite change, considered classical in adults, is highly variable in children. Thus polyphagia is as likely to be present as diminished appetite. In the preantibiotic era, infection was frequently found. Thus, furunculosis was described in earlier treatises. In our series, bacterial infections, including otitis media, streptococcal pharyngitis, and pneumonia, were found in about 20% of newly diagnosed diabetics. Presumed viral infections were found in 6.7% of admissions, while fungal infections, especially candidiasis involving the vulva in females, was observed in 2.7%. There was a total of 29.3% infections in our series of observations.

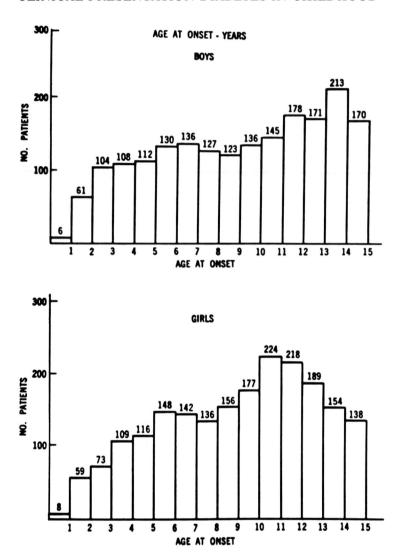

FIG. 1. Distribution of incidence of type 1 insulin-dependent diabetes by age and sex. From: Priscilla White, chapter 27 in The treatment of diabetes mellitus, eds Joslin EP, Root HF, White P, Marble A. Philadelphia: Lea & Febiger, 1959: 655–89, with permission.

Blurring of vision responds to correction of the hyperglycemia. Physicians unfamiliar with the problem may attempt correction of the visual derangement.

Parents may now be sufficiently informed to initiate the first diagnostic steps. The factors responsible for this in the USA are: 1. the widespread publicity given to diabetes by the American Diabetes Association and the Juvenile Diabetes Foundation International, 2. recognition of the significance of a positive family history, and 3.

TABLE 2. *Major manifestations at time of diagnosis*

	Pittsburgh pre-1957[a]	Rhode Island pre-1994
Total number	513	75
Polyuria	78.4%	93.3%
Polydipsia	75.8%	92.0%
Weight loss	57.5%	57.3%
Polyphagia	48.9%	16.0%
Anorexia	44.4%	20.0%

[a] Initially detected by onset of glycosuria

the availability of over-the-counter testing equipment. K.S. had two weeks of polyuria and polydipsia. Weight loss was suspected. Because a paternal grandmother had type 2 diabetes, the mother obtained a urine dipstick that was positive for glucose. On admission, the child's blood glucose was 58 mM (1047 mg/dl), serum sodium 122 mM, and total CO_2 22 mM. N.S., a 3-year-old boy, had polyuria and polydipsia of 3-days' duration. No weight loss was noted. His family history was noteworthy in that a paternal great-grandmother had type 2 diabetes, while a first cousin had type 1, and his 7-year-old sister had been diagnosed 16 days previously with symptoms and an initial blood glucose of 11.6 mM (209 mg/dl). His admission glucose concentration was 22.2 mM (400 mg/dl).

BLOOD SUGAR AT DIAGNOSIS

In the era before specific enzymatic methods were available for glucose determination, Danowski (6) reported that in approximately 85% of newly discovered diabetics blood sugar values were above the highest concentrations seen in healthy nondiabetic children, that is, in the shaded area in Fig. 2. These values were taken from newly discovered glycosuric children who ultimately proved to have diabetes, although with the currently accepted National Diabetes Data Group Criteria (4) a significant number of these children would not now be classified as diabetic initially. The distribution over ages 1–16 years is similar for the Pittsburgh and Rhode Island populations (Fig. 3). In particular, there is no trend toward higher values either in the very young or in adolescent groups.

HYPEROSMOLAR COMA

This diagnosis is more common in adults and is rarely found in children. Interestingly, using a blood glucose concentration of more than 44.4 mM (800 mg/dl) as indicative of increased risk, Danowski reported only six cases out of 513, while we found 14 out of 75 (18.7%). These were distributed over all ages. Rulein *et al.* (7) first reported this diagnosis in children in 1969. Six subjects were newly diagnosed

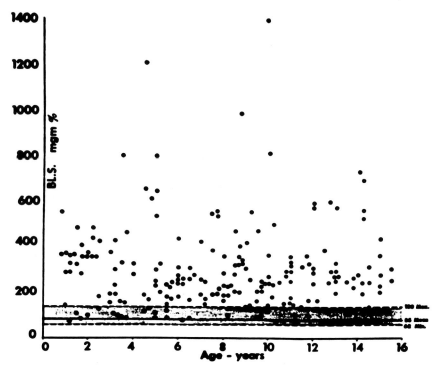

FIG. 2. Fasting venous blood sugar levels in newly discovered untreated diabetic children. Danowski reported a large series of blood sugar values at the time of diagnosis. Patients were selected initially by glycosuria. Eighty-five percent of the values were above those found in healthy nondiabetic children *(shaded area).* Reproduced with permission from Danowski TS. *Diabetes Mellitus.* Baltimore: Williams and Williams, 1957: 128.

diabetics. Although rare, this problem is of concern because of the ominous outcome. Special attention is required because of the possibility of cerebral edema.

METABOLIC ACIDOSIS AND COMA

This is an ominous presentation in a newly onset type 1 diabetic. Danowski (6) reported that 18.1% of his patients (93 in total) developed either acidosis or coma. He did not define these 93 children in terms of total CO_2 or pH. Acidosis has been arbitrarily classified as mild or absent (CO_2 18–30 mM), moderate (CO_2 8–18 mM), and severe (CO_2 <8 mM). In our series 10.4% had severe diabetic ketoacidosis (Fig. 4). Within this group over half were under 2 years of age. Two-thirds of our patients had no or only mild acidosis on admission.

Another variable on admission is pH. Kety *et al.* (8) elegantly showed the relationship of respiratory minute volume to pH (Fig. 5). At pH values below 7.1, respiration

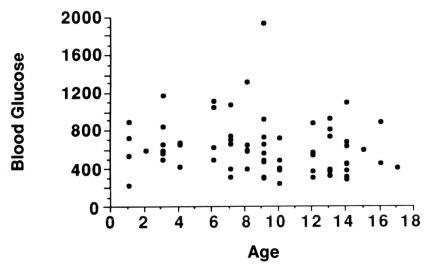

FIG. 3. Blood glucose concentrations at diagnosis of type 1 insulin-dependent diabetes shown relative to age (1990–1994).

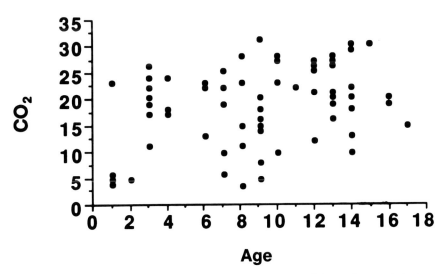

FIG. 4. Total CO_2 content at diagnosis of type 1 insulin-dependent diabetes shown relative to age (1990–1994).

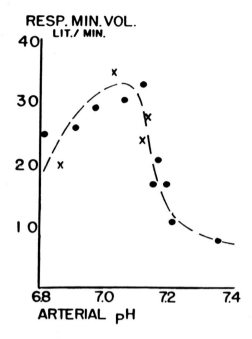

FIG. 5. Pulmonary ventilation in diabetic acidosis in adults plotted as a function of the arterial pH. From Kety SS, Polis BC, Nadler CS, Schmidt CF. Blood flow and oxygen consumption of human brain in diabetic acidosis and coma. *J Clin Invest* 1948: 27: 500–10, with permission.

is depressed so that respiratory compensation is reduced. This is an important criterion for initial sodium bicarbonate therapy to restore pH and respiratory center sensitivity.

The clinical presentation of ketoacidosis is highly variable. Thus abdominal pain and vomiting may be found. These are followed by headache and drowsiness and then by stupor and coma. Daughaday (9) has commented that the incidence of diabetic ketoacidosis cannot be expressed in any meaningful way. "The frequency of this condition among hospital admissions reflects the general level of medical care in the community and the spectrum of clinical interest of the attending staff. Where medical care is readily available and interest in diabetes is high, acidosis is rare." In our patients, ketoacidosis occurs in known subjects who develop an intercurrent infection or who reject the diagnosis, are noncompliant, and omit insulin. Daughaday states, "The occurrence of diabetic acidosis in a recognized case should be looked upon as a serious failure in diabetic education or lapse in doctor to patient interrelationship."

Although the diagnosis is not difficult in the older child or adult, in the young child it may be mistaken for salicylate intoxication. Hyperventilation is present in both, but dehydration is minimal in the latter. The diagnosis depends on a toxicology screen.

UNUSUAL PATIENTS: PERMANENT NEONATAL DIABETES (10)

Mother's History

In one particular case, the patient's mother herself was an insulin-dependent diabetic with diagnosis at 3 months of age. At the time her diagnosis was made, she was being evaluated for fever associated with poor weight gain, polydipsia, and polyphagia. The mother's birth weight had been 2835 g after a 42 week gestation (between the 10th and 25th percentile). The course of the mother's diabetes had been punctuated by innumerable hospital admissions for ketoacidosis as well as hypoglycemia. One such episode at age 5 years resulted in mild developmental delay. Although progression in school was slow, she was independent as regards self-care by the age of 16 years. She left home by 18 years and became pregnant by 20 years. She had this terminated by a medical interruption of pregnancy without event. By 24 years she met Charlie who devoted his subsequent life to her care. In addition, she had developed proliferative retinopathy at 24 years of age, at about the same time as proteinuria was noted. Her blood urea nitrogen and serum creatinine levels, however, were normal while she was pregnant.

A positive family history of diabetes included a maternal great-grandmother with maturity onset diabetes (type 2), and a paternal grandmother of American Indian and Irish descent who had been treated with insulin for 10 years before her death at the age of 42. The mother's parents were Jewish and the paternal grandmother was of Irish extraction. The patient's father had one nondiabetic half-brother. The mother had three normal brothers. She herself went on to develop many of the major complications of diabetes so that by the age of 34 she had lost vision and developed renal failure. Hemodialysis was begun, and she died when aged 37 years.

Infant's History

The infant was born when his mother was 27 years old. Premature delivery was needed because of an exacerbation of the mother's proliferative retinopathy (White class F/R), before which she had been treated with twice-daily insulin injections. The maternal HbA1c level was 6.4% of total hemoglobin two weeks after delivery. Delivery was complicated by an incision through an anterior placenta. Because of the mother's history of diabetes and her course during pregnancy, the diverse morbidities expected in an infant of an insulin-dependent mother were anticipated. Gestational age was 36 weeks. Apgar scores were 3 and 5 at one and five minutes, respectively. A venous packed red cell volume of 31% was obtained within the first hour of life. A Dubowitz neonatal examination was in agreement with the mother's dates. He was not macrosomic and weighed 2100 g (between the 10th and 25th percentile). The infant's head circumference at birth was 32 cm (just above the 25th percentile) and his length was 43 cm (just above the 10th percentile). His condition improved rapidly after intravenous therapy with volume expanders, which included packed red blood cells. There was no evidence of hypoglycemia in the first days after birth. Mild respiratory distress, which was noted shortly after birth, resolved by the second day of life. A minor abnormal finding noted on the initial chest radiograph was a hemivertebra at T11. The placenta weighed 461 g, had two grossly evident infarcts less than 2.5 cm in diameter, and had microscopic features consistent with prematurity.

Surprisingly, during the first days of life, Dextrostix determinations on whole blood were increased to more than 11 mM (200 mg/dl). This estimate was confirmed by a plasma glucose value of 13.4 mM (242 mg/dl) on the fifth day of life, during which time the intravenous dextrose infusion rate was 6 mg/kg/min. As the overall clinical condition improved and the intravenous fluids were reduced and the oral intake increased, hyperglycemia persisted in the range of 13.9–19.4 mM (250–350 mg/dl). Insulin treatment was withheld since the infant was growing well with respect to weight, length, and head circumference, and was neither dehydrated nor acidotic.

While in hospital, several diagnostic studies were carried out to evaluate his hyperglycemia. Mixed umbilical cord serum insulin antibodies were 3–4 U/liter; islet cell surface antibodies were undetectable; and at 2 weeks of age, glucose turnover rate using stable D-[U-^{13}C] glucose was determined to be 5.8 mg glucose/kg/min (normal range: 3.0–4.0). At 35 days of age, after a 4-hour fast, an intravenous tolbutamide tolerance test (20 mg/kg) was performed: plasma C-peptide concentration was 0.36 pmol/ml prior to the stimulus and increased approximately sixfold to 1.76 pmol/ml by 40 minutes; as the infant's plasma glucose concentration fell, there was a slight rise in plasma glucagon concentration from 125 to 340 pg/ml. During the study, plasma cortisol and growth hormone levels both rose by 40 minutes from 5.6 to 11.8 μg/dl and from 19 to 25 ng/ml, respectively. The infant was retested 7 days later after a 3-hour fast without tolbutamide stimulation during which his plasma glucose fell from 22.2 to 13.9 mM (400 to 250 mg/dl). During this fast, plasma β-hydroxybutyrate concentrations were normal at 0.06 mM (basal) and 0.09 mM by the end of the additional 90-minute fasting period.

Because of adequate weight gain and the absence of ketonuria, the infant was sent home at 8 weeks of age without insulin therapy. Before discharge, blood glucose concentrations had been in the range of 19.4–30.5 mM (350–550 mg/dl). The patient did well at home for one month until, at 13 weeks of age, he developed an upper respiratory tract infection associated with ketonuria. He was readmitted to the hospital, and insulin therapy was begun. At the time of his admission he had a head circumference at 37 cm, crown-heel length of 55 cm, and weight of 3600 g.

A repeat tolbutamide tolerance test three weeks later (after an overnight fast and 12 hours after the last insulin dose) showed a diminution in the plasma C-peptide response compared with the first study. At this time *in vitro* studies with rat adipocytes incubated in the presence or absence of exogenous insulin and the infant's serum showed that glucose was normally oxidized to carbon dioxide (courtesy of Dr. Michael P. Czech). The intravenous tolbutamide tolerance test was repeated for a third time at 16 months of age, and during it the plasma glucose concentration fell from 23.6 to 15.2 mM (425 to 273 mg/dl) over 100 minutes. Again, C-peptide levels were present but depressed. During the latter test, plasma free fatty acid levels fell slightly from 1.10 mM at time zero to 0.75 and 0.75 mM at 15 and 40 minutes, respectively.

Tissue typing was carried out on the patient and his parents when he was 3 months of age. This included histocompatibility leukocyte antigen (HLA) lymphocyte typing (courtesy of Dr. Edmund Yunis, Sidney Farber Cancer Center, Boston) as well as complement protein typing for properdin factor B (courtesy of Dr. Chester A. Alper,

Center for Blood Research, Boston). Tissue antigens DR3 and DR4 were not found in the HLA typing, and BF*F1 and C2*B were not found in complement typing.

Tests of insulin receptor binding were carried out. Four months postpartum, erythrocyte binding for the infant and his mother showed a specific binding of 14% and 5% respectively, in the absence of cold insulin (courtesy of Dr. Simeon Taylor, NIH). The normal range for adults is 6.7 ± 0.6%, mean ± SEM). Although no standards for 4-month-old infants are available, erythrocytes from neonates have been reported to have higher specific insulin binding than from adults. Cultured B lymphocytes drawn at that time also had normal insulin binding. Insulin binding done on cultured fibroblasts from maternal and infant skin biopsies taken at 6 months of age was normal for specific binding as well as for half maximal displacements (courtesy of Dr. Judy Podskalny, NIH).

Serum autoantibodies to a variety of tissue antigens were studied in the patient and his parents (courtesy of Dr. G. Bottazzo, Middlesex College, London, England). These included islet cell cytoplasmic antibodies, thyroglobulin hemagglutinins, thyroid microsomal hemagglutinins, gastric parietal cell antibodies, and others (antinuclear, antimitochondrial and anti-smooth-muscle antibodies); none was found.

His diabetes has not been well controlled up to 14 years of age. He has had behavioral problems and school delay. His growth has been slow and a significant scoliosis required orthopedic surgery. His most recent glycohemoglobin was 10.9%. His urinary microalbumin was 7 μg/mg creatinine after 14 years of diabetes. He has no ophthalmologic abnormalities.

RESULTS OF DELAYED ONSET OF INSULIN THERAPY

Second Patient

KS was a 10-year-old preadolescent female who had polyuria and polydipsia for three weeks before her father, an osteopathic physician, checked her urine and blood. She had no ketonuria but had 2 g/dl urinary sugar and a blood glucose of 20.4 mM (386 mg/dl). Because of his background, her father was convinced that she could be controlled by diet alone without insulin. Over the next 6 months, she was given a diet low in energy and carbohydrate.

Her growth ceased, in fact her weight fell from the 50th percentile to well below the 5th percentile. She finally developed ketonuria in association with an upper respiratory infection. On admission, she was markedly undernourished and mildly dehydrated. She had Kussmaul respirations. Retinal examination showed marked lipemia retinalis. Hepatomegaly was significant. Upon drawing blood, gross lactescence was observed. Initial laboratory studies indicated an unanalyzable hemoglobin, a grossly low serum sodium of 100 mM, potassium 2.5 mM, chloride 76 mM, and CO_2 3.7 mM. Her blood urea nitrogen was 3.3 mM while creatinine was 106.1 μM. Her admission serum glucose was 19.1 mM (344 mg/dl). The magnitude of her lipid concentrations was unexpected (Table 3), and the values represented some of the highest reported.

TABLE 3. *Plasma lipids in new onset diabetic (type 1)*

Date	Total lipids	Phospholipids (all results expressed in mg/100 ml)	Sphingomyelin	Cholesterol
NORMAL	400–800	150–250	15–60	150–270
5-2-56	25,200	1220		1612
5-5	10,000	658	229	610
5-8	7,750	645		
5-11	4,380	532	161	
5-14	2,120	402	119	
5-29	1,500	285	35	
6-26	330	127		208

Despite the factitiously abnormal electrolyte values, she was treated conservatively with fluid, electrolytes and insulin. Her course was uneventful. She was kept in hospital until the family was educated and her lipids were improving toward normal (Table 3). She showed catch-up growth and resumed her previous rate of weight gain. Her subsequent course was unremarkable.

CONCLUSION

The diagnosis of type 1 insulin-dependent diabetes is rarely difficult in the older child or adult. Virtually all have recognizable polyuria and polydipsia of several days to a month's duration. Other significant symptoms include weight loss and variable change in appetite. Family history is helpful only when it is positive in close family members.

In the young infant under two years, the classical symptoms of polyuria and polydipsia may go unrecognized for several days. As a result, weight loss may be significant. Ultimately, dehydration and ketoacidosis may occur. The physician unfamiliar with diabetes mellitus in the young infant may mistake Kussmaul hyperventilation for pneumonia or bronchiolitis. In the era before insulin therapy, weight loss was often advanced so that marasmus was an important sign.

Recognition and prompt correction of the metabolic derangement can avoid a fatal outcome and can initiate a management program with an optimistic prognosis.

REFERENCES

1. Davidson JK, ed. Historical perspective: the discovery of insulin. In: *Clinical diabetes mellitus.* New York: Thieme, 1991: 2–10.
2. Castiglione A. *A history of medicine.* New York: Alfred E Knopf, 1941: 89.
3. White P. *Diabetes in childhood and adolescence.* Philadelphia: Lea & Febiger, 1932: 2.
4. National Diabetes Data Group. Classification and diagnosis of diabetes mellitus and other categories of glucose tolerance. *Diabetes* 1979; 28: 1029–57.
5. White P. Diabetic children and their later lives. In: Joslin EP, Root HF, White P, Marble A. *The treatment of diabetes mellitus.* Philadelphia: Lea & Febiger, 1959: 655–89.

6. Danowski TS. *Diabetes mellitus*. Baltimore: Williams and Wilkins, 1957: 128.
7. Rulein HM, Kramer R, Drash A. Hyperosmolality complicating diabetes mellitus in childhood. *J Pediatr* 1969; 74: 177–86.
8. Kety SS, Polis BC, Nadler CS, Schmidt CF. Blood flow and oxygen consumption of human brain in diabetic acidosis and coma. *J Clin Invest* 1948; 27: 500–10.
9. Daughaday WH. Diabetic acidosis. In: Williams R, ed. *Diabetes*. Paul B Hoeber, Inc., Medical Division of Harper and Brothers, 49 East 33rd Street, New York, NY, USA. 1960; 516–48.
10. Widness JA, Cowett RM, Zeller WP, Susa JBS, Rubenstein AH, Schwartz R. Permanent neonatal diabetes in an infant of an insulin-dependent mother. *J Pediatr* 1982; 100: 926–9.

DISCUSSION

Dr. Dakou: I am disappointed that advances in therapy stopped at 1992. You did not add anything after that.

Dr. Schwartz: There is one thing that I didn't emphasize. The advent of antibiotics made a major change in patient survival. Before penicillin, in fact, furunculosis and carbunculosis were major problems, and we don't see these anymore. In terms of the larger picture, I agree we haven't made any major changes. Until we understand the etiology and can prevent the disease there is unlikely to be any further major progress.

Dr. Drash: I don't agree with you at all. There have been some very major advances. Patients don't understand what it was like 20 years ago. It has made a big difference that it is now easy to measure glycosylated hemoglobin, monitor blood glucose in the home, and have access to purified insulin; and what about the recent observations on ACE inhibitors and their possible effect on renal disease? I think we have made extraordinary advances in the last decade.

I would like to make some comments on your observations. It may well be that your distribution curve is truer than ours. Marian Rewers who spent a couple of years with us, has shown that by using appropriate statistical maneuvers you can usually identify two super-imposed curves in terms of the age of onset, and that there is an earlier peak at about 5 or 6 years of age. These look like your curves. From a clinical point of view, there do seem to be differences of a very major kind between the younger and the older onset groups. In the child under 6 or 7 at onset there seems to be a much more malignant early course. This group of patients very rarely goes into remission, either partial or complete. The older the age of onset the milder the course up to the time of diagnosis, and the greater the likelihood of clinical remission under appropriate management.

I have a couple of other comments. We are still seeing about 40% of new admissions with ketoacidosis, mild, moderate or severe. It is fascinating that in studies we have done with colleagues around the world there appears to be geographic variation in terms of the severity of the disease at presentation. These data have been published in several forms, but in general the greater the distance from the equator the greater the severity at presentation. For example in the Scandinavian countries you tend to see patients presenting with more severe disease and a higher frequency of ketoacidosis, while in Israel there is very little ketoacidosis. The other comment I would like to make is that there is a strong move around the world for outpatient initiation of therapy in the newly diagnosed diabetic child. We have avoided that in Pittsburgh, maybe because we are slow and recalcitrant, but our system is set up for inpatient evaluation and teaching. On the other hand, half of our new patients have ketoacidosis, and I am very concerned about trying to manage those patients from home. I think all of us who have been involved in the management of diabetic ketoacidosis respect it greatly;

I don't sleep well when a new case comes in, and management of these patients is very worrying.

Dr. Schwartz: We also have been concerned about outpatient management. We just don't think it is safe in our environment. So we are not going to do it until we are forced to.

Dr. Dakou: Our experience as far as mode of presentation is concerned is coma in 6% (which you did not mention at all), acidosis in 34%, polyuria/polydipsia in 84%, and a purely incidental finding in 6%. A few people make the diagnosis themselves from the symptoms.

Dr. Swift: I would like to make one or two supportive comments about outpatient management of children with diabetes. Of course whether or not this is appropriate depends upon the health of the child at presentation, but if the child is not acidotic, has a pH above 7.2, and is not vomiting, then they can be managed out of hospital just like adults. However, this depends entirely on the level of community care available. I also agree with Drash that we have made major advances in the last decade or so in the overall management of children with diabetes, particularly in countries in which we have been able to enlist the help of nurses. One of the major advances in the past decade is the enlistment of nurses who can work not only in the hospital but also in the home and in the community.

Dr. Schwartz: As far as outpatient therapy is concerned, I think we have to discriminate between new patients and a patient with known disease who, for example, gets an infection and develops ketoacidosis. I think Drash and I are in agreement that new patients have to be admitted, whether they walk in or are carried in, because they have to be educated. I am less concerned about giving them insulin than I am about teaching them all the things they have to learn in order to take care of themselves subsequently. That is the real problem. In our group, the patient who is a known diabetic and who develops an infection with acidosis will be seen in the emergency room and given appropriate intravenous fluids. If vomiting stops and symptoms improve over the course of several hours, they can go home and we communicate by phone. If vomiting persists, they have to be admitted.

Dr. Dakou: We do the same. We admit newly diagnosed cases to hospital and we try to keep out of hospital those who come up with complications. I would like to ask those who handle their patients on an outpatient basis whether they have evidence that the families are better adapted afterwards, or whether the children are better able to accept the disease. Such data would give support to outpatient treatment of new diabetics, at least those who come in walking.

Dr. Swift: There are very few units that do not admit children to hospital but there is no evidence of detriment in not admitting to hospital. I agree absolutely with Schwartz's comment that the most important thing in the first week or two after the diagnosis is good education, and in my view that can be done on an outpatient basis better than on an inpatient basis because once a child is admitted to hospital the parents and children meet at least 20 or 30 different people, all of them giving slightly different messages. If you can do the education on an outpatient basis with a small team of perhaps three people, a doctor, a nurse, and.a dietician, then a consistent message can be given.

Dr. Chiumello: I completely agree with you, but you have to consider the different realities. Israel is a small country and you can organize everything much better than one can, for instance, in big cities such Milan.

Dr. Crofford: Dr. Michael May of the Faculty of Medicine in Vanderbilt has analyzed data on factors influencing how long patients admitted to Vanderbilt hospital with diabetic ketoacidosis had to stay at the hospital. It was interesting that one of the major influences was whether they were cared for by a diabetes specialist or a general internist: there was a clear reduction in the duration of stay if they were cared for by a diabetes specialist. The presumed interpretation of this is that the specialist was more familiar with the system for providing outpatient education and training. When I have outpatient nurses and a good outpatient organization, it is unnecessary to keep the patient in the hospital longer than the time required to treat the emergency aspects of diabetic acidosis. As soon as that is over, the educational process can be done much more effectively in an outpatient setting than in an inpatient one.

Dr. Siadati: What is the most common cause of diabetic ketoacidosis in your experience? In my country stopping insulin and infection are the most common causes.

Dr. Schwartz: I would say infection with secondary vomiting is the most likely cause in our known diabetics. In the newly diagnosed diabetics I think it is delay in making the diagnosis.

Dr. Drash: I think a lot of our secondary cases are due to lack of insulin administration: many teenagers were simply not giving the appropriate doses over long periods of time.

Dr. Hoet: I think that for about 75% of the world the most common cause is the nonavailability of insulin. From a study we did a few years ago, that was quite obvious.

Diabetes, edited by Richard M. Cowett,
Nestlé Nutrition Workshop Series,
Vol. 35. Nestec Ltd.,
Vevey/Raven Press, Ltd., New York © 1995.

Long-Term Consequences of Diabetes and Its Complications May Have a Fetal Origin: Experimental and Epidemiological Evidence

B. Reusens, S. Dahri, A. Snoeck, N. Bennis-Taleb, C. Remacle, and J. J. Hoet

Cell Biology Laboratory, Catholic University of Louvain, 1348 Louvain-la-Neuve, Belgium and WHO-Collaborating Center for the Development of Biology of Endocrine Pancreas

Patients with insulin-dependent diabetes may suffer from major vascular disease leading to retinopathy, glomerulonephropathy and hypertension as well as to neuropathy, especially in the presence of poor metabolic control. Recently, the DCCT study (Diabetes Control and Complication Trial) reported the prevention or delay of these complications by normalization of blood sugar with intensive insulin treatment (see chapter by Crofford). The reason why not all patients develop vascular complications, even in the presence of poor control of long duration, is not apparent (1,2) but predisposing factors should contribute. Reduced weight at birth and at 1 year of age are predictive for vascular disease and hypertension in adult life in diabetic and nondiabetic subjects (3). Adult onset diabetes and insulin resistance is also associated with abnormal development during intrauterine life and in the early postnatal period (4). These observations are based on retrospective studies but suggest that adverse metabolic conditions in the intrauterine environment may disturb the normal development of fetal target tissues involved in complications of non-insulin-dependent as well as insulin-dependent diabetes. Metabolic pathways in target tissues may not be able to adapt or compensate, or may have become sensitive to adverse metabolic conditions. They may be prone to further deterioration in the presence of adverse conditions later in life, such as poorly controlled diabetes, which would accelerate the process. Target tissues such as blood vessels or nephrons with developmental alterations may react inappropriately to trigger mechanisms, for example, raised blood glucose, and this would initiate the chain of events leading to vascular or renal complications. The issue of the fetal origin of vascular complications, which is apparent for the population in general, should also be examined in subjects with non-insulin-dependent or insulin-dependent diabetes. A fetal origin of predisposing factors would explain susceptibility to the development of vascular anomalies, leading to retinal and renal pathology in a subset of patients.

The objective of this chapter is to present experimental and epidemiological evidence relating deleterious events during fetal life to the occurrence of degenerative pathology later in life. A striking relationship of this kind has already been shown for fetal alterations in the endocrine pancreas inducing diabetes in later life.

MATERNAL NUTRITION IN PREGNANCY AND CONSEQUENCES FOR THE OFFSPRING IN LATER LIFE

High blood sugar levels resulting from maternal diabetes or from the administration of glucose during pregnancy can impair organ performance in the fetus (5). The effects on the endocrine pancreas are especially important. The composition of pancreatic tissues and the proliferative and secretory functions of the β cells are affected (6).

Other disturbances dating from the fetal period may also have metabolic consequences in later life. For example, a low-protein, isocaloric diet given to the mother during pregnancy affects the development of the fetal pancreas (7). Current results from studies in rats show how variations in maternal protein intake can induce metabolic anomalies in both the pregnant dams and their fetuses. In pregnant rats fed a low-protein (8% instead of 20%), isocaloric diet throughout pregnancy, there are striking alterations in metabolism. More adipose tissue accumulates in the peritoneum of protein-restricted mothers than in control dams, and the plasma becomes lipidemic in the second half of pregnancy (Fig. 1), although glucose and insulin levels in maternal and fetal serum and in the amniotic fluid remain unchanged (8). Although total serum amino acids as well as pooled essential and nonessential serum amino acids are also unchanged at 21.5 days of gestation in the protein-restricted group (Table 1), the low-protein diet induces changes in the concentration of several specific amino acids in maternal and fetal serum (Table 2). The concentrations of histidine, isoleucine, phenylalanine, and valine are significantly reduced in the serum of dams fed the low-protein diet, and the histidine concentration is significantly lower in fetuses from dams fed the low-protein diet than in the controls. The amino acids α-amino butyric acid and taurine, which are derived from metabolic pathways, are significantly reduced in maternal and fetal serum in the protein-restricted group. In contrast, citrulline concentration is raised in both maternal and fetal serum in the protein-restricted group. The concentrations of all amino acids remain higher in the fetus than in the mother, whether or not the mother is fed the protein-restricted diet. These results indicate that a low-protein, isocaloric diet given during pregnancy modifies the levels of specific amino acids such as taurine and citrulline in the mother and the fetus. Taurine, which is particularly involved in development (9), is reduced in the fetus. Considerable amounts of taurine are necessary for normal development. In taurine-deprived pregnant animals, large rates of fetal loss occur. Live, full-term births are rare and surviving progeny even more so. Taurine deficiency during pregnancy in cats affects fetal growth as well as brain and retinal development and induces limb alterations (9).

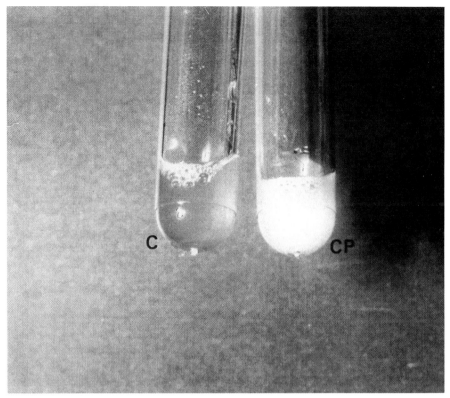

FIG. 1. Plasma of the mother fed with 20% protein **(C)** and with 8% protein **(CP)** at 21.5 days of gestation.

TABLE 1. *Pooled amino acids concentrations (AA) in the serum of mother and fetus at 21.5 days of gestation (MEAN (nmol/ml)* ± *SEM, n = 4); differences between the low-protein and control groups are not significant*

	Control	Low protein
AA mother	2158 ± 126	1964 ± 130
AA fetus	6209 ± 327	5607 ± 707
Essential AA		
Mother	1406 ± 116	1159 ± 56
Fetus	3832 ± 219	3312 ± 457
Nonessential AA		
Mother	751 ± 30	805 ± 75
Fetus	2377 ± 141	2295 ± 257

TABLE 2. *Individual amino acid concentrations in maternal and fetal serum at 21.5 days of gestation*

| | Control | | Low protein | |
	Mother	Fetus	Mother	Fetus
Histidine	35 ± 3	106 ± 11	25 ± 2[a]	63 ± 12[b]
Isoleucine + leucine	205 ± 23	545 ± 36	137 ± 1[a]	412 ± 66
Phenylalanine	70 ± 3	266 ± 42	57 ± 3[a]	238 ± 37
Valine	114 ± 19	415 ± 39	85 ± 7[a]	300 ± 50
α-Aminobutyric acid	75 ± 18	160 ± 23	32 ± 4[a]	74 ± 15[a]
Taurine	181 ± 12	356 ± 32	112 ± 19[a]	234 ± 31[c]
Citrulline	102 ± 5	115 ± 2	149 ± 15[c]	179 ± 15[c]

Differences between control and low protein mothers or control and low-protein fetus: [a] $p = 0.014$, [b] $p = 0.057$, [c] $p = 0.029$. Values are means (nmol/ml) ± SEM, n = 4.

Weight gain during pregnancy is also of interest in our experiment. There is a reduced weight gain in the low protein group during the last 48 hours of gestation, the final weight gain being 85.4 ± 1.7 g (n = 39) *versus* 95.7 ± 3.7 g (n = 29) in the control group, despite a similar energy intake in the two groups. This isocaloric, low-protein diet affects weight gain only in pregnancy and not in the nonpregnant state; in nonpregnant rats, a similar diet caused no reduction in normal weight gain over 22 days when compared with a control group on normal diet (8).

The isocaloric, protein-restricted diet given to the mother also affects weight gain and organ composition in the fetus. A significant reduction in fetal weight at 21.5 days and in newborn weight is observed in the protein-restricted group: fetal body weight was 4.09 ± 0.03 g (n = 175) for the low-protein fetus *versus* 4.18 ± 0.03 g (n = 134) for the control fetus; birthweight was 4.86 ± 0.04 g (n = 118) in the low-protein newborn *versus* 5.14 ± 0.04 g (n = 97) in the control newborn. Values at both ages are significantly different ($p < 0.0001$).

The structure and function of the endocrine pancreas are disturbed in the low-protein group. Islet cell proliferation, islet size, and pancreatic insulin content are significantly reduced by 18%, 21%, and 30%, respectively, in newborns of mothers fed the isocaloric, low-protein diet (7). When islets from the fetuses of protein-deprived mothers are challenged *in vitro* with amino acids such as leucine and arginine in the presence of glucose, their insulin response is significantly reduced compared with islets from fetuses from the control group (10). Cyclic adenosine monophosphate (cAMP) content is also lower in the islets of fetuses from mothers fed the isocaloric, low-protein diet and does not increase to normal levels following a challenge with insulin secretagogues such as glucose or amino acids (11).

Pathological findings in human infants suffering from primary malnutrition have also shown a reduction of total pancreas weight and pancreatic endocrine tissue weight (12).

These experimental and pathological observations illustrate the adjustments that are required in the structure and function of the endocrine pancreas when metabolic and nutritional alterations occur in the intrauterine milieu.

Besides the effect on the endocrine cells, the most obvious additional effect of the low-protein diet on the fetal pancreas is reduced vascularization of the endocrine pancreas. This is substantial, vessel density being reduced to 62% of that in the controls (7). Developing blood vessels thus seem to be sensitive to the metabolic modifications of the intrauterine milieu induced by protein restriction in the mother.

Moreover, the developing kidney is also affected. An acquired nephron deficit of 40% has been reported in the fetal rat when the mother is fed a low-protein diet (5% protein) during pregnancy (13). A hereditary deficit of nephron numbers in rats has been shown to be associated with functional alterations that enhance susceptibility to hypertension and cause acceleration of glomerular sclerosis in later life (14). In infants, malnutrition reduces kidney weight and reduced the number of glomeruli (12). The same findings are apparent in infants with a birthweight below the 10th percentile (15).

It is apparent from these observations that a low-protein diet given to a pregnant mother reduces the numbers of pancreatic islet cells and nephrons and affects the proliferation of vascular endothelial cells in the fetus of both the human and the rat. It is possible that later catch-up growth could be compromised, and this is likely to have consequences in adult life. Long-term studies of the functional and structural development of the endocrine pancreas and the kidney may reveal pathological features.

Study of the development of the endocrine pancreas may reveal more about the consequences of intrauterine events. To investigate this further, we studied three groups of rats: a control group (C) fed a normal (20%) protein diet during intrauterine life, during the suckling period, and after weaning; a low-protein diet group (LP) fed a low-protein diet (8%) during intrauterine life, during the suckling period, and after weaning; and a recuperation group (R) fed a low-protein diet only during fetal life and a normal (20% protein) diet during the suckling period, and after weaning.

Results showed that there was a reduction in glucose tolerance by adult age in the LP and R groups when compared with the C group. Insulin response was lower in the LP and R groups (10). Further data showed that female adult animals from the R group were more affected than male (16). The insulin content of the endocrine pancreas was significantly lower in the LP group than in the C and R groups. The *in vitro* insulin response of the β cells to glucose and amino acids (leucine and arginine) was significantly lower in the LP and R group (11,17). The reduction in the secretory function of the β cells already observed in the neonatal period persisted in the adult offspring and especially in the progeny of mothers fed an isocaloric, low-protein diet and receiving the same diet until adulthood (LP group). The β cells of the R group retained a deficiency in their insulin response to stimulation by arginine with or without theophylline, (11,17). This indicates that a normal diet postnatally does not completely restore the lesions induced by a low-protein diet during pregnancy.

We have verified the lack of adaptation of the endocrine pancreas to a physiological challenge such as pregnancy in the low birth weight progeny of mothers fed an isocaloric, low-protein diet during pregnancy (17). The progeny are unable to regain an appropriate insulin secretory response to a glucose challenge even when given a normal protein diet throughout postnatal life. The imprint of metabolic changes acquired during the developmental stage and relating to the secretory function of the endocrine pancreas persists and prevents this function from adapting properly to a physiological challenge such as pregnancy, even with normal feeding postnatally.

The vascular density of the endocrine pancreas, which was reduced at birth when the mother had received a low-protein diet, normalizes by adult age when the offspring are fed a normal diet after birth. This normalization does not occur when a low-protein diet is given until adult age (16). Therefore these vessels are capable of proliferating postnatally with proper nutrition. However, the functional characteristics of the vessels are unknown. Preliminary results also show a reduction in blood vessel density of adult brain in rats in the low-protein group, although vessel density in the liver is not affected at birth and shows a 10% increase by adult age (data not shown). Angiogenesis during fetal life thus seems to be affected in different ways depending on the type of organ. These data emphasize the sensitivity of the blood vessel proliferation process to metabolic changes in the intrauterine milieu induced by protein deprivation.

Low birthweight offspring possessing fewer nephrons at birth develop glomerulosclerosis prematurely (14). This implies that progressive glomerular pathology results from an acquired deficit in nephron numbers, assuming normal kidney function during postnatal life. The loss of nephrons is accelerated by additional renal injury or aging (18).

The experimental data presented above show that a single identifiable factor such as a low-protein, isocaloric diet given during pregnancy may explain not only low birthweight but also changes in the structure and function of specific cells such as β cells, endothelial cells, and glomeruli that are determinants for later morbidity in the offspring.

EPIDEMIOLOGICAL EVIDENCE

Epidemiological evidence should confirm the relationship between metabolic changes in the mother and alterations in fetal tissues that are targets for diabetic complications.

Atherosclerotic fatty streaks and the gradual formation of fibrous plaques are already evident before the age of 3 years. In infants, risk factors for adult vascular disease may appear soon after birth. These pathological changes occur more often in small-for-dates infants and in infants from underprivileged communities where thinness at birth is frequent (19,20). Low birthweight subjects are also prone to develop syndrome X, insulin resistance, and aberrations of coagulation factors later in life (3,4). Since there is a continuum of risk factors from early infancy through to adult life, it is important to realize that disturbances of fetal development caused by maternal ill health or inappropriate diet may result in pathological events in later life. Poor physique of the mother is often associated with reduced birthweight of the offspring, who are in turn then made susceptible to life-threatening events such as stroke, cardiovascular disease, hypertension, and diabetes (3,4).

Even among normal infants in a prospective study, subsets classified by lower (<3.100 g) or higher (>3.700 g) birthweights already have higher blood pressures by 4 years of age, although there are different regulatory patterns during growth (21). The late occurrence of syndrome X is also significantly more common in a cohort of subjects of low birthweight (4,20,22). A similar trend relating low birthweight to later diabetes has already been emphasized.

Both the experimental and the epidemiological data highlight how the intrauterine environment, which is influenced by maternal health and nutrition, determines the development of risk factors for later chronic vascular disease.

DISCUSSION AND IMPLICATIONS

The experimental results described here emphasize the role of maternal metabolism in determining the number of fetal β cells and their proliferative capacity and secretory function. Metabolic consequences such as diabetes in the offspring may ensue if the mother has experienced high blood glucose levels or low dietary protein intake during pregnancy. A low-protein diet during pregnancy also appears to impair the growth of the kidney such that the number of nephrons in the neonate is reduced (13). Protein deprivation interferes specifically with renal development in the primate fetus: kidney weights are reduced by 25% when pregnant mothers are fed diets with adequate energy but reduced protein but not when they are fed a low-energy, protein-sufficient diet (23). Hypoxia due to experimental intrauterine growth retardation in the rat also causes a reduction of the number of β cells (24) and nephrons (13). Similar observations have been made in the human (12,25,26). These experimental and pathological observations indicate that the β cells and the renal glomeruli are very sensitive to disturbed intrauterine metabolism. Both tissues have a limited capacity to increase their cell numbers after birth. The number of nephrons also tends to decrease after the age of 40 years (14). This decrease results in alterations in glomerular function that may cause hypertension and ensuing damage to the vascular system. This has been shown in individuals known to have a critical decrease in nephron number and also in experimental studies (14). On the basis of our observations, it seems likely that the development of blood vessels in specific target tissues may also be impaired by intrauterine metabolic derangements, although postnatal recovery seems possible (17). Further study is required to establish whether the restored vasculature is functionally normal.

Patients with type 1 and type 2 diabetes have a similar risk of nephropathy (2) and in both types some subjects are susceptible but others are resistant to the development of hypertension. Susceptibility seems to have a familial origin, since diabetic patients who develop renal complications are more likely to have a parental history of essential hypertension (14). The hypothesis of a congenital nephron deficiency that may contribute to hypertension in the parents and to the susceptibility to hypertension and glomerular injury in the diabetic offspring has been raised (14). The prevention of hypertension in spontaneously hypertensive rats *in utero* by early treatment of the mother with an angiotensin-converting enzyme inhibitor is an example of the influence of environmental factors on fetal development. Primary prevention was possible only *in utero,* and the normalizing effect was maintained after withdrawal of the inhibitor from the offspring after birth. The untreated second generation was also devoid of hypertension (27).

The mechanisms by which maternal events affect the developing fetus and specifically how protein deprivation affects the tissues that are responsible for the occurrence of late diabetic complications are unknown. The low levels of serum taurine that we observed in protein-deprived rats might predispose developing renal tissue to disease later on, when trigger mechanisms such as poorly controlled diabetes intervene. Taurine is known to play an essential role in brain development but is found in almost all mammalian tissues and constitutes over 50% of the free amino acids in many tissues (9).

Although no specific studies seem to have been reported on taurine and the developing kidney, the potential importance of taurine is emphasized by recent observations in streptozotocin (STZ) diabetic rats (28). In this model, the severity of diabetic glomerulonephropathy is significantly reduced by treatment with taurine. Improvement in function also occurs, with creatinine clearance doubling and albuminuria decreasing by 30% in the taurine-treated group compared with untreated diabetic animals. Renal taurine concentrations and the pattern of localization of taurine within the renal parenchyma are altered in STZ diabetic rats and may be restored with taurine administration (28). The increase in serum triglycerides observed in STZ diabetic rats is also attenuated by taurine (29).

Taurine metabolism is presumably involved in several tissues that are targets for diabetic complications. Taurine is reduced in the peripheral neural tissues of STZ diabetic animals, although taurine supplementation does not restore taurine levels or neural function to normal (30). In STZ diabetic animals, the retina shows a reduced uptake of taurine (31), and the heart has an increased taurine content (32). Taurine also has a blood pressure lowering action in spontaneously hypertensive rats and attenuates the hypercholesterolemia that occurs in these animals (33). In normal rats, taurine lowers serum, liver, and aortic cholesterol (29).

Being a zwitterion, taurine penetrates cell membranes and prevents the intracellular production of oxygen free radicals that seem to be implicated in the development of pathological lesions of the kidneys (9). A reduction in tissue taurine would be expected to hinder the normal effect of taurine in preventing the intracellular accumulation of oxidative stress molecules. The increased citrulline we observed in our animals may have been liberated through the arginine pathway following the accumulation of oxygen free radicals.

In the human, serum taurine levels have been analyzed in several situations, such as in vegetarians (34) and in patients with cystic fibrosis or hypertension (35). Alterations in taurine concentrations in tissues and urine as well as in plasma have been detected in hypertensive patients. Taurine concentrations are also very low in the breast milk of vegans. These data show that taurine metabolism is modulated by the reduction in total protein intake and by the changes induced in specific protein biosynthesis or transport in these conditions.

CONCLUSION

Experimental and epidemiological evidence highlights the importance of maternal metabolic and nutritional disturbances for intrauterine development. These influence the development of tissues that are targets for diabetes or its later complications. Alterations in the endocrine pancreas, blood vessels, and nephrons have been identified. Diabetes developing postnatally may aggravate an inherited deficit in the numbers of glomeruli and blood vessels, and this may set the scene for the later development of hypertension and vascular disease. In such circumstances, diabetes and poor diabetic control may initiate a chain of events leading to major deterioration of vascular function and renal function, both already predisposed to impairment by prenatal events.

Poor nutrition during pregnancy can be shown to compromise normal development and birthweight in the offspring. Taurine biosynthesis and transport may play a key role during development and in later life. Intrauterine events other than nutrition and leading, for example, to low birthweight should be suspected as well. A fetal origin of late diabetic complications and their progression may explain why only a subset of persons with diabetes is susceptible to developing major complications. This implies the need to search for early predisposing factors favoring the progression of late complications when there is poor diabetic control. Additional experimental, clinical and epidemiological studies are needed. The DCCT data and other studies may reveal factors in early development that could explain why high blood glucose levels induce degenerative complications only in a subset of persons with diabetes.

REFERENCES

1. Hasslacher C, Ritz E, Terpstra J, *et al*. Natural history of nephropathy in type 1 diabetes. Relationships to metabolic control and blood pressure. *Hypertension* 1985; 7 (suppl II): 74–8.
2. Hasslacher C, Wahl P, Ritz E. Similar risks of nephropathy in type 1 and 2 diabetes. *Kidney Int* 1988; 133: A193. (Abstract).
3. Hales CN, Barker DJP. Type 2 (non-insulin dependent) diabetes mellitus: the thrifty phenotype hypothesis. *Diabetologia* 1992; 35: 595–601.
4. Phillips DIW, Barker DJP, Hales CN, Osmond C. Thinness at birth and insulin resistance in adult life. *Diabetologia* 1994: 37: 150–4.
5. Reusens-Billen B, Remacle C, Hoet JJ. The development of the fetal rat intestine and its reaction to maternal diabetes. II. Effect of mild and severe maternal diabetes. *Diabetes Res Clin Pract* 1989; 6: 213–9.
6. Holemans K, Aerts L, Verhaeghe J, Van Assche FA. Maternal diabetes: consequences for the

offspring. An experimental model in the rat. In: *Diabetes* The 35th Nestlé Nutrition Workshop. New York: Raven Press, Vevey: Nestec Ltd. in press.

7. Snoeck A, Remacle C, Reusens B, Hoet JJ. Effect of a low protein diet during pregnancy on the fetal rat endocrine pancreas. *Biol Neonate* 1990; 57: 107–18.

8. Snoeck A. *Perturbations du pancréas endocrine pendant la gestation sous l'effet de la carence en protéines chez le rat. Conséquences sur le développement foetal et post-natal.* Louvain-la-Neuve, Belgium: UCL, Faculté des Sciences, 1993. Doctoral thesis.

9. Sturman JA. Taurine in development. *Physiol Rev* 1993; 37: 119–47.

10. Dahri S, Snoeck A, Reusens B, Remacle C, Hoet JJ. Islet function in offspring of mothers on low protein diet during gestation. *Diabetes* 1991; 40 (suppl 2): 15–20.

11. Dahri S, Cherif H, Reusens B, Remacle C, Hoet JJ. Effects of an isocaloric low protein diet during gestation in rat on in vitro insulin secretion by islets of the offspring. *Diabetologia* 1994; 37 (suppl): A 80.

12. Naeye RL. Malnutrition, probable cause of growth retardation. *Arch Pathol* 1965; 79: 284–91.

13. Merlet-Benichou C, Lelièvre-Pegorier M, Gilbert T, Muffat-Joly M, Leroy B. Intra-uterine growth retardation (IUGR) and inborn nephron deficit in rat. *J Am Soc Nephrol* 1992; 3: 49P. (Abstract)

14. Brenner BM, Garcia DL, Anderson S. Glomeruli and blood pressure. Less of one, more the other? *Am J Hypertens* 1988; 1: 335–47.

15. Leroy B, Josset P, Morgan G, Costil J, Merlet-Benichou C. *Pediatr Nephrol* 1991; 5: C21. (Abstract)

16. Dahri S, Snoeck A, Reusens B, Remacle C, Hoet JJ. Low protein diet during gestation in rats: its relevance to human non-insulin dependent diabetes. *J Physiol* (Lond) 1993; 467: 292P. (Abstract)

17. Dahri S, Reusens B, Remacle C, Hoet JJ. Nutritional influences on pancreatic development and potential links with non insulin dependent diabetes. *Proc Nutr Soc* 1995; 54 (in press).

18. Brenner BM. The etiology of adult hypertension and progressive renal injury: an hypothesis. *Bull Acad R Belg Med* 1994; 149: 1–2.

19. Blonde CV, Webber LS, Foster TA, Berenson GG. Parental history and cardiovascular disease, risk variables in children. *Prev Med* 1981; 10: 25–37.

20. King H, Finch C, Zimmet P, Alpers M. Plasma glucose and insulin responses in young Papua New Guineans (aged 10–19 years). *Diabetes Res Clin Pract* 1990; 10: 153–9.

21. Launer LJ, Hofman A, Grobbee DE. Relation between birth weight and blood pressure: longitudinal study of infants and children. *BMJ* 1993; 307: 1451–4.

22. Valdez R, Athens MA, Thompson GH, Bradshaw BS, Stern MP. Birthweight and adult health outcomes in a biethnic population in the USA. *Diabetologia* 1994; 37: 626–31.

23. Cheek DB, Hill DE. Changes in somatic growth after placental insufficiency and maternal protein deprivation. In: Cheek DB, ed. *Fetal and postnatal cellular growth hormones and nutrition.* New York: John Wiley & Sons, 1975: 299–310.

24. De Prins F, Van Assche A. Intrauterine growth retardation and development of the endocrine pancreas in the experimental rat. *Biol Neonate* 1982; 41: 16–21.

25. Van Assche FA, Aerts L. The fetal endocrine pancreas. *Contrib Gynecol Obstet* 1979; 5: 44–57.

26. Milner RDG. Metabolic and hormonal response to glucose and glucagon in patients with infantile malnutrition. *Pediatr Res* 1971; 5: 33–9.

27. Wu J-N, Berecek KM. Prevention of genetic hypertension by early treatment of spontaneously hypertensive rats with the angiotensin converting enzyme inhibitor captopril. *Hypertension* 1993; 22: 139–46.

28. Trachman H, Lu P, Sturman JH. Immunohistochemical localization of taurine in rat renal tissue: studies in experimental disease states. *J Histochem Cytochem* 1993; 41: 1209–16.

29. Goodman HO, Shihabi ZK. Supplemental taurine in diabetic rats: effects on plasma glucose and triglycerides. *Biochem Med Metab Biol* 1990; 43: 1–9.

30. Stevens MJ, Lattimer SA, Kamijo M, Van Huysen C, Sima AAF, Greene DA. Osmotically-induced nerve taurine depletion and the compatible osmolyte hypothesis in experimental diabetic neuropathy in the rat. *Diabetologia* 1993; 36: 608–14.

31. Caputo S, Di Leo MAS, Lepore D, et al. Reduction of taurine uptake in retina of streptozotocin diabetic (STZ-D) rat. *Diabetes* 1994; 43 (suppl 1): A352. (Abstract)

32. Atlas M, Bahl JJ, Roeske W, Bressler R. In vitro osmoregulation of taurine in fetal mouse hearts. *J Mol Cell Cardiol* 1984; 16: 311–20.

33. Yamori Y, Nara Y, Horie R, Ooshima A, Lovenberg W. In: Schaffer SW, Baskin SI, Koesis JJ, eds. *The effects of taurine on excitable tissues.* New York: Spectrum, 1981: 391.

34. Rana SK, Sanders T. Taurine concentrations in the diet, plasma urine and breast milk of vegans compared with omnivores. *Br J Nutr* 1986; 56: 17–27.

35. Thompson GN, Thomas FM. Protein metabolism in cystic fibrosis: responses to malnutrition and taurine supplementation. *Am J Clin Nutr* 1987; 46: 606–13.

DISCUSSION

Dr. Steenhout: If your rat model is correct and has some similarities with the human, how do we explain the epidemiological studies, for example, the studies of Drash showing a decrease in frequency from north to south? Finland, for example, is certainly not a country where malnutrition occurs in mothers during pregnancy.

Dr. Hoet: The north-to-south gradient is mainly applicable to type 1 diabetes, and my presentation was really concerned with type 2 diabetes. In order to comment further on your question and with regard to complications that may have an origin *in utero,* why should type 1 cases not inherit complications similar to type 2? One of the factors we have analyzed during fetal development is a low-protein diet affecting the development of fetal blood vessels, but this does not mean there are no other factors predisposing the individual to complications.

Dr. Drash: I should like to make some comments from a pediatric perspective. As practicing pediatricians, we are now faced with a dilemma, which is the widespread concept that bigger is better. Everybody wants boys to grow up to be tall, so we are under pressure to give growth hormones to children who are a little below average in size, and performance-enhancing drugs are being used indiscriminately to produce bigger muscles. But what about the longstanding data in animals showing that chronic, moderate malnutrition results in longer life? If length of life is an important index, there must be some middle ground between what our current Western society is doing, with all the problems of arteriosclerosis, etc., and the severe malnutrition that I think your model may represent. We need some real guidance in terms of public health policy as to how to attain that middle road.

Dr. Hoet: There are certainly reasons for believing that bigger is not better. It is clear for example that the macrosomic infants of the Pima Indians are going to become diabetic, and presumably, although we don't know this yet for certain, they will have vascular anomalies. But what is also of interest is that the low-birthweight infants of the Pima Indians are also at risk. I would remind you as well about the paper published in *British Medical Journal* in 1993 (1) in which it was shown that, at 4 years of age, blood pressure was higher in children of low birthweight (<3100 g) *and* in those weighing more than 3700 g at birth than in children of normal birthweight. The point is that a child may be predisposed to major aberrations by low birthweight and by high birthweight. What this type of data indicates is that public attention must be shifted away from diet and exercise at age 40 and toward health promotion in younger individuals and in mothers.

Dr. Assan: Does your malnutrition syndrome in rats have some correspondence with the two main malnutrition diabetic syndromes in humans, I mean kwashiorkeo and calcific pancreatitis with diabetes of nonalcoholic origin?

Dr. Hoet: Malnutrition diabetes is still a matter of much discussion. Presumably it exists, and I definitely agree with you that calcification in the pancreas of these individuals has been observed. In general, we did not see calcification, but what we did observe in our animals, as soon as we put them on a low-protein diet, was a great reduction in their pancreatic insulin content during pregnancy, so malnutrition diabetes may be a consequence of the low-protein diet these people are taking, and the calcification may have other causes.

Dr. Catalano: In the low-protein-diet group what was the remainder of the diet? Does it make any difference whether it is a low-protein/high-fat diet or a low-protein/high-carbohy-drate diet?

Dr. Hoet: This is a very important question. In our study, the low-protein, isocaloric diet was a high-carbohydrate diet. Your question gives the opportunity of underlining observations that were made as long as 30–35 years by Tejning (2), who analyzed the endocrine pancreas in male and female adult rats that were fed either with high-carbohydrate, high-fat, or high-protein diet. The high-fat diet induced the lowest endocrine pancreatic mass when compared with a natural diet. A high-protein diet increases the endocrine tissue by 25% in male and 36% in female, while a high-carbohydrate diet enhances the pancreatic tissue by 51% in male and 76% in female. These results indicate the greater plasticity of the β cells in females. The high-carbohydrate, low-protein, isocaloric diet used in our investigation, which is administered to the mother, results in an abnormal oral glucose tolerance (OGT) and low insulin levels in the female but not in the male offspring when fed a normal diet after birth. Therefore, there is already a different effect of a low-protein diet on the β cell of female when compared with the male offspring. It indicates the greater sensitivity of β cells in female animals as well as the greater plasticity of female *versus* male β cells.

Dr. Carrascosa: As you know, insulin growth factors play an important role in growth proliferation and differentiation during fetal and postnatal life. Do you have any data about the levels of insulin growth factor (IGF) I or II in your experimental animal model?

Dr. Hoet: Yes we do. There are no major changes in this model, either in the mother or in the neonate for the IGF-I, but binding proteins have not been verified as yet in our model. We don't really know about the fetal stage but, at time of birth, there do not seem to be major changes.

Dr. Scott: You mentioned declining taurine and increasing citrulline. Would you expand on those findings?

Dr. Hoet: Taurine is an amino acid derived from methionine and cysteine. Taurine may improve the pathological observations in the kidney of streptozotocin diabetic rats. Taurine distribution is decreased in the renal parenchyma of streptozotocin diabetic rats and taurine administration to these animals restores the pattern (3) Moreover, a lessening of the glomerular-sclerotic lesion and tubulo-interstitial damage of streptozotocin diabetic rats is observed when the animals are treated with taurine. Functional improvement is also achieved as stated in the text.

REFERENCES

1. Launer LJ, Hofman A, and Grobbee DE. Relation between birth and blood pressure: longitudinal study of infants and children. *Brit Med J* 1993; 307: 1451–4.
2. Tejning S. Dietary factors and quantitative morphology of the islets of Langerhans. *Acta Medica Scandinavica.* Suppl 1947: 1–154.
3. Trachman H, Lu P, and Sturman JH. Immunohistochemical localization of taurine in rat renal tissue: studies in experimental disease states. *J Histochem Cytochem* 1993; 41: 1209–16.

Diabetes, edited by Richard M. Cowett,
Nestlé Nutrition Workshop Series,
Vol. 35. Nestec Ltd.,
Vevey/Raven Press, Ltd., New York © 1995.

The Effect of Intensive Diabetes Management on the Complications of Insulin-Dependent Diabetes Mellitus: Results of the Diabetes Control and Complications Trial

Oscar B. Crofford

*D-3100 Medical Center North, Vanderbilt University,
Nashville, Tennessee 37232-2358, USA*

The Diabetes Control and Complications Trial (DCCT) was designed to assess the value of intensive treatment in patients with insulin-dependent diabetes mellitus (IDDM). The study was conducted under the auspices of the National Institute of Diabetes, Digestive and Kidney Diseases (NIDDK), one of the 13 institutes of the National Institutes of Health in the United States. Studies in animal models of diabetes (1–3) and epidemiologic studies (4–6) had implicated hyperglycemia in the pathogenesis of the long-term complications of IDDM. Although previous clinical trials had suggested that a large-scale, long-term clinical trial in the United States and Canada was feasible (7–10), the NIDDK and the DCCT Study Group did not believe that a beneficial effect of intensive treatment had been conclusively demonstrated or that the risks and burdens of intensive treatment had been well documented (11). Thus the DCCT was designed with sufficient size and duration to test the glucose hypothesis definitively and to aid in clinical decision making by estimating the magnitude of the postulated benefits and risks. The first patient was enrolled in August, 1983, and the study ended in June, 1993, one year ahead of schedule. The results were summarized in the *New England Journal of Medicine* in October, 1993, (12).

METHODS

Design Features

The design and methodologic considerations for both the feasibility and full-scale phases of the DCCT have been published previously (13,14). Briefly, the DCCT was a randomized clinical trial conducted in 29 clinical centers in the United States and Canada. Specimens were collected, and examinations were performed locally in a standardized way by trained and certified personnel and transported to central units for analysis or grading by persons who were masked to patient identifiers and treatment-group assignment. The data were maintained and analyzed by the central data coordinating center, and outcome data were revealed only to an independent data monitoring committee (15). The sample size and trial duration estimates were based upon diabetic retinopathy as the principal study outcome. Patients were recruited into two cohorts; Primary Prevention and Secondary Intervention, on the basis of certain baseline characteristics as specified in the protocol. Patients in the Primary Prevention cohort had duration of IDDM ranging from 1–5 years and no evidence of background retinopathy or microalbuminuria. Patients in the Secondary Intervention cohort had duration of IDDM ranging from 1–15 years, early background retinopathy, and possible microalbuminuria. Within each cohort, patients were randomly assigned to receive either Conventional (Conv) or Intensive (Int) treatment. The basic analyses were conducted within each cohort and compared the two treatment groups with respect to the cumulative incidence of the outcome of interest using life table methods (16,17). Only one variable showed significant treatment-group imbalance at baseline, and analyses were carried out with and without adjustment for this imbalance (16).

Study Population

Over a period of 66 months, 1441 patients were enrolled, approximately 50 patients per clinical center. All patients had IDDM as defined by clinical criteria and C-peptide assay. The baseline characteristics of the patients have been published previously (12). They had the following general characteristics: youth (13–39 years of age, median age of 27); excellent general health (no known illness other than IDDM without major complications), 1–15 years of IDDM (mean of 5.7 years); physically fit (8% overweight and 19% sedentary); above average education (mean of 14 years); lack of racial diversity (96% Caucasian); and good gender balance (47% female).

Treatment Regimens

Conventional treatment consisted of one or two daily injections of insulin, including mixed intermediate and rapid-acting insulins, daily self-monitoring of urine or blood glucose, and education about diet and exercise. Conventional treatment did not usually include daily adjustments in the insulin dosage. The goals of conventional treatment included the absence of symptoms attributable to glycosuria or hyperglycemia; the absence of ketonuria; the maintenance of normal growth, development, and ideal body weight; and freedom from severe or frequent hypoglycemia. Women who became pregnant or were planning pregnancy received intensive treatment until the time of delivery, after which they resumed conventional treatment. Patients in the conventional treatment group were examined every three months.

Intensive treatment included the administration of insulin three or more times daily by injection or an external pump. The dosage was adjusted according to the results of self-monitoring of blood glucose, performed at least four times per day, to dietary intake, and to anticipated exercise. The goals of intensive treatment included preprandial blood glucose concentrations of between 3.9 and 6.7 mmol/liter (70 and 120 mg/dl), postprandial concentrations of less than 10 mmol/liter (180 mg/dl), a weekly 3 AM measurement greater than 3.6 mmol/liter (65 mg/dl), and hemoglobin A_{1c} (HbA_{1c}), measured monthly, within the normal range (<6.05%). The patients initially chose either multiple injections or pump treatment and could subsequently change to the other method if their glycemic goals were not achieved or if such was their preference. The patients in the intensive treatment group visited their study center each month and were contacted even more frequently by telephone to review and adjust their regimens.

RESULTS

Adherence and Metabolic Control

The entire cohort of 1441 patients was followed for a mean of 6.5 years (range, 3–9), a total of more than 9300 patient-years. Ninety-nine percent of the patients completed the study, and more than 95% of all scheduled examinations were completed. Eleven patients died, and eight patients were lost to follow-up. Overall, 97% of the patients on average received their assigned treatment. This includes 95 women assigned to conventional treatment who received intensive treatment during pregnancy or while planning a pregnancy.

The adherence to assigned treatment and the effectiveness of intensive treatment in lowering blood glucose concentrations were reflected in the substantial difference over time between the HbA_{1c} values of the intensive treatment group and those of the conventional treatment group (7.23 ± 0.96% versus 9.11 ± 1.31%, mean ± SD; $p < 0.001$). Although 44% of the patients receiving intensive treatment achieved the goal of a glycosylated hemoglobin value of 6.05% or less at least once during the study, fewer than 5% maintained an average value in this range. The blood glucose concentrations achieved with each treatment were measured with quarterly 7-point capillary blood glucose profiles. The mean (±SD) value for all glucose profiles in the intensive treatment group was 8.6 ± 1.7 mmol/liter (155 ± 30 mg/dl), compared with 12.8 ± 3.1 mmol/liter (231 ± 55 mg/dl) in the conventional treatment group ($p < 0.001$).

Retinopathy

Primary Prevention Cohort

The cumulative incidence of retinopathy, defined as a change of three steps or more on fundus photography that was sustained over a 6-month period, was similar in the two treatment groups until approximately 36 months, when the incidence

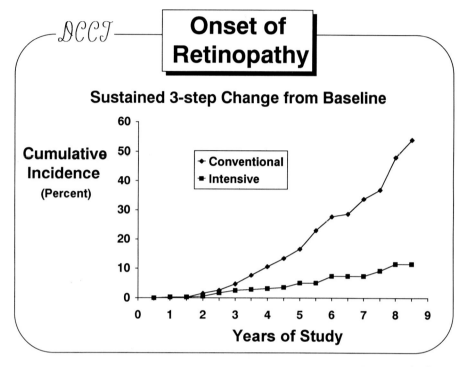

FIG. 1. Cumulative incidence of a sustained 3-step change from baseline in the onset of retinopathy in patients with insulin-dependent diabetes mellitus receiving conventional or intensive treatment.

curves began to separate (Fig. 1). From five years onward, the cumulative incidence of retinopathy in the intensive treatment group was approximately 50% less than in the conventional treatment group. During a mean of 6 years of follow-up, retinopathy as defined above developed in 23 patients in the intensive treatment group and in 91 patients in the conventional treatment group. Intensive treatment reduced the adjusted mean risk of retinopathy by 76% (95% confidence interval, 62–85%). For meaningful analyses, too few patients in the primary prevention cohort had proliferative or severe nonproliferative retinopathy (two in the intensive treatment group and four in the conventional treatment group) or clinically important macular edema (one and four, respectively), or required photocoagulation (three and two patients, respectively).

Secondary Intervention Cohort

The patients in the intensive treatment group had a higher cumulative incidence of sustained progression of retinopathy by three steps or more during the first year than did those in the conventional treatment group, but a lower cumulative incidence

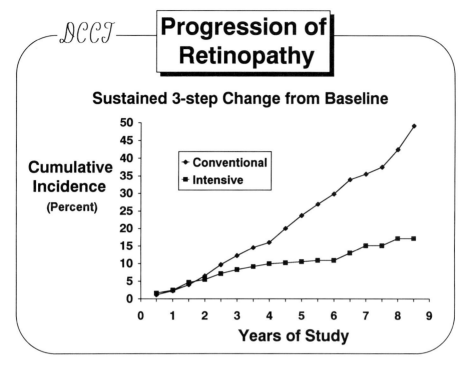

FIG. 2. Cumulative incidence of a sustained 3-step change from baseline in the progression of retinopathy in patients with insulin-dependent diabetes mellitus receiving conventional or intensive treatment.

beginning at 36 months and continuing for the rest of the study (Fig. 2). Intensive treatment reduced the average risk of such progression by 54% (95% confidence interval, 39–66%) during the entire study period (77 patients in the intensive treatment group and 143 patients in the conventional treatment group). Intensive treatment reduced the adjusted risk of proliferative or severe nonproliferative retinopathy by 47% (Fig. 3) and that of treatment with photocoagulation by 56% ($p = 0.011$ and 0.002 respectively).

One of the most important observations was that the beneficial effect of intensive treatment increased over time. Patients in the conventional treatment group showed the expected increase in the rate of progression of retinopathy with increasing duration of diabetes. In contrast, patients in the intensive treatment group showed stable or even decreasing rates of progression (Figs. 1–4). Accordingly, the best estimate of the long-term efficacy of intensive treatment would be a risk reduction of 80% or more.

Nephropathy

In both cohorts, microalbuminuria (defined as urinary albumin excretion, measured annually, of ≤28 μg/min) or albuminuria (urinary albumin excretion of ≤209 μg/min)

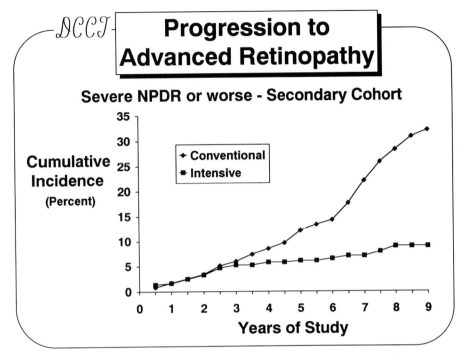

FIG. 3. Cumulative incidence of progression to severe nonproliferative diabetic retinopathy (NPDR) or worse in patients with insulin-dependent diabetes mellitus receiving conventional or intensive treatment.

developed in fewer patients in the intensive treatment group than in the conventional treatment group (Fig. 5). Intensive treatment reduced the mean adjusted risk of microalbuminuria by 34% ($p = 0.04$) in the primary prevention cohort and by 43% ($p = 0.001$) in the secondary intervention cohort. The risk of albuminuria was reduced by 56% ($p = 0.01$) in the secondary intervention cohort. Advanced nephropathy, as defined by urinary albumin excretion of ≤209 μg/min and a rate of creatinine clearance below 70 ml/min/1.73 m² of body surface area, developed in very few patients (two in the intensive treatment group and five in the conventional treatment group).

The cumulative incidence of microalbuminuria was analyzed among selected subgroups in the 1368 patients in both cohorts in whom urinary albumin excretion was less than 40 mg/24 h at baseline. The effect of intensive treatment in reducing risk was maintained with the subgroups defined according to age, sex, duration of IDDM, mean blood pressure, baseline glycosylated hemoglobin value, dietary protein intake, and history of smoking. In the secondary cohort, 73 subjects (38 treated intensively, 35 treated conventionally) had AER (albumin excretion rate) levels ≤28 μg/min at the time of entry into the study. In each treatment group, eight developed AER ≤208 μg/min during the course of the study. In the intensively treated group,

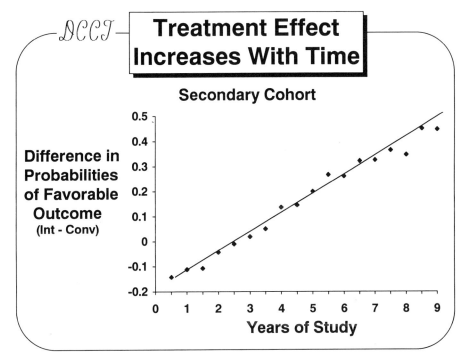

FIG. 4. Slopes of the Mann-Whitney differences at 6-monthly visits over time (differences in the estimated probabilities that participants in the intensive treatment group would have a more favorable outcome, *i.e.* fewer steps of worsening or more steps of improvement, than those in the conventional treatment group) in the secondary intervention cohorts.

AER levels returned to normal in 22 subjects, 12 maintained levels in the microalbuminuric range, and four subjects developed sustained clinical albuminuria. In the conventionally treated subjects, AER levels returned to normal in 18, 11 maintained levels in the microalbuminuric range, and six subjects developed sustained clinical albuminuria. These proportions were not significantly different.

Neuropathy

Clinical neuropathy was defined as an abnormal neurologic examination that was consistent with the presence of peripheral sensorimotor neuropathy plus either abnormal nerve conduction in at least two peripheral nerves or unequivocally abnormal autonomic nerve testing. In the patients in the primary prevention cohort who did not have neuropathy at baseline, intensive treatment reduced the appearance of neuropathy at 5 years by 69% (to 3% *versus* 10% in the conventional treatment group; $p = 0.006$). Similarly, in the secondary intervention cohort, intensive treatment reduced the appearance of clinical neuropathy at 5 years by 57% (to 7% *versus* 16% $p < 0.001$). All three components of the definition of clinical neuropathy were reduced similarly by intensive treatment (Fig. 6).

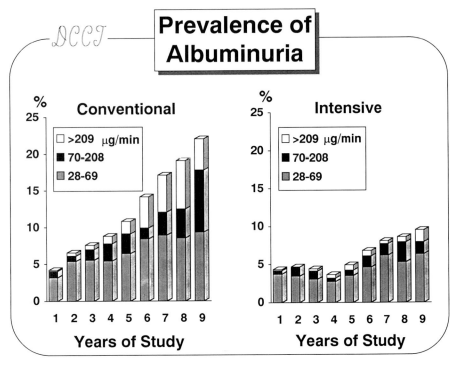

FIG. 5.   Point prevalence of 3 degrees of albuminuria in patients receiving conventional or intensive treatment.

Macrovascular Disease

The relative youth of the patients made the detection of treatment-related differences in rates of macrovascular events unlikely. However, intensive treatment reduced the development of hypercholesterolemia, defined as a serum concentration of low-density lipoprotein cholesterol greater than 4.14 mmol/liter (160 mg/dl), by 34% (95% confidence interval, 7–54) in the combined cohort ($p = 0.02$). When all major cardiovascular and peripheral vascular events were combined, intensive treatment reduced (albeit not significantly), the risk of macrovascular disease by 41% (to 0.5 events *versus* 0.8 events per 100 patient-years; 95% confidence interval, –10 to 68).

Adverse Events and Safety

Mortality did not differ significantly between the treatment groups (seven deaths in the intensive treatment group and four in the conventional treatment group) and was less than expected on the basis of population-based mortality studies (18). The incidence of severe hypoglycemia, including multiple episodes in some patients, was

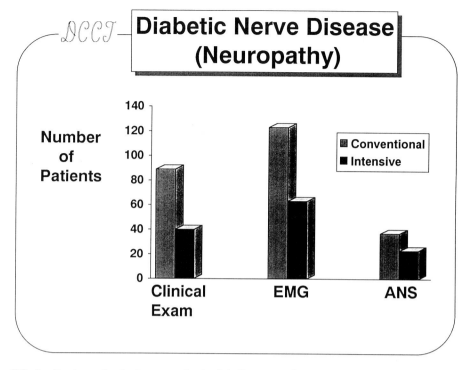

FIG. 6. Numbers of patients progressing to diabetic neuropathy assessed by clinical examination or by electrophysiological or autonomic testing.

approximately three times higher in the intensive treatment group than in the conventional treatment group ($p < 0.001$). In the intensive treatment group, there were 62 hypoglycemic episodes per 100 patient-years in which assistance was required in the provision of treatment, as compared with 19 such episodes per 100 patient-years in the conventional treatment group. This included 16 and five episodes of coma or seizure per 100 patient-years in the respective groups. There were no deaths, myocardial infarctions, or strokes definitely attributable to hypoglycemia, and no significant differences between groups with regard to the number of major accidents requiring hospital admission (20 in the intensive treatment group and 22 in the conventional treatment group). However, there were two fatal motor vehicle accidents, one in each group, in which hypoglycemia may have had a causative role. In addition, a person not involved in the trial was killed in a motor vehicle accident involving a car driven by a patient in the intensive treatment group who was probably hypoglycemic. Since the treatment phase of the trial ended in June, 1993, two additional deaths have occurred, one in each group. There were 54 hospital admissions, usually brief, to treat severe hypoglycemia in 40 patients in the intensive treatment group, as compared with 36 admissions in 27 patients in the conventional treatment group, including seven and four admissions, respectively, to treat hypoglycemia-related injuries.

Despite the higher risk of severe hypoglycemia with intensive treatment, there was no difference between the two treatment groups in the occurrence of clinically important changes in neuropsychological function (19). In addition, there were no significant differences in the mean total scores in a quality-of-life questionnaire (20), despite the added demands of intensive treatment. Weight gain was a problem with intensive treatment, with an increase of 33% in the mean adjusted risk of becoming overweight, a condition defined as a body weight more than 120% above the ideal (12.7 cases of overweight per 100 patient-years in the intensive treatment group versus 9.3 in the conventional treatment group). At 5 years, patients receiving intensive treatment had gained a mean of 4.6 kg more than patients receiving conventional treatment. The event rates of diabetic ketoacidosis were 1.8 and 2.0 episodes per 100 patient-years in the conventional-treatment and intensive-treatment groups, respectively ($p > 0.7$).

Economic Evaluation

An economic analysis has indicated that intensive treatment, as practiced in the DCCT (with research costs excluded), was two-and-a-half to three times more costly than conventional treatment (21,22). The major components of the increased cost were greater frequency of clinic visits and increased usage of blood glucose monitoring strips, insulin syringes, and pump supplies. When accumulated over a lifetime, the increased cost of intensive treatment is substantial. Nevertheless, disease progression models indicate that the lifetime benefits of intensive treatment are also substantial. This is true when the lifetime benefits are expressed as symptom-free years, quality-adjusted life years (QALYs), or money saved from lesser cost of treatment of major microvascular and neuropathic complications. On balance, the analysis has established beyond reasonable doubt that intensive treatment as practiced in the DCCT is cost effective from an economic as well as from a human perspective. Calculations derived from the treatment recommendations of the American Diabetes Association indicate that approximately 400,000 patients with IDDM currently living in the United States should be considered as candidates for intensive treatment. The thoughtful implementation of intensive treatment for suitable patients would have an enormous impact in reducing the overall cost of health care in the United States.

DISCUSSION AND CONCLUSIONS

Intensive treatment of patients with IDDM delays the onset and slows the progression of clinically important retinopathy, including vision-threatening lesions, nephropathy, and neuropathy, by between 35 and 70%. The large number of patients studied, the inclusion of a primary prevention cohort, and the long follow-up period in this study provided the opportunity to demonstrate the effects of treatment in patients with a range of ages, durations of diabetes, degrees of severity of retinopathy, and baseline glycosylated hemoglobin values.

In contrast to the clear-cut efficacy of intensive insulin treatment in reducing long-term complications, the risk of severe hypoglycemia was three times higher with such therapy. Relatively few patients required hospital admission or medical attention for hypoglycemia or resultant injuries, and serial neuropsychological testing showed no changes in cognitive function. Although we are mindful of the potential for severe injury, we believe that the risk of sever hypoglycemia with intensive treatment is greatly outweighed by the reduction in microvascular and neurologic complications.

On the basis of these results, we recommend that most patients with IDDM be treated with closely monitored intensive regimens, with the goal of maintaining their glycemic status as close to the normal range as safely possible. Because of the risk of hypoglycemia, intensive treatment should be implemented with caution, especially in patients with repeated severe hypoglycemia or unawareness of hypoglycemia. The risk-benefit ratio with intensive treatment may be less favorable in children under 13 years of age and in patients with advanced complications, such as end-stage renal disease or cardiovascular or cerebrovascular disease. Patients with proliferative or severe nonproliferative retinopathy may be at higher risk for accelerated progression of their retinopathy after the start of intensive treatment (23) and should be followed closely by their ophthalmologists. Finally, although we did not study patients with non-insulin-dependent diabetes mellitus (NIDDM), hyperglycemia is associated with the presence or progression of complications in NIDDM (24,25), as it is in IDDM. If the main conclusions of this trial with regard to the benefits of reducing glycemia are extended to patients with NIDDM, then careful regard for age, capabilities, and coexisting diseases will be necessary. We therefore advise caution in the use of treatments other than diet that are aimed at achieving euglycemia in patients with NIDDM.

Most of the detailed results of the DCCT are now in press or have been submitted for publication. The data tapes and analysis plans will soon be made available to the scientific community and general public. A long-term follow-up of the patients who participated in the DCCT has been approved and will be funded by the NIDDK. This study, "The Epidemiology of Diabetes Intervention and Complications" (EDIC) is currently in progress.

REFERENCES

1. Engerman R, Bloodworth JM, Nelson S. Relationship of microvascular disease in diabetes to metabolic control. *Diabetes* 1977; 26: 760–9.
2. Engerman RL, Kern TS. Progression of incipient diabetic retinopathy during good glycemic control. *Diabetes* 1987; 36: 808–12.
3. Cohen AJ, McGill PD, Rossetti RG, Guberski DL, Like AA. Glomerulopathy in spontaneously diabetic rat: impact of glycemic control. *Diabetes* 1987; 36: 944–51.
4. Klein R, Klein BE, Moss SE, Davis MD, DeMets DL. The Wisconsin epidemiologic study of diabetic retinopathy. II. Prevalence and risk of diabetic retinopathy when age at diagnosis is less than 30 years. *Arch Ophthalmol* 1984; 102: 520–6.
5. Klein R, Klein BE, Moss SE, Davis MD, DeMets DL. Glycosylated hemoglobin predicts the incidence and progression of diabetic retinopathy. *JAMA* 1988; 250: 2964–71.
6. Chase HP, Jackson WE, Hoops SL, Cockerham RS, Archer PG, O'Brien D. Glucose control and the renal and retinal complications of insulin-dependent diabetes. *JAMA* 1989; 261: 1155–60.

7. Kroc Collaborative Study Group. Blood glucose control and the evaluation of diabetic retinopathy and albuminuria: a preliminary multicenter trial. *N Engl J Med* 1984; 311: 365–72.
8. Lauritzen T, Frost-Larsen K, Larsen H-W, Deckert T. Two-year experience with continuous subcutaneous insulin infusion in relation to retinopathy and neuropathy. *Diabetes* 1985; 34(suppl): 74–9.
9. Brinchmann-Hansen O, Dahl-Jorgensen K, Hanssen KF, Sandvik L. The response of diabetic retinopathy to 41 months of multiple insulin injections, insulin pumps, and conventional insulin therapy. *Arch Ophthalmol* 1988; 106: 1242–6.
10. Reichard P, Nilsson B-Y, Rosenqvist U. The effect of long-term intensified insulin treatment on the development of microvascular complications of diabetes mellitus. *N Engl J Med* 1993; 329: 304–9.
11. DCCT Research Group. The Diabetes Control and Complications Trial (DCCT): Are continuing studies of metabolic control and microvascular complications in insulin-dependent diabetes mellitus justified? *N Engl J Med* 1988; 318: 246–50.
12. DCCT Research Group. The Diabetes Control and Complications Trial (DCCT): The effect of intensive treatment of diabetes on the development and progression of long-term complications in insulin-dependent diabetes mellitus. *N Engl J Med* 1993; 329: 977–86.
13. DCCT Research Group. The Diabetes Control and Complications Trial (DCCT): Design and methodologic considerations for the feasibility phase. *Diabetes* 1986; 35: 530–45.
14. DCCT Research Group. The Diabetes Control and Complications Trial (DCCT): Update. *Diabetes Care* 1990; 13: 427–33.
15. Siebert C, Clark DM. Operational and policy considerations of data monitoring in clinical trials: the Diabetes Control and Complications Trial experience. *Controlled Clin Trials* 1993; 14: 30–44.
16. Lee ET. Statistical methods for survival data analysis. Belmont, California: Lifetime Learning 1980: 88–92, 127–9, 306–12.
17. Snedecor GW, Cochran WG. *Statistical methods*. 6th ed. Ames: Iowa State University Press, 1967.
18. Dorman JS, Laporte RE, Kuller LH, *et al*. The Pittsburgh insulin-dependent diabetes mellitus (IDDM) morbidity and mortality study: mortality results. *Diabetes* 1984; 33: 271–6.
19. DCCT Research Group. A screening algorithm to identify clinically significant changes in neuropsychological function in the Diabetes Control and Complications Trial. *J Clin Exp Neuropsychol* 1994; 16: 303–16.
20. DCCT Research Group. Reliability and validity of a diabetes quality-of-life measure for the Diabetes Control and Complications Trial (DCCT). *Diabetes Care* 1988; 11: 725–32.
21. DCCT Research Group. Resource utilization and costs of intensive and conventional therapies in the Diabetes Control and Complications Trial. Personal communication.
22. DCCT Research Group. Lifetime benefits of intensive therapy as practiced in the Diabetes Control and Complications Trial: an economic evaluation. Personal communication.
23. Lawson PM, Champion MC, Canny C, *et al*. Continuous subcutaneous insulin infusion (CSII) does not prevent progression of proliferative and preproliferative retinopathy. *Br J Ophthalmol* 1982; 66: 762–6.
24. Klein R, Klein BE, Moss SE, Davis MD, DeMets DL. The Wisconsin epidemiologic study of diabetic retinopathy. III. Prevalence and risk of diabetic retinopathy when age at diagnosis is 30 or more years. *Arch Ophthalmol* 1984; 102: 527–32.
25. Nathan DM, Singer DE, Godine JE, Harrington CH, Perlmuter LC. Retinopathy in older type II diabetics: association with glucose control. *Diabetes* 1986; 35: 797–801.

DISCUSSION

Dr. Dakou: Have you broken down the data for the age group 13 to 17 years, which is a very interesting one?

Dr. Crofford: We have done a limited number of subgroup analyses. The results I have shown you are consistent across age and gender and among the participating clinics. The results are similar when comparing adult to adolescent patients. In general, the adolescent patients came in with glycohemoglobin values about 1 unit higher than the adults, but the magnitude of the fall in glycohemoglobin was approximately the same as in the adults, and the magnitude of the treatment effect was about the same. The youngest patient was 13 at entry, so most were young adults at the time the study was over. There was no significant difference between the adolescents whom we followed and the rest of the study cohort.

Dr. Schwartz: You did not tell us what the actual hemoglobin A_{1c} results were. How close to normal did you get?

Dr. Crofford: I left that out when I presented the data because this was not a trial designed to stratify patients according to glycohemoglobin but an intervention trial. We were comparing two interventions, a standard intervention and an intensive intervention. One may speculate that the treatment effects can be attributed exclusively to changes in glycemic control between the groups but that can never be proved with certainty, so the difference in effects was attributed to the different treatment regimens. To answer your question specifically, mean glycohemoglobin at the time of entry was about 9 units for the conventionally treated group and it stayed at 9 throughout the study. For the intensively treated group the value fell to about 7.2 and remained between 7.0 and 7.2 throughout the study, so the separation was between 1.5 and 2 glycohemoglobin units. Since the upper limit of normal in our assay was 6.5, these values were not in the normal range. If you look at blood sugar profiles, the patients came in with an average blood sugar throughout the day of about 13 mM (240 mg/dl). In patients receiving conventional treatment, the value stayed at about 13 mM; in those receiving intensive treatment it was perhaps 5 mM (90 mg/dl) lower, but the values were not in the normoglycemic range. About 10% of the patients were able to achieve and maintain normal blood sugar levels throughout the period, but most patients were not able to do this without an excessive frequency of hypoglycemia. It is my belief that if one could lower the glycohemoglobin to normal and keep it there, the risk of developing complications would be reduced to virtually zero, but that is not achievable with the technologies used in the context of a multicenter trial.

Dr. Dakou: Would you like to speculate whether the continuous contact may in fact have been one of the most important influences?

Dr. Crofford: In most clinical trials you think that you are studying an isolated variable but in fact you are not, you are comparing two different treatment regimens. You don't know for sure that the patients do what you tell them to, you just hope they do. So you can never, or only very rarely, attribute your effect to a single variable. We studied two different philosophies of treatment, and I attribute the effect to some, perhaps multiple, components of those philosophies. I speculated that the most important factor was the glycemic separation, and I think most people would agree that that may reflect the entire spectrum of metabolic and hormonal arrangements associated with insulin-dependent diabetes. However, we cannot prove that point specifically.

Dr. Cowett: Some of these individuals got pregnant. Would you discuss what happened to them and how the intensively treated group differed from what is generally considered optimal management of the pregnant diabetic patient currently. What happened to the fetus, what was the outcome?

Dr. Crofford: I think that the patients in intensive treatment who became pregnant received treatment that was equivalent to that given by the best obstetricians experienced in caring for people with diabetes. We haven't finished the analysis as to whether there were any differences in outcome. I don't expect there to be large differences because we did not have a poorly controlled group of patients. If you believe that pregnancy causes acceleration of diabetic retinopathy, then the question has always existed, is it the pregnancy that accelerates the retinopathy or is it the rapid institution of tight control? Since half of our patients were always under intensive control and half were rapidly switched to intensive control when they became pregnant, we have an excellent opportunity to determine whether it is the pregnancy *per se* or the rapid institution of tight control that contributes to the progression of retinopathy.

Dr. Guesry: Have you quantified the amount of insulin used in the two groups, and what were the differences?

Dr. Crofford: There was no substantial difference. The total daily amount of insulin was about the same between the two treatment groups, so it was not that intensive patients got more insulin, but it was given at different time periods through the day. The total daily dose was about 0.7 units/kg body weight in both groups.

Dr. Guesry: You mentioned that intensive care could be expensive but I suspect on the other hand that it produced large savings overall. Have you done a cost-benefit analysis? This will be very important to convince the health authorities of the need for this intensive care.

Dr. Crofford: We have done a very extensive economic evaluation of both the cost and the benefit. We have not completed it yet, but it will be published shortly. I can summarize by saying that the total cost for *standard* treatment, not the cost related to research but just the delivery of standard treatment in the United States, would be about $2000 per patient per year, and for *intensive* treatment it is a little more than twice that, *i.e.*, around $4000 per patient per year. If one does disease progression modeling and looks at the savings that eventually occur, they are substantial. The crossover point occurs at about 20 years, so you have got to put 20 years of money up front before you start showing a financial saving. Our nation is not noted for long-term planning, so that is a difficult obstacle.

Dr. Guesry: I suspect that you already had statistically significant differences before the ninth year. Why have you continued the study, with the risk of retinopathy?

Dr. Crofford: The whole process of sequential data monitoring, as you are well aware, is a very complex one. It involves a decision by a committee that has to look at the risks, the benefits, and the outcomes and make a decision as to whether the study question has been definitively answered. We had two problems: first, we thought we would probably never be able to do the study again, so it must be done right this time; second, the results needed to be sufficiently compelling to result in a change in clinical practice. Just proving that something has a nominal p value of 0.001 may not be enough to persuade providers that their behavior needs to be modified. One technical point that gets directly to your question is that not all the patients were followed for 9 years. This is not clear from the cumulative incidence curves. At about 5 years, we thought we were getting a significant treatment effect, but because of the early worsening effect, there were more patients who got worse at that time than got better. Under the circumstances, the results were not very compelling. Thus we wanted to be sure that the absolute number of patients that improved in response to intensive treatment was greater than the number who improved with conventional treatment. That is a different consideration from a nominal p value that can be calculated from the cumulative incidence curves. We stopped the study as soon as we thought we could. This decision was made by a totally independent data monitoring committee with no members of the study group involved in making the decision.

Dr. Nattrass: Could I ask you a question relating to macrovascular disease? One of the things against intensive regimens has always been the worry that intensive insulin treatment might lead to hyperinsulinemia, arteriosclerosis, and an increase in mortality. From what you said in reply to a previous question, you have obtained better control without increasing the insulin dose, but the fact that these patients also gained weight must surely imply that they had higher circulating insulin. Can you give us your thoughts in this area?

Dr. Crofford: I can say that, even though the numbers were small, the absolute event rates for all measures of macrovascular disease were lower in the intensive treatment group, although this did not reach statistical significance. We do have in place a long-term, 10–20 year additional follow-up because of the fact that these patients had a median age of 27 years at entry, and we did not expect to observe many major macrovascular events, but we are hopeful that the long-term follow-up may give us a better feel for this as time progresses. We have no evidence that in insulin-dependent diabetes intensive treatment *increased* the risk for macrovascular events, but, if it has a beneficial effect, the benefit does not yet reach statistical significance.

Dr. Katsilambros: You have shown that you had three vehicle accidents with deaths in the intensive treatment group while there was only one in the other group. How can you know these were not caused by hypoglycemia?

Dr. Crofford: The total number of deaths was seven in the intensive-treated group and four in the conventionally treated group, so there was a total of 11 deaths. Subsequently there have been two additional deaths, one in each treatment group and incidentally one of these was a woman. One cannot exclude hypoglycemia with absolute certainty because most of the time you don't have data sufficiently close to the time of the accident to know for sure. Our independent data monitoring groups had a special committee called the Morbidity and Mortality Classification Committee that was totally independent of the study group. This committee reviewed all the available evidence, everything from the necropsy to the police report, all the witness statements, in fact everything they had, and then came to a decision as to whether the death was attributable to hypoglycemia. There were three cases in which hypoglycemia could not be totally excluded, but there were none in which they thought that hypoglycemia was the most likely cause of death. You are all right, however, that you can never exclude this with certainty. We did have one fatality associated with hypoglycemia, although the dead person was not a patient. A study patient had a hypoglycemic attack while driving and a person in another car was killed. So there was definitely one fatality attributed to hypoglycemia.

Diabetes, edited by Richard M. Cowett,
Nestlé Nutrition Workshop Series,
Vol. 35. Nestec Ltd.,
Vevey/Raven Press, Ltd., New York © 1995.

Exercise in Diabetes Mellitus: Clinical Aspects

Nicholas Katsilambros and Vassiliki Rabavila

First Department of Propedeutic Medicine, Athens University Medical School, Laiko General Hospital, Athens, Greece

The treatment of diabetic patients for the past 70 years has been based on drugs (insulin or oral hypoglycemic agents), diet, and exercise.

The influence of exercise (beneficial or otherwise) on the metabolism of diabetic patients has been recognized for many years, and numerous contradictory opinions have been expressed (1). For almost 50 years after the discovery of insulin, the predominant opinion was that exercise was the cornerstone of treatment for diabetic patients (2,3). Our knowledge of the physiology of exercise and of its effects in diabetic patients has expanded during recent years (4,5), and the view that exercise constitutes a special form of treatment for diabetic patients has been partially revised (5–8).

We know today that physical exercise has different effects in insulin-treated and non-insulin-treated diabetic patients. Many investigations have shown that physical activity has a beneficial influence on metabolic control in non-insulin-treated (type 2) patients. Opinions concerning insulin-treated diabetic patients are less positive (1). All diabetic patients should, however, be encouraged to exercise for the same reasons as healthy people but with due care because, in diabetes, vigorous exercise may be accompanied by complications such as hypoglycemia and coronary events (1).

PHYSIOLOGICAL CONSIDERATIONS

Fuel Sources

During exercise, the working muscles require an increase of energy and oxygen supply. Increased respiration and cardiac output provide the necessary oxygen supply. The major sources of energy for resting and working muscles are glucose and free fatty acids. These substrates are derived from the circulation and from depots contained in muscle, liver, and adipose tissue. Amino acids and ketone bodies may

TABLE 1. *Fuel sources during muscular exercise*

Glucose
Free fatty acids
Amino acids
Ketone bodies

---

also be used as fuel to a lesser extent, especially when the available glucose and free fatty acid supply is limited (Table 1).

The contribution of the different fuels to the energy needs of the muscle depends on the intensity and duration of exercise and on the state of nutrition. Resting muscles mainly use free fatty acids derived from adipose tissue (9). During the transition from rest to exercise, the muscles use a mixture of glucose, glycogen, and free fatty acids. At the beginning of exercise, the glycogen stores in the working muscles supply the necessary glucose. As exercise continues, glycogen stores in the working muscles are depleted, and the contribution of circulating glucose and free fatty acids becomes increasingly important. Circulating glucose is derived from hepatic glucose output, which slowly shifts from the initial hepatic glycogenolysis to gluconeogenesis as hepatic glycogen stores are consumed. In a healthy person, the glucose uptake by the contracting muscles and the hepatic glucose production are balanced; consequently, blood glucose remains stable, at least during moderate exercise of 60- to 90-minutes duration. When exercise is prolonged, hepatic gluconeogenesis may not be able to maintain a sufficient glucose production to meet the needs of the exercising muscles and blood glucose begins to decline (10). After 2 hours of exercise, free fatty acids become the fuel that supplies the greater proportion of energy needed by the muscles, and thus their energy contribution is especially significant (9).

Hormonal Changes

Under physiologic conditions, the interactions of insulin, glucagon, catecholamines, cortisol, and growth hormone (Table 2) regulate the fuel supply to the working muscles and simultaneously preserve glucose homeostasis (5,11). The increase in hepatic glucose production during exercise is regulated by the combined effects of

TABLE 2. *Hormonal changes during muscular exercise*

Decrease of insulin
Increase of catecholamines
Increase of glucagon
Increase of cortisol
Increase of growth hormone

---

insulin, glucagon, catecholamines, and, to a lesser extent, of cortisol and growth hormone (5,7). During exercise, insulin secretion decreases while glucagon, catecholamines, cortisol, and growth hormone increase (5–7).

During physical activity, insulin and muscle contraction seem to be the most important stimuli for increased glucose uptake. Insulin secretion is decreased from the start of exercise. This results in portal and peripheral hypoinsulinemia with a consequent relative hyperglucagonemia. The change in the ratio of glucagon to insulin is important for increased hepatic glucose production. In addition, exercise results in an increase in the insulin sensitivity of muscles and other tissues. This occurs even with mild exercise and lasts beyond the exercise period (12). The increase in insulin sensitivity may be due to an increase in insulin binding to its skeletal muscle receptor or to an increase in the number of insulin receptors. The fall of serum insulin during exercise stimulates lipolysis, and the liberation of free fatty acids from muscle and adipose tissue.

Glucose uptake by working muscles is also regulated by catecholamines. Experiments in animals and humans have shown that epinephrine inhibits insulin-mediated glucose uptake in skeletal muscle by inhibiting glucose phosphorylation. During prolonged exercise, epinephrine mobilizes glucogen from inactive muscles, and the produced lactate can then be used as fuel for working muscles through gluconeogenesis in the liver. The increase in hepatic glucose production during exercise is dependent not only on a change in the glucagon/insulin ratio but also on the activation of the sympathetic nervous system. Recent investigations have shown that sympathetic neural norepinephrine seems to be the operative catecholamine in stimulating glucose production during exercise, while epinephrine has no particular significance in this process (13). In addition, the increased circulating catecholamines stimulate lipolysis and the release of free fatty acids from muscles and adipose tissue through a β-adrenergic mechanism.

INSULIN-DEPENDENT DIABETES MELLITUS AND INSULIN-TREATED NON-INSULIN-DEPENDENT DIABETES MELLITUS

Metabolic Consequences of Exercise

Insulin-dependent diabetes mellitus (IDDM) is characterized by a lack of endogenous insulin secretion. Neither traditional insulin treatment nor the modern methods of exogenous insulin administration (intensified insulin treatment or pump therapy) can fully substitute for or imitate physiological insulin secretion. This may result in unacceptably low or high insulin levels in portal or peripheral venous blood. Therefore, either an abnormally low or an abnormally high blood sugar may occur during exercise (Table 3), reflecting the prevailing insulin concentrations.

In cases of insulin deficiency, intensive insulin treatment may result in metabolic disorientation that may even lead to overt ketoacidosis. In such cases, hepatic glucose

TABLE 3. *Possible metabolic effects of exercise in IDDM*

---

1. Aggravation of diabetic control (hyperglycemia, ketoacidosis, hypoglycemia)
2. Improvement of metabolic control

---

production exceeds peripheral utilization. Different studies conducted in both insulinopenic diabetic patients (14) and pancreatectomized dogs (15) have shown that exercise during a state of insulin deficiency causes an increase in glucose production in the liver, while the uptake of glucose by muscle tissue is considerably reduced. This further increases the preexisting hyperglycemia. Glycemic control is further disturbed by the large increases in glucagon, catecholamines, cortisol, and growth hormone. The lack of insulin and the increased hormone levels also cause increased liberation of free fatty acids and ketone bodies.

Insulin administration may result in hyperinsulinism that is aggravated when insulin absorption is accelerated by giving the insulin injection into an exercising limb (16). An additional factor contributing to the possible induction of hypoglycemia is the increased insulin sensitivity of the peripheral tissues observed during exercise (14).

Clinical Significance

Exercise has been encouraged as an adjuvant to antidiabetic treatment (2,3) since it was realized that injected insulin could cause hypoglycemia. However, as mentioned above, this view is nowadays not considered to be entirely valid, since under certain circumstances ill-considered exercise may give rise to serious problems. Furthermore, the long-term effect of exercise, if any, on metabolic control is not always beneficial (17; and see below), while very good glycemic control may be achieved through intensive insulin treatment alone (18).

Unfortunately, the net effect of exercise on blood glucose concentrations in insulin-dependent diabetes cannot be predicted because of the large variety of confounding factors, such as the degree of metabolic control before the initiation of exercise, the duration and the intensity of the effort, the physical state of the patient, and the type, dose, and site of the injected insulin (Table 4). Therefore the patient who uses exercise as an adjunct to antidiabetic treatment must coordinate insulin injections, meals, and

TABLE 4. *Effect of exercise in insulin-dependent diabetes—factors influencing metabolic control*

---

1. The nutritional status of the patient
2. The degree of metabolic control before exercise
3. Training of the patient
4. Time of the day when exercise is performed
5. Duration and intensity of exercise
6. Type, dose, and site of insulin injection

---

exercise. In spite of these difficulties, exercise should be encouraged, even in unstable diabetes, because physical activity represents an important part of social life and because exercise has multiple positive effects on general health unrelated to glucose metabolism.

People with insulin-dependent diabetes who are going to take exercise must know about the preventive measures they should undertake to avoid aggravating their metabolic state. Blood glucose concentrations in the range of 300 mg/dl accompanied by ketonuria indicate that there is a real lack of insulin. If muscular exercise is performed under these circumstances, the situation may be aggravated (19), and therefore exercise must be avoided.

NON-INSULIN-DEPENDENT DIABETES MELLITUS

Non-insulin-dependent diabetes mellitus (NIDDM) is characterized by hyperglycemia, insulin resistance, and a relative defect in insulin secretion. In addition, there is an increased frequency of cardiovascular risk factors such as hypertension and hyperlipidemia. The main predisposing factors for NIDDM are the presence of a positive family history of diabetes and obesity, especially when there is a central type of fat distribution and physical activity is restricted. This situation represents a state of apparent insulin resistance. One of the main goals of treatment is therefore to increase insulin sensitivity, and this can be achieved through a reduction in body weight and through exercise.

In spite of the increasing incidence of NIDDM in the population, studies related to the effects of exercise on metabolic control in this condition are relatively sparse. A study of obese patients with NIDDM who presented with a moderate degree of postprandial hyperglycemia (about 200 mg/dl) and normal basal plasma insulin levels showed that exercise resulted in a decrease of glucose concentrations (by about 50 mg/dl) while there was no change in the insulin levels (20). It was also observed that in subjects who presented with NIDDM, hyperinsulinemia, and moderately high fasting glucose levels, prolonged muscular activity reduced plasma glucose levels and, to a moderate extent, insulin concentrations (20).

It seems that the reduction in blood glucose that accompanies exercise is due to the fact that the exercise-induced increase in the hepatic glucose output is relatively small, while at the same time there is a normal increase in glucose consumption by the peripheral tissues. The factors responsible for the relative decrease in hepatic glucose production are the preexisting hyperglycemia combined with the presence of sustained plasma insulin concentrations. The latter may be due to sulfonylurea administration but possibly also to the presence of hyperglycemia, or even to an insufficient control in insulin secretion.

TRAINING: ITS CLINICAL SIGNIFICANCE AND USE IN PREVENTION OF NIDDM

Various different studies have dealt with the question of whether physical training can improve glucose tolerance or glycemic control. Data obtained on middle-aged subjects with impaired glucose tolerance (21) as well as on patients with NIDDM (22) have shown that a 6-month training program results in only a small improvement in glucose tolerance. A similar study on men with NIDDM who followed a program of systematic physical activity for more than 2 years failed to show any effect on the degree of the glucose tolerance (23), while another study (24) showed only a temporary improvement in intravenous, but not oral, glucose tolerance. In further studies (25,26), however, systematic physical activity was followed by a decrease in fasting blood glucose levels and glycated hemoglobin. According to these investigators, muscular training is indicated as a therapeutic approach to improve metabolic control in NIDDM. This positive effect is related to an increase in tissue sensitivity to insulin, which is observed mainly during the period of training. These studies (25,26) showed that training resulted in an increased glucose uptake from peripheral tissues.

Apart from the improvement in metabolic control shown in at least some studies, systematic physical exercise also leads to other beneficial effects including loss of weight (which is followed by a decrease in tissue insulin resistance), decreased hyperinsulinemia, better glycemic control, reduction of high arterial pressure and blood lipid levels, and an increase in high density lipoprotein (HDL) cholesterol. Even in cases where, in spite of training, body weight remains unchanged, insulin resistance can be improved. This is apparently due to a reduction in body fat mass combined with a parallel increase in the mass of muscle tissue.

It has also been shown that systematic exercise is associated with a decrease in the frequency of coronary heart disease, at least in the general population (27), although there are no definitive data for persons with NIDDM. However, as mentioned above, many important risk factors for coronary heart disease are substantially reduced by exercise (27). The protective effect of exercise against macroangiopathy is most pronounced in early life. It is also important to emphasize that exercise tends to improve the sense of well-being and the quality of life (28).

Systematic muscular exercise may protect against the appearance of NIDDM. This has been shown in some prospective studies (27) and may be particularly true in high-risk subjects, such as persons with a positive family history for NIDDM or hypertriglyceridemia, in women with indications of glucose intolerance during pregnancy, and probably in all subjects with the central type of obesity.

RISKS OF EXERCISE AND HOW TO AVOID THEM

Before the initiation of a training program, the doctor must obtain a full clinical history and must thoroughly examine the patient, looking for signs of micro- and macroangiopathy as well as for neurological complications. Blood tests for glucose and blood urea nitrogen and a resting ECG are also essential (29). Because silent ischemia is relatively frequent in NIDDM, all persons aged more than 35 years must have an exercise ECG (28,29). This may also help in identifying patients with an excessive blood pressure response to exercise and those who develop orthostatic

TABLE 5. *How to avoid hypoglycemia during or after exercise*

Frequent measurement of blood glucose before, during and after exercise
Start exercise 1–2 hours after a meal
Intake of extra carbohydrates before as well as each hour during exercise
Reduce insulin dose (in insuli-treated patients)
Inject insulin in a nonexercising limb
Avoid intense exercise at the time when the injected insulin exerts its maximum effect
Reduce dose of sulfonylureas (in non-insulin-treated patients)

hypotension after the end of exercise (28). Before starting a training program, hypertension must be effectively treated. In addition, laser eye therapy, if required, must be done because the exercise-induced increase in arterial blood pressure may further aggravate preexisting retinopathy (1).

Hypoglycemia is the most frequent complication of exercise in insulin-treated diabetic patients. In cases where the time, duration, and intensity of a course of exercise are known in advance, hypoglycemia can be avoided by a reduction in insulin dosage. If, however, the regular insulin injection has already been given before exercise has begun, an increased intake of carbohydrates is strongly recommended both during and after the end of the physical activity (Table 5).

The so called *Monday effect* represents the probability that a hypoglycemic attack will occur many hours after exercise or even on the next day. This is due to the replenishment of glycogen stores after a protracted course of exercise.

The amount by which insulin dosage should be decreased or carbohydrate intake increased is not the same in all cases. It depends on the intensity and duration of exercise as well as on the prevailing level of glycemia (1,27). Usually the dose of insulin is reduced by 30–40%. If more than one type of insulin is being used, the decrease in dose should be confined to the insulin type that has its peak activity coinciding with the time of exercise (27). The amount of additional carbohydrate to be taken by mouth is 20–40 g per hour of exercise. Each patient can, however, determine his or her needs on an individual basis since the variation from person to person is considerable. Therefore only general advice can be given.

The time of the day when exercise is performed is also important. It has been shown that the risk of hypoglycemia is less when physical activity is taken before the morning insulin injection, when the insulin levels are low. Intense exercise in the late evening increases the risk of nocturnal hypoglycemia. It is worth remembering that during the night the output of glucose by the liver is a very important factor in glucose homeostasis. It has also been shown that the overall glycemic effect of a meal is less when exercise precedes food ingestion (30). In insulin-treated subjects, certain sports such as diving, climbing, or motor racing are best avoided because of the very serious consequences of a hypoglycemic attack.

In patients on continuous subcutaneous insulin infusion (CSII), hypoglycemia can usually be avoided by reducing the premeal bolus insulin dose by 50% as well as by interrupting the basal insulin infusion during exercise (31).

TABLE 6. *Possible untoward events due to muscular exercise in diabetic subjects*

Hypoglycemia
Hyperglycemia
Ketoacidosis
Arrhythmias (often due to ischemia, possibly silent)
Excessive arterial blood pressure increase during the exercise
Orthostatic hypotension after exercise
Retinal hemorrhage (in association with proliferative retinopathy)
Proteinuria
Foot ulcers (in cases of peripheral diabetic neuropathy)

Patients with NIDDM on sulfonylurea treatment may also decrease the dosage of the oral agent before exercise (1), although it may be more practical for these patients to eat extra carbohydrate (Table 5).

Apart from hyperglycemia or hypoglycemia, diabetic patients are also at risk of other health problems (28) that may appear during exercise under certain specific circumstances (Table 6). Active forms of proliferative retinopathy are in general a contraindication for exercise (32). Jogging must be restricted in patients with peripheral neuropathy (28,32). In general, appropriate types of exercise for diabetic persons are walking, bicycling (including stationary bicycling), swimming, dancing, skiing, skating, tennis, squash, and volley ball. Exercise should be in the range of 50–70% of the VO_{2max}. This may be easily achieved by regular walking. The duration of exercise should be 20–60 minutes, three to five times per week (28,29,33). Patients with autonomic neuropathy must ingest sufficient amounts of water (and electrolytes) if they exercise in high temperatures.

It is clear, therefore, that exercise must be individualized according to the needs and circumstances of any given patient. Education of the patient and special courses on exercise in diabetes appear also to be necessary.

REFERENCES

1. Kemmer FW, Berger M. Exercise. In: Alberti KGMM, De Fronzo RA, Keen H, Zimmet P, eds. *International textbook of diabetes mellitus.* New York: John Wiley & Sons, 1992: 725–43.
2. Joslin EP. The treatment of diabetes mellitus. In: Joslin EP, Root HF, White P, Marble A, eds. *Treatment of diabetes mellitus.* 10th ed. Philadelphia: Lea & Febiger, 1959: 243–300.
3. Katsch G. Arbeitstherapie der Zuckerkranken. *Erg Physikal Diat Ther* 1939; 1: 136.
4. Vranic M, Berger M. Exercise and diabetes mellitus. *Diabetes* 1979; 28: 147–57.
5. Kemmer FW, Berger M. Exercise and diabetes mellitus: physical activity as a part of daily life and its role in the treatment of diabetic patients. *Int J Sports Med* 1983; 4: 77–88.
6. Kemmer FW, Berger M. Exercise in therapy and the life of diabetic patients. *Clin Sci* 1984; 67: 279–83.
7. Kemmer FW, Berger M. Therapy and better quality of life: the dichotomous role of exercise in diabetes mellitus. *Diabetes Metab Rev* 1986; 2: 53–68.
8. Berger M, Kemmer FW. Discussion: exercise, fitness and diabetes. In: Bouchard C, Shepart RJ, Stepehens T, Sutton JR, McPherson BD, eds. *Exercise, fitness and health: a consensus of current knowledge.* Champaign, IL.: Human Kinetics Books, 1990: 491–5.

9. Ahlborg G, Felig P, Hagenfeldt L, Hendler R, Wahren J. Substrate turnover during prolonged exercise in man. *J Clin Invest* 1974; 53: 1080–90.

10. Ahlborg G, Felig P. Lactate and glucose exchange across the forearm, legs and splanchnic bed during and after prolonged exercise. *J Clin Invest* 1982; 69: 45–54.

11. Hoelzer D, Dalsky G, Clutter W, *et al.* Glucoregulation during exercise: hypoglycemia is prevented by redundant glucoregulatory systems during exercise: sympathochromaffin activation and changes in hormone secretion. *J Clin Invest* 1986; 77: 212–21.

12. Koivisto VA, Yki-Jarvinen H, De Fronzo RA. Physical training and insulin sensitivity. *Diabetes Metab Rev* 1986; 1: 445–81.

13. Hoelzer DR, Dalsky GP, Schwartz NS, *et al.* Epinephrine is not critical to prevention of hypoglycemia during exercise in humans. *Am J Physiol* 1986; 251: E104–10.

14. Zinman B, Murray FT, Vranic M, *et al.* Glucoregulation during moderate exercise in insulin treated diabetics. *J Clin Endocrinol Metab* 1977; 45: 641–52.

15. Vranic M, Kawamori S, Pek S, Kovcevic N, Wrenshall GA. The essentiality of insulin and the role of glucagon in regulating glucose utilization and production during strenuous exercise in dogs. *J Clin Invest* 1976; 57: 245–55.

16. Koivisto V, Felig P. Effefcts of leg exercise on insulin absorption in diabetic patients. *N Engl J Med* 1978; 298: 77–83.

17. Zinman B, Zuniga-Guajardo S, Kelly D. Comparison of the acute and long-term effects of exercise on glucose control in type 1 diabetes. *Diabetes Care* 1984; 7: 515–9.

18. Muhlhauser I, Bruckner I, Berger M *et al.* Evaluation of an intensified insulin treatment and teaching program as routine management of Type 1 (insulin dependent) diabetes. The Bucharest-Dusseldorf Study, *Diabetologia* 1987; 30: 681–91.

19. Berger M, Berchtold P, Cuppers HJ, *et al.* Metabolic and hormonal effects of muscular exercise in juvenile type diabetics. *Diabetologia* 1977; 13: 355–65.

20. Minuk HL, Hanna AK, Marliss EB, Vranic M, Zinman B. Metabolic response to moderate exercise in obese man during prolonged fasting. *Am J Physiol* 1980; 238: E322–9.

21. Saltin B, Lindgarde F, Housten M, Horlin R, Nygaard E, Gad P. Physical training and glucose tolerance in middle-aged men with chemical diabetes. *Diabetes* 1979; 28(suppl 1): 30–2.

22. Saltin B, Lindgarde F, Lithell H, Erisson KF, Gad P. Metabolic effects of long term physical training in maturity onset diabetes. In: Waldhausl WK, ed. *Diabetes.* Amsterdam: Excepta Medica, 1980: 345.

23. Skarfors ET, Wegener TA, Lithell H, Selinus I. Physical training as treatment for Type 2 (non-insulin-dependent) diabetes in elderly men. A feasibility study over 2 years. *Diabetologia* 1987; 30: 930–3.

24. Ruderman NB, Ganda OP, Johansen K. The effects of physical training on glucose tolerance and plasma lipids in maturity onset diabetes. *Diabetes* 1979; 28(suppl 1): 89–92.

25. Reitman JS, Vasquez B, Klimes I, Nagulesparan M. Improvement of glucose homeostasis after exercise training in non-insulin-dependent diabetes. *Diabetes Care* 1984; 7: 434–41.

26. Bogardus C, Ravussin E, Robbins DC, Wolfe RR, Horton ED, Sims EAH. Effects of physical training and diet therapy on carbohydrate metabolism in patients with glucose intolerance and non-insulin-dependent diabetes mellitus. *Diabetes* 1984; 33: 311–8.

27. Koivisto VA. Diabetes and exercise. *Diabetes Rev* 1993; 2: 5–7.

28. Schneider SH, Ruderman NB. Exercise and NIDDM. *Diabetes Care* 1991; 14(suppl 2): 52–6.

29. Katsilambros N. Diabetes and exercise. *Proceedings of 3rd Course on Biochemistry and Exercise.* Eptalofos SA, Athens: 1987: 267–73.

30. Koratzanis G, Rontoyannis GP, Katsilambros N, Phillippides Ph, Frangaki D, Pournaras N. Should exercise precede or follow a meal in type-2 diabetics? *Diabetes* 1983; 32(suppl 1). (Abstract)

31. Sonnenberg GE, Kemmer FW, Berger M. Exercise in type 1 (insulin dependent) diabetic patients treated with continuous subcutaneous insulin infusion: prevention of exercise induced hypoglycemia. *Diabetologia* 1990; 33: 696–703.

32. Koivisto VA. Exercise and diabetes mellitus. In: Pickup J, Williams G, eds. *Textbook of diabetes,* vol 2. Oxford: Blackwell Scientific Publications, 1991: 795–802.

33. ADA Position Statement. Diabetes mellitus and exercise. *Diabetes Care* 1991; 14(suppl 2): 36–7.

DISCUSSION

Dr. Schwartz: Some of us say that our patients should exercise without quantifying what we are doing. I was impressed by how rapidly the fall in muscle and liver glycogen occurs with exercise compared with basal conditions. Can you define how much exercise a patient should tolerate?

Dr. Katsilambros: You cannot easily use our data to do that; it has to be individualized because you cannot generalize about glycogen stores in muscle and liver. As you have seen, it very much depends on the previous diet. However, I believe that patients themselves can have a clear idea of their exercise tolerance on an empirical basis.

Dr. Assan: In daily practice, how do you advise your young adult type 1 patients, and how many of them comply over the long term?

Dr. Katsilambros: Here in Greece, I'm afraid compliance is poor. Most people take taxis or buses. There are some people who exercise regularly, especially younger people in the villages, but I am afraid that in general compliance is not good enough.

Dr. Marliss: Your well-balanced review is a little bit more optimistic than previously. I think one must try to instill a commitment to exercising, just like blood glucose self-monitoring and so on. If it is sold as part of the package and monitored as we monitor all the other things, then I think there is a greater chance of its actually working. At least in cases of obesity, with or without diabetes, the evidence seems to be that those individuals who introduce exercise as a part of their change in lifestyle are more successful at weight reduction and sustaining weight loss. Clearly the benefits are there, and enough people manage to undertake exercise programs on a long-term basis for us to know that the idea is practicable. I wanted particularly to bring to the attention of this audience the differences that you have already underscored between mild-to-moderate exercise and highly intense exercise, defined as greater than 85% VO_2 max. After 15 minutes of exercise at 100% VO_2 max in normal individuals, there is a marked rise in blood glucose both during the exercise and in the minutes following exercise to exhaustion, which means the inability to cycle any more. The hyperglycemic response may be sustained for as long as 40 to 60 minutes postexercise and is accompanied by a very considerable rise in plasma insulin, which is sustained for approximately the same length of time. The relevance of this is, first, that people with type 1 diabetes cannot do it, and, second, that this is the one kind of exercise in which the hyperinsulinemic response is not predictable. Sometimes it occurs but not always. In moderate- and high-intensity exercise, there is a slight rise in plasma glucagon that is insufficient to account for the eightfold rise in glucose production that occurs in that kind of exercise, but the catecholamines rise by 15- to 20-fold, which is well within the range that is likely to cause increased glucose production. Then what happens in people with type 1 diabetes is the following. If you start with euglycemia in type 1 diabetic individuals, following an overnight insulin infusion, a period of exercise without a change in the insulin infusion rate either during or after the exercise results in a hyperglycemic response that is maintained for around 2 hours after the end of exercise. If, under the same circumstances, these individuals are rendered slightly hyperglycemic, about 8 mM, they have an almost equivalent rise after exercise, and it is also sustained. This could very well explain the predictability you pointed out earlier in the responses of plasma glucose in such individuals. It is hard to imagine in this setting how one would adjust either diet or insulin at this point to render this kind of glycemic response normal.

Dr. Dakou: My main difficulty is with children who practice competitive sports, I guess because the catecholamines go so high.

Dr. Katsilambros: I believe that the general psychological and physical benefits to a child's participating in sports are more important than the temporary failure of regulation of blood sugar.

Dr. Nattrass: Can I ask Dr. Marliss whether, in view of the massive increase in catecholamines that occurs with a ketogenic stimulus, he thinks it is a sensible suggestion that people with insulin-dependent diabetes should undertake intensive exercise?

Dr. Marliss: In fact, and to our great surprise, both fatty acid levels and ketone body levels decrease by 50% or more during this kind of exercise, in both normal and diabetic individuals. Thus, the physiologic response of the reasonably well-controlled individual under these circumstances is not likely to be an important factor in ketosis, surprisingly enough.

Dr. Swift: From a practical point of view, prescribing exercise is not the right way to go about things in childhood and adolescence because an adolescent doesn't listen to prescriptions. I agree totally with your conclusion that exercise needs to be individualized. In children on intensive exercise—camps and skiing trips—your comments about training are very important, because those youngsters who go skiing, for instance, and are not used to much exercise all have quite a considerable fall in their insulin requirements. To try to link this with Crofford's work, could I ask a question on the DCCT trial? With so many motivated young people involved, there must have been a subgroup that undertook very heavy regular exercise, and I wonder whether he has any comments to make about their control and outcome in both groups, conventional and intensive.

Dr. Crofford: We did not prescribe different levels of exercise, although we tried to monitor it. We have not yet done a subgroup analysis to see whether there was any difference in the exercising group.

Dr. Guesry: We have discussed mainly the effect of acute exercise. I wonder what would be the effect of long-term exercise, I mean, repeated exercise that would increase muscle mass.

Dr. Katsilambros: Muscle mass increases with regular exercise, and it is considered that in the general population the incidence of non-insulin-dependent diabetes mellitus decreases with systematic exercise. Trained persons require relatively less glucose and can utilize free fatty acids better than untrained individuals, and free fatty acid mobilization occurs earlier in trained people, either diabetic or nondiabetic. From my literature search, I have not been able to discover any very positive effects on glucose tolerance itself unless obesity decreases.

Dr. Girard: There is one very important point about training: you must not stop. If you stop exercise for 2 or 3 days you completely lose the positive effects. I would like to ask Dr. Marliss a question. Is the fact that, during acute intense exercise, you have an increase in blood glucose concentration without any increase in plasma, free fatty acids, and ketones the result of stimulation of α-adrenergic receptors and not β receptors? It has been suggested that the fall in plasma insulin during exercise could be due to recruitment of $\alpha2$ receptors and that could also explain the fact that the mobilization of free fatty acids is also not stimulated during acute exercise.

Dr. Marliss: I didn't say they weren't mobilized, and I think that in fact they probably are, although it is likely that they are taken up somewhat more rapidly than they are mobilized. But the point of the question is well taken. We have exercised normal people and people with type 1 diabetes while infusing a β-blocker (which makes it a little more difficult for them to exercise although they can nevertheless do it moderately intensively) or an α-blocker (phentolamine). The evidence clearly suggests that there is an α-adrenergic component that is more important in the stimulation of hepatic glucose production.

Dr. Katsilambros: Does this α-stimulatory effect appear only in the liver or in the muscles as well?

Dr. Marliss: We have no evidence that glucose disposal during radiolabeled glucose administration is affected by α-adrenergic receptors at the level of muscles, but during β-blocade—probably by virtue of its effect in inhibiting muscle glycogenolysis—there is a considerably greater uptake of circulating glucose into the muscle, presumably because of a lesser provision of glucose-6-phosphate within the muscle due to reduced glycogenolysis.

Dr. Crofford: One clinical observation is that, when diabetic patients are in good control and are then put on programs of intensive control, they often feel better. They have more energy. That is one of the reasons why they take more exercise.

Diabetes, edited by Richard M. Cowett,
Nestlé Nutrition Workshop Series,
Vol. 35. Nestec Ltd.,
Vevey/Raven Press, Ltd., New York © 1995.

New Approaches to the Prevention of Insulin-Dependent Diabetes

Edwin A.M. Gale

St. Bartholomew's Hospital, London ECIA IAA, UK

Insulin-dependent diabetes mellitus (IDDM) remains an incurable disease. The metabolic lesion resulting from β cell destruction cannot be reversed, and insulin replacement therapy remains palliative at best. It is true that, as the Diabetes Control and Complications Trial (DCCT) has shown, intensified insulin therapy can lead to a major reduction in risk of progression to microvascular complications, but this treatment option is demanding and expensive. At our current level of technology, and with major constraints upon health care costs throughout the world, sustained near-normoglycemia is likely to remain an unattainable goal for the great majority of patients. Although advances in insulin therapy and ultimately restoration of endogenous insulin secretion by islet transplantation or genetic engineering may confidently be expected, prevention of IDDM remains the most rational and cost-effective long-term objective. Recent progress in our understanding of the pathogenesis of the disease and in our ability to predict its onset suggest that this long-term goal could potentially be achieved.

IS IDDM POTENTIALLY PREVENTABLE?

The argument for this could be set out as follows:

1. Although there is a genetic basis for disease susceptibility, the majority of susceptible individuals do not develop the disease. The most direct evidence for this comes from the study of IDDM in identical twins, in whom only around 30% show concordance for the disease (1).

2. There is evidence for involvement of one, or possibly several, environmental agents in the pathogenesis of the disease. Without pausing to consider this in detail, we may note that the steady rise in incidence of childhood diabetes in genetically stable populations in Europe and elsewhere appears susceptible to no other explanation (2).

3. There is an autoimmune basis to the disease. Intervention with immunosuppressive agents after diagnosis can prolong residual insulin secretion, presumably by

prolonging survival of the minority of β cells that are still functioning at clinical presentation (3).

4. There is a long preclinical prodrome, readily identifiable by the presence of islet cell antibodies and other autoantibodies in the circulation. These are often detectable 5 years or more before clinical onset (4). This phenomenon means that there is adequate time for screening and intervention to be attempted in the prediabetic period.

5. A variety of interventions can reduce disease incidence in animal models of spontaneous autoimmune diabetes and, thus, potentially also in humans.

Taken together, these considerations seem sufficient to establish that a potential for disease prevention exists. There is, however, a wide gap between a theoretical possibility and the reality of clinical evaluation. Can we—or should we—attempt to intervene in prediabetes at our *current* level of understanding?

AUTOIMMUNITY AND IDDM

The evidence that autoimmune processes are involved in type 1 diabetes is now overwhelming and includes: 1. its association with certain immune response genes in the histocompatibility leukocyte antigen (HLA) region, 2. the overlap with other organ-specific autoimmune disorders, 3. the description of lymphocytic infiltration of the islets "insulitis" in patients who died soon after diagnosis, 4. the presence of a variety of circulating autoantibodies in newly diagnosed patients, 5. the demonstration of lymphocytic activation directed against islet autoantigens, and 6. the prolongation of β cell function after diagnosis by immunosuppressive agents such as cyclosporin.

ANIMAL MODELS OF TYPE 1 DIABETES

Only two other creatures apart from humans develop a spontaneous autoimmune insulin-requiring form of diabetes. These are both rodent strains, the BB (bio-breeding) rat and the NOD (non-obese diabetic) mouse. While these animal models have stimulated a tremendous amount of useful research, it is important to remember that they are valuable analogies, rather than a direct equivalent of the human disease. Important differences exist—for example, the fact that female NOD mice are very much more likely to develop diabetes than males.

Some areas of comparison between these animal models and humans are of potential clinical relevance. For example, in rodent models, most of the susceptible animals develop insulitis, but only a minority go on to develop the disease. Further, insulitis appears within a few weeks of birth. By analogy, the human disease might be expected to be initiated relatively soon after birth but to progress only in a minority. Another point of note is that the development of diabetes in, for example, the NOD mouse is a highly vulnerable process. The risk of progression is modified by diet and even by ambient temperature, as well as by a wide variety of immunological manipulations.

It has been argued that this diminishes the value of animal models as a guide to intervention in humans, but it may at the same time be telling us that intervention at several points in the natural history of the disease might be equally effective (5). Alternatively, it should be noted that most successful interventions have been attempted at or around the time that insulitis develops, whereas in human prediabetes we are confronted with a well-established and amplified immune response directed against many islet constituents. Intervention at this stage might well be much more difficult than at first inception of the disease process. Clinical trials will be needed to establish whether this is the case.

STRATEGIES FOR DIABETES PREVENTION

Diabetes prevention could be attempted at the level of environmental manipulation, for example, exclusion of cow's milk from the diet of infants (primary prevention), or could be designed to interrupt progression to diabetes in individuals in whom an autoimmune process has already been activated (secondary prevention). The latter must depend on our ability to recognize the disease process at a subclinical level and thus to identify those individuals who are at greatest risk of clinical disease. The level of risk at which intervention could be considered could then be related to the potential hazards of treatment. A relatively safe form of therapy could reasonably be used in lower-risk populations (or earlier in the disease process) even in the knowledge that many of those treated may never develop the disease. In contrast, a potentially toxic agent could be used only when diabetes appears almost inevitable, that is, in those who already have substantial β cell damage.

Predicting IDDM

Siblings of a child with IDDM are some 20 times more likely to develop the disease than a child of the same age and from the same population but with no immediate family history of the disease. Parents and children of an individual with IDDM have similarly increased levels of risk. Prospective family studies have therefore provided the basis for our ability to predict disease onset. Measurement of islet cell antibodies remains the basis of current attempts to predict IDDM, even though repeated workshop meetings have shown test results to be poorly reproducible except in the most expert hands (6). Islet cell antibody screening identifies around 2–2.5% of relatives as strongly positive ($\geq$20 JDF units), and of these some 35% will progress to insulin treatment within 5 years (7,8). This risk is modified by age; a child of 10 with a high titer of islet cell antibodies is some five times more likely to develop diabetes than an adult of 45 with the same titer. Analysis of islet cell antibodies in combination with other autoantibody markers such as insulin autoantibodies or glutamic acid decarboxylase antibodies (GADA) shows that this difference in risk can be accounted for by the higher frequency of multiple autoantibody specificities in children; age itself is not an independent predictor of risk (9,10).

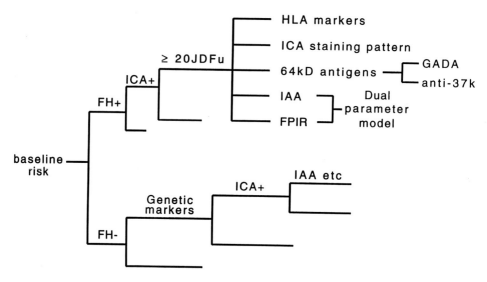

FIG. 1. The decision tree approach allows risk of IDDM to be built up in incremental stages, offering progressively increasing probability that a given outcome will or will not occur.

Risk of progression to diabetes can be set out in the form of a decision tree analysis (Fig. 1). This provides a stepwise selection procedure with progressively increasing probability that a given outcome will or will not occur. The first two steps in the sequence provide a very solid platform for prediction; a first-degree relative aged less than 40 years with a titer of islet cell antibodies of ≥20 JDF units is more likely than not to be on insulin within 10 years. Additional specificity can be obtained as further markers are deployed. Insulin autoantibodies and GADA have already been mentioned, and antibodies to a 37K fragment of the 64K antigen also look extremely promising, although technically difficult to measure. Combined analysis of islet cell antibody-positive relatives using these three additional markers shows that 75% of future cases will be contributed by the 25–30% of islet cell antibody-positive individuals who carry multiple autoantibodies; 10-year risk levels in excess of 80% can be identified within this subgroup without recourse to metabolic testing (9).

Another well-established way of improving specificity of prediction is by testing insulin secretion in the intravenous glucose tolerance test (IVGTT). Loss of the first-phase insulin response (FPIR) to below the first centile of a control population is highly predictive not only of diabetes development but also of early progression to the disease. A first-degree relative with islet cell antibody titers >80 JDF units and loss of the FPIR below the first centile has an 80–100% risk of progression within 5 years, but this very high degree of specificity has to be set against the fact that the first-phase response is lost at a very advanced stage of the disease process—what could be called end-stage prediabetes. The predictive power of the test is excellent, but the scope for intervention is limited. Ideally, we would not need to wait for β cell function to decline to this level before we offer therapy.

Most studies of diabetes prediction have drawn upon family members, and, although impressive levels of risk estimation can now be achieved in this population, we should not lose sight of the fact that some 85–90% of future cases of IDDM will manifest in individuals with no family history of the disease. The future prevalence of IDDM will not be materially affected until population-based screening and intervention becomes a practical proposition. Several studies have now considered the risk of islet cell antibodies in healthy children with no immediate family history of IDDM. One study has suggested that these children carry the same level of risk as islet cell antibody-positive first-degree relatives (11), but this observation has not been confirmed by other studies. For example, we have found a prevalence of 2.8% in healthy British children with no family history of IDDM; 0.8% had islet cell antibody titers ≥20 JDF units. This level of islet cell antibodies would, in family members, be associated with a 35% risk of progression to IDDM within 5 years, but we estimated the risk in our population of unrelated children to be only 5–10% (12). If confirmed, the implication from this observation is that the majority of islet cell antibody-positive individuals in the general population, even at titers of ≥20 JDF units, will not progress to IDDM within 10 years and that a proportion will never do so. Would a lower prognostic significance of islet cell antibodies imply that accurate diabetes prediction will not be possible in the general population? Happily, the indications are that this is not the case. We have seen that genetic markers have only a modest role to play in risk estimation in families, but they are likely to have a much more useful discriminant function in those without a family history. At present, this type of analysis is largely theoretical, but confirmation (or disproof) from research studies should be available in the near future.

Important lessons do, however, emerge from consideration of risk assessment, both in first-degree relatives and in the general population. These are that current methods can identify increased risk in 70–80% of those first-degree relatives who will progress to diabetes and are theoretically capable of identifying a substantial proportion of future cases from within the general population, but that risk can be visualized as a pyramid. Highly specific risk prediction is in this view possible only in a minority of the at-risk population; the majority of future cases will come from those in lower-risk categories (for example, with low titers of islet cell antibodies). It will be appreciated that relatively low levels of risk will need to be treated if we are to have any hope of a major quantitative reduction in the future incidence of diabetes. This in turn means that individuals in some categories of risk will be offered treatment even though only a minority would be expected to develop diabetes over the initial treatment period. There is nothing unusual about this approach. For example, we routinely offer antihypertensive therapy to middle-aged men with mild hypertension even though only 2–3% are expected to suffer a stroke in the course of the next 10 years, and therapy will only lower this risk by around 40%. The clear implication from this is that a favorable ratio of benefit to risk can only be maintained under these circumstances if the treatment offered is no more hazardous than, for example, antihypertensive therapy.

POTENTIAL THERAPIES FOR PREVENTION OF IDDM

Several issues need to be taken into consideration before a form of treatment can be taken into human intervention trials. Ideally, the therapy should be effective in animal models of spontaneous diabetes and after clinical diagnosis in humans. It should not have adverse metabolic effects, and (since we shall need to treat children) it should not affect growth or reproductive capacity. The ideal would perhaps be a form of selective immunotherapy, targeted only against those limbs of the immune response that are involved in β cell damage. Although it seems likely that such "magic bullets" will one day become available, they are probably several years in the future.

What interim options are available? Powerful immunosuppressive agents, such as azathioprine and cyclosporin (13,14), have been shown to prolong β cell survival after clinical diagnosis of type 1 diabetes in humans, but these agents are generally considered to be too toxic for use in prediabetes. Subcutaneous (15), or even oral (16), insulin therapy is effective in animal models, and the combination of intermittent intravenous insulin infusions with continuous subcutaneous therapy has produced promising results in a small pilot study (17). Oral insulin, or other forms of therapy designed to induced immune tolerance such as oral or injected glutamic acid decarboxylase, holds some promise for the future. Above all, these forms of prevention appear potentially safe and could be given early in life to large numbers of at-risk individuals. Subcutaneous insulin therapy should be reasonably safe at low dose, but otherwise healthy individuals are only likely to consider taking regular injections if they can be assured that diabetes is a virtual certainty. Safer or more acceptable treatments will need to be developed before intervention therapy could be extended to include those with a better-preserved β cell mass and less immediate risk of diabetes.

Oral nicotinamide has also produced promising results in one published pilot study (18), and at present many see nicotinamide as the most promising option for more widespread use in the prediabetic population. Nicotinamide (nicotinic acid amide or niacinamide) is a water-soluble group B vitamin, derived from nicotinic acid. Its effect in prevention of toxin-induced models of diabetes has been known since it was first shown to inhibit the development of diabetes in alloxan-treated rats in 1947 (19), and it is also effective in preventing streptozotocin-induced diabetes (20). It appears to act in the final stage of β-cell damage, preventing the cytotoxic effects of cytokines. There are two proposed mechanisms for its action: 1. that it acts as a free radical scavenger to reduce DNA damage and 2. that it restores the islet cell content of NAD (shown to be reduced in both animal models) toward normal. Nicotinamide inhibits poly ADP-ribose, a major route of NAD metabolism (10) and the enzyme NADase (21). It increases intracellular NAD and is a free radical scavenger in its own right.

Nicotinamide given well in advance of the usual time of clinical onset is also effective in preventing spontaneous diabetes in the NOD mouse (21) in which free radicals are implicated in autoimmune β-cell destruction. It also inhibits transplant allograft insulitis in other animal models of immune β-cell damage (22). Nicotinamide preserves residual β cells in partially pancreatectomized rats (23) and enhances their regeneration; it also promotes the growth of cultured human islet cells (24). These effects may result from the inhibitory effect of nicotinamide upon poly (ADP-ribose), which might disinhibit DNA replication (25) and promote islet DNA synthesis.

Further effects of nicotinamide have been demonstrated. These include suppression of major histocompatibility complex (MHC) class II antigen expression on murine islet cells, implying that nicotinamide might reduce presentation of autoantigens to helper T cells by islet β cells in human type 1 diabetes. Nicotinamide has also been shown to inhibit macrophage-mediated cytoxicity directed against rat islet cells (26). This may be of particular importance since macrophages constitute an early and prominent feature of the insulitis seen in the BB rat, and silica, another agent specifically toxic to macrophages, prevents the onset of spontaneous diabetes in both the NOD mouse and the BB rat. There is therefore good evidence to suggest that nicotinamide could offer a protective effect to human β cells, particularly if the drug were given at an early stage of the disease process (27).

Safety of Nicotinamide

Nicotinamide has a good safety record, and therefore constitutes an excellent model drug for a large-scale collaborative prospective placebo-controlled intervention trial in islet cell antibody-positive relatives. Nicotinic acid and nicotinamide have been used widely in the treatment of patients with schizophrenia, in coronary artery disease, and in the treatment of granuloma annulare. Over several years of treatment with doses ranging from 3–12 g daily, the only reported side effects have been rashes, nausea, and vomiting, and headaches. From previous studies, the incidence of liver toxicity has been estimated at 1/6,000 cases (28), although in the Coronary Drug Project minor increases in glutamic-oxaloacetic transaminase (GOT) and serum alkaline phosphatase were observed in subjects receiving nicotinic acid medication, 3 g daily for 5 years (29). These doses correspond to 50–200 mg/kg body weight, which is significantly more than the dose proposed in the present study (30 mg/kg). Thus, nicotinamide at the proposed dose seems reasonable and safe.

Nicotinamide appears to have no oncogenic potency if given alone, although in combination with streptozotocin and alloxan, it has been reported to potentiate the development of islet cell tumors in rats (30). Since human IDDM is not associated with islet cell tumors and nicotinamide alone does not induce tumors in animal models of IDDM, this does not appear to constitute a problem. In New Zealand, a substantial number of nondiabetic first-degree relatives and normal school children have been treated with nicotinamide for 6–40 months without any recognizable side effects (Dr. R. B. Elliott, personal communication). In three recent studies, 28 patients with newly diagnosed or established IDDM were treated with nicotinamide for 1.5–12 months, with daily doses ranging from 1–3 g. The reported side effects were no different from those in the placebo groups. The risks associated with use of nicotinamide at this dosage level thus appear minimal, and the ratio of risk to benefit is entirely favorable for use in a controlled trial.

THE EUROPEAN NICOTINAMIDE DIABETES INTERVENTION TRIAL (ENDIT)

More than 20 national study groups in Europe and Canada have collaborated in setting up this multinational trial. This will be a 5-year prospective placebo-controlled trial requiring participation by 420 first-degree relatives aged 5–40 years with a confirmed level of islet cell antibodies of ≥20 JDF units. This in turn will require screening of around 30,000 first-degree relatives. The first patients were scheduled to be randomized to therapy in the summer of 1994. The international group that has been formed for this trial will provide the basis for a longer-term program aimed at prevention of childhood diabetes.

FUTURE STRATEGIES

Intervention should be considered only in relatives and in the context of approved, controlled clinical trials. Such trials must necessarily be on a very large scale to produce conclusive results. Since only the United States is sufficiently large to recruit for and support such large trials from its own resources, other groups worldwide must look to multinational studies. Several consequences follow from this. One is the need for careful standardization of assays and clinical procedures, through such means as the IDW meetings and the ICARUS registry. ICARUS (islet cell antibody register user's study) arose from the conviction that research into the pathogenesis of childhood diabetes was being held back because the many clinical and population studies that are currently under way lack the power individually to evaluate new genetic or immune markers rapidly and definitively or to provide the basis for intervention trials designed to delay onset of the disease. The basic concept of the register has been to treat islet cell antibody positivity in a nondiabetic as a rare disease, to establish standard methods of investigation and follow-up, and to set up a shared database and bank of serum, served by international reference laboratories. One achievement has been a new international standard for performance of the IVGTT (31) and for routine clinical follow-up of high-risk, prediabetic individuals. The first workshop report on the large joint database was generated early in 1994 (10). Successful collaborative resources such as this are a promising indication of the potential that exists for tackling ambitious projects on a collaborative basis.

CONCLUSION

Our ability to screen for risk of IDDM has developed rapidly over the past few years and with it the ability to apply predictive tests such as GADA on a very large scale. One consequence of this is that haphazard screening programs may spring into existence, without adequate safeguards and counseling. Such schemes could easily create more misery than benefit. The possibility that such tests might be used in a discriminatory fashion by independent agencies such as employers or insurance companies also seems very real. This is perhaps no more than a reminder that there is a price to pay for all advances in medical technology; our responsibility does not cease with the introduction and evaluation of novel predictive tests. Random treatment with untested agents is potentially an even more harmful consequence. Whatever the outcome of intervention trials currently under way, we are entering a new era of diabetes therapy. On the other hand, it now seems clear that there is a real possibility that strategies for diabetes prevention will be validated and move on to the clinical agenda within a few years. Effective international cooperation could do a lot to bring that day closer.

REFERENCES

1. Barnett A, Eff C, Leslie RDG, Pyke DA. Diabetes in identical twins: a study of 200 pairs. *Diabetologia* 1981; 20: 87–93.
2. Bingley PJ, Gale EAM. Rising incidence of IDDM in Europe. *Diabetes Care* 1989; 12: 289–95.
3. Assan R, Debray-Sachs M, Laborie C, *et al*. Metabolic and immunological effects of cyclosporin in recently diagnosed Type 1 diabetes mellitus. *Lancet* 1985; i: 67–71.
4. Gorsuch AN, Spencer KM, Lister J, *et al*. Evidence for a long prediabetic period in Type 1 (insulin-dependent) diabetes mellitus. *Lancet* 1981; ii: 145–7.
5. Gale EAM, Bingley PJ. Can we prevent IDDM? *Diabetes Care* 1994; 17: 339–44.
6. Bonifacio E, Boitard C, Gleichman H, *et al*. Assessment of precision, concordance, specificity, and sensitivity of islet cell antibody measurements in 41 assays. *Diabetologia* 1990; 33: 731–6.
7. Bonifacio E, Bingley PJ, Dean BM, *et al*. Quantification of islet-cell antibodies and prediction of insulin-dependent diabetes. *Lancet* 1990; 335: 147–9.
8. Riley WJ, Maclaren NK, Krischer J, *et al*. A prospective study of the development of diabetes in relatives of patients with insulin-dependent diabetes. *N Engl J Med* 1990; 323: 1167–72.
9. Bingley PJ, Christie MR, Bonifacio E, *et al*. Combined analysis of autoantibodies improves prediction of insulin-dependent diabetes in islet cell antibody positive relatives. *Diabetes* 1994; 43: 1304–10.
10. Bingley PJ. Prediction of diabetes: interaction of risk markers in islet cell antibody positive family members: the first analysis of the ICARUS dataset. (Abstract) *Diabetologia* 1994; 37 Suppl 1 :A55.
11. Schatz D, Krischer J, Horne G, *et al*. Islet cell antibodies predict insulin dependent diabetes in United States school age children as powerfully as in unaffected relatives. *J Clin Invest* 1994; 93: 2403–7.
12. Bingley PJ, Bonifacio E, Shattock M, *et al*. Can islet cell antibodies predict IDDM in the general population? *Diabetes Care* 1993; 16: 45–50.
13. Johnston C, Raghu PK, McCulloch DK, *et al*. B-cell function and insulin sensitivity in non-diabetic HLA-identical siblings of insulin-dependent diabetics. *Diabetes* 1987; 36: 829–37.
14. Paul TL, Hramiak JL, Mahon JL, *et al*. Nicotinamide and insulin sensitivity. (Abstract) *Diabetologia* 1993; 36: 369.
15. Atkinson MA, Maclaren NK, Luchetta R. Insulitis and insulin dependent diabetes in NOD mice reduced by prophylactic insulin therapy. *Diabetes* 1990; 39: 933–7.
16. Davies JL, Kawaguchi Y, Bennett ST, *et al*. A genome wide search for human type 1 diabetes susceptibility genes. *Nature* 1994; 371: 130–6.
17. Keller RJ, Eisenbarth GS, Jackson RA. Insulin prophylaxis in individuals at high risk of type 1 diabetes. *Lancet* 1993; 341: 927–8.
18. Elliott RB, Chase HP. Prevention or delay of Type 1 (insulin-dependent) diabetes mellitus in children using nicotinamide. *Diabetologia* 1991; 34: 362–5.
19. Lazarow A. Protection against alloxan diabetes. *Anat Rec* 1947; 97: 353.
20. Dulin WE, Wyse BM, Kalamazoo MS. Studies on the ability of compounds to block the diabetogenic activity of streptozotocin. *Diabetes* 1969; 18: 459–66.
21. Yamada K, Nonaka K, Hanafusa T, Miyazaki A, Toyoshima H, Tarui S. Preventive and therapeutic effects of large-dose nicotinamide injections on diabetes associated with insulitis. *Diabetes* 1982; 31: 749–53.
22. Nomikos IN, Prowse SJ, Carotenuto P, Lafferty KJ. Combined treatment with nicotinamide and desferrioxamine prevents islet allograft destruction in NOD mice. *Diabetes* 1986; 35: 1302–4.

23. Yonemura Y, Takishima T, Miwa K, *et al*. Amelioration of diabetes mellitus in partially depancreatized rats by poly (ADP-ribose) synthetase inhibitors. *Diabetes* 1984; 33: 401–4.
24. Lipton RB, Atchison JJ, Dorman JS, *et al*. Genetic, immunological, and metabolic determinants of risk for type 1 diabetes mellitus in families. *Diabetic Med* 1992; 9: 224–32.
25. Hayaishi O, Ueda K. Poly (ADP-ribose) and ADP ribosylation of proteins. *Annu Rev Biochem* 1977; 46: 95–116.
26. Kroncke K-D, Funda J, Berschick B, Kolb H, Kolb-Bachofen V. Macrophage cytotoxicity towards oslated rat islet cells: neither lysis nor its protection by nicotinamide are β-cell specific. *Diabetologia* 1991; 34: 232–6.
27. Tuomilehto J, Lounamaa R, Tuomilehto-Wolf E, *et al*. Childhood Diabetes in Finland (DiMe) Group. Epidemiolgy of childhood diabetes mellitus in Finland—background of a nationwide study of Type 1 (insulin-dependent) diabetes mellitus. *Diabetologia* 1992; 35: 70–6.
28. Hoffer A. Safety, side effects and relative lack of toxicity of nicotinic acid and nicotinamide. *Schizophrenia* 1969; 1: 78–87.
29. The Coronary Drug Project Research Group. Clofibrate and niacin in coronary heart disease. *JAMA* 1975; 231: 360–81.
30. Yamagami Y, Miwa A, Takasawa S, Yamamota H, Okamoto H. Induction of rat pancreatic β-cell tumors by the combined administration of streptozocin or alloxan and poly (ADP-ribose) synthetase inhibitors. *Cancer Res* 1985; 45: 1845–9.
31. Bingley PJ, Colman PG, Eisenbarth GS, *et al*. Standardization of IVGTT to predict IDDM. *Diabetes Care* 1992; 15: 93–102.

DISCUSSION

Dr. Bergman: Your numbers were very small. Is it really possible to calculate probability on the basis of 2 out of 5 *versus* 7 out of 7? In statistical terms, these are very small numbers. Do we really know that one treatment was any better than the other with such a tiny number of events? I am not a statistician, but I remember the Framingham study in which small numbers of heart attacks caused an enormous change in the results and a lot of policies based on 22 or 23 patients were introduced that later turned out to be a false direction because of inadequate statistical power.

Dr. Gale: The pilot studies don't show anything definite, but they may indicate trends. The difficulty is how far you go with the pilot study. It takes as long to do a pilot study as it would take to do the full insulin trial, because you still need a large number of individuals over many years to do it. The studies are consistent with the idea that we need controlled trials but, in themselves, they prove nothing. That is why they are pilot studies.

Dr. Bergman: A pilot study is not designed to prove *nothing*. If we cannot assign any statistical power to a study, then it is not indicative of anything in my view. I am trying to see whether it is really indicative, and my own view is that it may not be.

Dr. Gale: I am trying not to let people get too carried away by such a small data set, although there are significant *p* values to the studies. We were looking at 100% progression against 40–50% progression and that may be enough to tell us clinically whether these forms of treatment ought to be investigated further.

Dr. Bergman: No one has really talked about resting the β cell by giving exogenous insulin. There has also been very little discussion on the possibility of inducing β-cell rest by other means, for example by reducing the need for insulin secretion by increasing insulin sensitivity, either with drugs or with exercise or with some other kind of intervention. Could you comment on this?

Dr. Gale: It is by no means clear to me that treatments of the type you are suggesting, for example 0.5 of a unit of insulin per kg/d with a free diet, will induce β-cell rest, but perhaps Dr. Crofford or others might want to comment on this.

Dr. Bergman: I think the best way to rest the β cell is to improve the utilization of carbohydrate without insulin, because a lot of carbohydrate utilization is insulin-independent. If you do a test on marathon runners, for example, they have almost no insulin response, and they take up enormous amounts of glucose, even at rest, because they are utilizing it at such a high rate, essentially without an insulin response. In my view, this is the best way to rest the β cell, *i.e.,* to generate a situation in which insulin is not required for glucose utilization rather than giving a little bit of insulin.

Dr. Gale: I am not contesting that at all. I was merely doubting whether we had evidence that β-cell rest is the effective component of insulin administration. I think it is a very interesting approach. As you know, the Seattle group has been interested in whether there is some sort of automatic increase or reduction in insulin resistance in the terminal phase of prediabetes. I rather believe this concept. In other words, these people are producing less insulin, but they manage to compensate temporarily by a period of enhanced sensitivity until they develop a virus infection or whatever it is that precipitates their diabetes.

Dr. Van Assche: If the β-cell rest hypothesis is true then we may expect that pregnancy would precipitate diabetes in those individuals who are prone to it. Is something known about this?

Dr. Gale: I know that there was one study from Denmark that found an increased incidence of classic type 1 diabetes in pregnancy. The model that I was talking about, where you have progressive β-cell failure together with the changes in insulin sensitivity that occur during pregnancy, would make it very likely that you will get more cases. This may be part of the reason why you get more cases during puberty, for example, with the changes in insulin sensitivity/resistance that occur at that time.

Dr. Drash: I might comment on that. We used the immunosuppressive agent FK 6 in the BB rat and completely prevented diabetes. We continued our observations for about 300 days, and the only time diabetes developed in these animals on continued immunosuppression was when they became pregnant.

Dr. Drash: I wonder whether antioxidants might be an appropriate form of management. There is evidence that different antioxidants get into cells in different ways. A recent study comparing vitamin E with probucol showed that they affect the antioxidant mechanism in different ways. I wonder about a pack of four or five different antioxidants, all with different routes of entry and action, as an approach to prevention. They have minimum toxic side effects from what we know about them.

Dr. Gale: I think that it is an interesting idea, but I would have some hesitation about it. First of all we are not sure whether nicotinamide is going to be effective in humans, and, in animal and isolated-cell models, more powerful antioxidants than nicotinamide are ineffective. The other hesitation I would have is that it is hard enough to assess the risks of *one* form of treatment given as monotherapy. If you are giving four or five together, quite how you would run your safety analysis and how you would know when something is going wrong is rather difficult to imagine. So I think we have to keep to very simple questions, using the agents on which we have at least some preliminary data.

Dr. Drash: Probucol is concentrated in the β cells and we showed that it was an effective drug in the baby rat in reducing but certainly not in preventing diabetes.

Dr. Scott: Clinical trials with anticancer agents seem to me to have more rigorous requirements than the type 1 diabetes trials. I would like to know how you decided to go ahead with these trials, what was the point that made you say they are worth doing.

Dr. Gale: I agree that the cancer trials are at a very advanced stage, but they have been going on for 20 years. If you look back at the early cancer trials, you will see that they were quite speculative and far more risky than the sort of interventions we are testing. We have to start somewhere, with some forms of intervention, and build up experience to enable us to go through a sequence of future trials with better-defined, predictive end points, with more rationally selected and more precise forms of intervention.

Dr. Scott: Wouldn't you agree that the models of type 1 diabetes are probably more advanced than the animal models of cancer and, in that respect, one would require more complete animal data in the type 1 diabetes trials than would be needed in cancer trials because the cancer models are not as good as the type 1 diabetes models?

Dr. Gale: I think there comes a point in the development of any drug at which you have to move out of animal models—they provide an analogy but not a blueprint, and there are a lot of differences between diabetes in the BB rat and the NOD mouse and diabetes in man. I think the particular problem we face in prediabetes is that we are coming up with very powerful and constantly improving predictive models. We can assign risk with much greater certainty than in most other diseases that I am familiar with. There is thus a kind of psychological pressure to do something about it once you have assigned the risk. One reason why I have pushed very hard to continue my trial is that I believe that one large trial with an agent that appears reasonably safe is a lot better than a dozen smaller trials with a lot of agents, some of which may not be safe, and where the results may be difficult to interpret. I believe it is very important that people should get together and work together, and we should start with the safest available agents. I fully believe we may be sitting on treatments that can reduce the risk of progression to insulin dependence. If giving something such as nicotinamide or insulin injections can stop people's getting diabetes, then I think it is worth going ahead to try to find out.

Dr. Nattrass: One of the problems seems to be that we tend to be black and white thinkers. We want to know whether a specific agent *prevents* type 1 diabetes, and because of the way we work we tend not to look much further ahead than 5 years. The trouble is that any agent you use may just delay the onset of type 1 diabetes. Once you start to think along those lines you run into very different considerations, for example, on the long-term safety of the agent you are using and considerations about what length of time is worthwhile to delay the onset of diabetes rather than to prevent it.

Dr. Gale: We tend to say "predict" rather than "risk assessment" and we say "prevent" when we mean "reduce risk within a defined time period." When people giving antihypertensive treatment say it prevents a stroke, that is all they mean; they don't mean that the people are not going to get a stroke the year after the end of the trial or 5 years further down the line. They mean that within the period of treatment the risk of a certain event happening is reduced. Until we have done the trial and come up with the magnitude of the effect and the data about the duration of the effect, we are not in a position to prejudge the issue. The hypertension comparison is one I use a lot. If you, as a middle-aged man, had moderate or mild hypertension, you would automatically be offered antihypertensive treatment. If antihypertensive treatment reduces the risk of stroke by around 40%, 900 people would have to be treated for 1 year to prevent 1 stroke. In prediabetes, if we are talking about an equivalent of 40% reduction in progression, you would have to treat only 30 people for 1 year to delay or prevent one episode of diabetes.

Dr. Nattrass: I agree with what you are saying but to continue that analogy, if all you did by treating my hypertension was move my stroke from 12 months hence to 24 months hence, then I would want to know what price I was going to pay for that extra year without a stroke, and if by treating me you are going to make me impotent I might choose not to have the antihypertensive medication.

Dr. Gale: That is the problem we face in every aspect of modern medicine. We are delaying risk, we are treating people for cholesterol, we are treating raised blood pressure, we are treating this and that risk factor, and at every point you have to do an analysis of benefit *versus* risk. It seems to me that, until we have done these trials, we can't find out what the benefit is, and indeed we will still be unclear as to what the risk is.

Dr. Drash: It is my understanding that the US insulin intervention study appears to be going forward on the basis that individuals will not be taken off treatment if they are well. I am very disturbed about this from a scientific point of view. What is the procedure going to be in the nicotinamide trial? Is there to be a definite end point when they come off treatment?

Dr. Gale: It is a clinical trial with a defined end point, and we reach an answer at 5 years. We will have to think very hard about what happens after that. As far as I am concerned at this stage of the study it is a 5-year protocol, but if there is a fairly dramatic effect of nicotinamide then it is going to be hard ethically to take people off it. We have no evidence that the autoimmune process in prediabetes will burn itself out. We may just be damping it down.

Dr. Crofford: If a new treatment becomes accepted by society before the treatment has been properly tested (*i.e.,* if, because of premature press reports, unrefereed papers, drug company promotions, and so on, the thinking of society is that a certain agent is good), then all the health care providers throughout the world will start using the agent, and you run into the ethical dilemma that it becomes impossible to do a randomized trial because you can't get anybody to be in the control group. We see this in many aspects of medicine, where therapies are given that have never been proved effective. If you delay doing a definitive study beyond a certain point, you are committed to using the treatment in the hope that it works but with no definite proof one way or the other. So there has to be a combination of technical decision making, biological decision making, and philosophical-social decision making. All these have to be put in the same context in order to decide when is the critical time to start intervention trials, and it is a very difficult decision in my opinion.

Dr. Marliss: I must say that I have the same kind of reservation as that already expressed by others, but for a couple of additional reasons. For example, while in the specific case of nicotinamide, one might be reasonably confident that the risk is small, the same may not be true for β-carotene and/or vitamin E, as shown by a recent cancer prevention study. I don't think it is necessarily obvious that reasonably large doses of nicotinamide over a protracted period will turn out to be as innocuous as we hope. The concern I have is that you are only postponing the inevitable. Also I am not at all sure that you will be justified in saying that this intervention that may be effective in familial diabetes will necessarily be effective in the other kind of type 1 diabetes, which may have a different pathophysiology.

Dr. Gale: It is a difficult area. I accept what you said about nicotinamide: we cannot assume it is absolutely safe. However, going back over 30 or 40 years during which high doses of nicotinamide have been given for different reasons, we don't have any evidence of harm apart from some changes in liver enzymes. With regard to extrapolation of results, I still think that if you could, for example, delay the onset of diabetes in a child by a few years that would be well worth doing, but that remains to be seen.

Diabetes, edited by Richard M. Cowett,
Nestlé Nutrition Workshop Series,
Vol. 35. Nestec Ltd.,
Vevey/Raven Press, Ltd., New York © 1995.

Protein Metabolism in Diabetes Mellitus: Implications for Clinical Management

Réjeanne Gougeon, Paul B. Pencharz,* and Errol B. Marliss

*McGill Nutrition and Food Science Centre, Royal Victoria Hospital, 687 Pine Avenue West, Montreal, Quebec H3A 1A1 Canada; *Hospital for Sick Children, Division of Clinical Nutrition, 555 University Avenue, Toronto, Ontario M5G 1X8 Canada*

Diabetes mellitus is characterized by derangements in the metabolism not only of glucose and fat but also of protein (1). However, protein has always received less attention than fat and glucose, both in terms of alterations in its metabolism and in its nutritional implications. Although hyperglycemia and its consequences have always been the hallmark of the disease and plasma glucose the main index of diabetic control, altered protein metabolism was recognized even in the preinsulin era because of the severe muscle and other protein depletion that occurred, even with an apparently adequate protein intake. In 1906, the German investigator Bernhard Naunyn observed an increase in glycosuria with increased dietary protein and recommended that protein intake as well as carbohydrate intake should be restricted (2). In the preinsulin era (1922), Marsh *et al.* addressed the issue as to whether "the laws that govern protein metabolism of non-diabetic subjects applied equally to those with diabetes" (3). These investigators concluded, in contrast to Benedict and Joslin [cited in (3)] who preceded them, that protein requirements for achieving nitrogen equilibrium were similar to those of nondiabetic persons. However, this was in a setting in which glycosuria had been eliminated by the high-fat, low-carbohydrate diet that was then the only way of achieving metabolic control.

There intervened a long period in which a disproportionately small amount of attention was paid to the question of protein metabolism. It is informative to trace the trends in nutritional recommendations for persons with diabetes from the preinsulin era to the present. With the advent of insulin and oral agents and with data emerging from clinical and experimental research, nutrition recommendations have evolved from low-carbohydrate, high-fat to high-carbohydrate, high-fibre, low-fat, low-cholesterol diets (4,5). From 1935 until the current decade, guidelines for protein intake had remained at 85–90 g/day or approximately 18% of energy intake. One report of intakes during World War II gave values of 68 g protein and 2150 kcal/d, which were associated with general improvement of "adult diabetes" (*diabète gras*) (6). The benefit was most likely to have been related to the energy restriction. The current dietary recommendations in many countries are meant to apply whether diabetes results from an absolute or a relative deficiency of insulin. Protein intakes of the order of 1.5 g/kg ideal body weight appear to be habitually consumed by the diabetic and nondiabetic populations alike in North America. This represents nearly twice the amount recommended for healthy diabetic and nondiabetic individuals, which, at 0.8 g of complete protein/kg/day, provides a margin of safety in the latter.

What remains uncertain at present is the appropriateness of either the usual *or* the recommended intakes, because the state of protein metabolism of both type 1 and type 2 diabetic persons receiving conventional treatment is not yet clearly defined. Various studies of fasting amino acid and protein kinetics using isotopic amino acid turnover methods have been done, beginning in the 1980s, and these are reviewed below. The integrated fasting-fed cycle has not been the subject of so much investigation, however, since methodological problems have precluded precise study of the fed state. It has been presumed that, since no specific clinical disorder in persons with diabetes can yet be ascribed to altered protein metabolism, the habitual intakes are safe. Clearly, the rates of accumulation of advanced glycosylation end products in structural and other proteins will be affected not only by the prevailing plasma glucose concentrations but also by the rates of turnover of proteins. For this and other reasons, definition of fed-fasted protein metabolism at different levels of diabetes control, as well as different protein intakes, is mandatory.

The goals of nutrition therapy for diabetes are to achieve and maintain a normal metabolic state. By attaining an optimal body weight and normal blood glucose, glycosylated proteins, and desirable plasma lipids, it is hoped that it will be possible to retard or reduce complications such as retinopathy, nephropathy, and neuropathy that are specific to the disease (4). In this regard, the recent Diabetes Control and Complications Trial (DCCT) results strongly support the value of intensive control in persons with type 1 diabetes (*see* Crofford in this volume). Of the estimated 14 million North Americans with diabetes mellitus, type 2 diabetes accounts for 90–95% of all cases. Since 70–80% of these are obese, treatment should include weight reduction through energy restriction. Energy restriction itself has an impact on the efficiency of utilization of dietary protein even in persons without diabetes, such that more is required as the energy deficit increases. This is another good reason for studying protein-energy relationships at different levels of diabetes control in obese subjects.

Furthermore, 25% of new-onset, chronic renal failure is related to diabetes, and protein restriction is now being recommended for both diabetic and nondiabetic persons with incipient renal failure (7). Some investigators have been concerned with the generous protein recommendations for diabetes because studies in experimental animals show that dietary protein contributes to the development of azotemia and renal failure (8), and there is a growing body of literature that suggests that dietary protein restriction is of value as a preventive or therapeutic measure for renal insufficiency (7). Protein intakes of 0.62 g/kg body weight, with associated reductions in phosphate, fat, and sodium, have been shown to retard the rate of decline of glomerular filtration rate in diabetic nephropathy (9). However, one study of protein intakes in a cohort of type 1 diabetic subjects compared by degree of nephropathy failed to show significant differences (10). It has been reported that protein consumption influences glomerular filtration rate but not microalbuminuria (11). One contributor to the present uncertainty is that diabetes control is likely to be a major regulator of the disposition of ingested protein, a variable that has not been controlled for systematically. This makes it even more important to determine the extent to which the relative or absolute reduction in insulin action in diabetes alters protein metabolism, and if optimal control of diabetes (as indicated by normoglycemia, glycated hemoglobins, or fructosamine) will normalize protein metabolism in the setting of the current standards of diabetes practice.

Other settings in which the appropriate levels of protein intake in relation to level of diabetic control need to be defined include infancy, childhood, and adolescence, when there is a need for rapid rates of body protein accretion. Likewise, during pregnancy and lactation, the changed physiological demands have well-defined effects on nutrient requirements, but, with either pregestational or gestational diabetes, these may well be altered, in particular the requirements for protein.

There is clear experimental evidence dating from the 1950s (12) that the diabetic state affects protein metabolism and that insulin is an important regulator of the response of protein metabolism to nutrient intake in achieving net protein retention. Thus a deficiency of insulin or insulin action may be associated with an abnormal handling of dietary protein such that minimum requirements may differ from those in normal persons if they are to be considered safe. Concern has been expressed (7,13,14) as to what the safe levels of protein intake are in diabetes and to what extent restrictions can be recommended in the establishment of a prudent nutrition plan. Such concerns are supported by the work of the group of Hoffer, who showed an 18% increase in obligate minimum nitrogen excretion in very intensively treated type 1 diabetic subjects compared with normal controls, using the protein-free diet technique (15). A significant correlation between average plasma glucose and minimum nitrogen excretion was found even in a range of plasma glucoses that spanned the normal and minimally elevated range. These authors suggest that even with rigorous glycemic control, optimal protein metabolism might require higher protein intakes, and these could be even higher in patients treated with conventional insulin regimes. Proof that the concern is justified was provided by the recent study by Brodsky *et al.* that clearly showed that protein restriction to 0.6 g/kg/d in type 1 diabetic subjects with early nephropathy compromised their protein metabolism (16).

Data obtained from nitrogen (N) balance studies have shown that insulin withdrawal is associated with an increase in urinary nitrogen loss, which is reversed by restoration of insulin therapy. However, nitrogen balance studies do not distinguish between changes in the rates of protein synthesis and breakdown, and total insulin withdrawal is a very coarse stimulus that does not necessarily give clinically relevant information applicable to conventionally controlled diabetic persons (13). Because of the limitations of the nitrogen-balance method, studies carried out during the past decade particularly have estimated whole body protein turnover using the ^{13}C-labeled essential amino acid leucine (or occasionally other amino acids and other labels) as a tracer. Recent studies of protein metabolism inferred by leucine kinetics (flux, synthesis, and breakdown) have shown that it is the cooperative action of the increases in plasma concentrations of insulin and amino acids (branched chain amino acids, possibly leucine) that mediates the response of protein metabolism to food intake. The combination of increased insulin along with exogenous amino acids enhances the rate of protein synthesis and decreases the rate of whole body protein breakdown, resulting in a net retention of amino acids in body protein (17). Such observations have been made in humans (17,18) and in dogs (19) with infused insulin and/or amino acid mixtures that would result in an increase in endogenous insulin (17,18).

Controversy exists as to whether insulin alone can increase protein synthesis (20). Studies by Garlick and Grant [reported in (20)] in postabsorptive rats indicate that infused insulin producing concentrations well above those found in the normally fed animal stimulated protein synthesis but had a maximal effect on muscle protein synthesis at concentrations within the physiological range when given in combination with amino acids. The authors concluded that the response of muscle protein synthesis to feeding arises from an increase in the sensitivity to insulin brought about by amino acids. *In vitro* studies in skeletal muscle of the effects of amino acid and insulin treatment on protein synthesis and breakdown suggest that myofibrillar protein degradation may be inhibited by dietary protein but not by circulating insulin (21) [the inhibition possibly being brought about by the α-keto acid of leucine (22)], and that insulin stimulates protein synthesis. In contrast, *in vivo* postabsorptive studies of insulin infusion (in the absence of an exogenous source of protein) have shown that the primary effect of insulin is to restrain whole-body proteolysis, as assessed by a decrease in leucine release from protein. Such studies have not shown an effect of insulin on synthesis or leucine incorporation into protein (23–25). In the absence of exogenous amino acids, insulin, by inhibiting proteolysis, decreases the release of many amino acids from insulin-sensitive tissues, thereby decreasing the substrate available for protein synthesis. This would appear to be responsible for the apparently paradoxical whole-body *decrease* in protein synthesis found in such experiments. Insulin deficiency has also been associated with a decrease in the albumin fractional synthetic rate (25).

Taken together, the *in vivo* and *in vitro* experiments are conclusive that amino acids, as well as insulin, elicit responses in protein synthesis and breakdown similar to those resulting from feeding, these two factors acting cooperatively (20). What modifications must be made in one factor when the other is deficient (such as insulin in diabetes), to ensure the maintenance of normal body composition and function? What modifications are also indicated when energy restriction is superimposed on the relative insulin deficiency, such as during weight reduction in the obese type 2 diabetic population? Conventional, energy-restricted diets for weight reduction, providing 1500 kcal with 18% of energy derived from protein, would supply only 67 g of protein. Recent recommendations for low-energy balanced diets, *e.g.*, less than 1200 kcal/day, have included as much as 28% of energy from protein to provide 0.8–1.2 g protein/kg body weight. We have shown a return to nitrogen equilibrium and maintenance of rates of whole-body N flux in nondiabetic obese subjects with a 93 g protein, 400 kcal/d diet (26, and detailed below). It may be, therefore, that in obese persons with type 2 diabetes the protein requirement to maintain equilibrium will rise more steeply than in nondiabetic persons as energy intake is decreased below isoenergetic values.

Altered postabsorptive-state amino acid metabolism has been well documented in type 1 diabetic human subjects using isotopic tracer techniques: rates of leucine turnover and oxidation are reported to be increased during insulin withdrawal (27–31) and are not completely corrected by conventional insulin therapy (28,29,31,32). The lowering of plasma glucose to normal levels by intensive insulin therapy reduced leucine turnover and oxidation rates (28–31). These observations indicate that, in type 1 diabetes, poor glycemic control is associated with altered leucine kinetics, suggesting increases in protein breakdown greater than those in protein synthesis; the consequent net protein loss can be returned toward normal with optimized insulin therapy, a result of a reduction in protein breakdown. The apparently paradoxical increase in protein synthesis is thought to be caused by greater availability of amino acids (from the increased catabolism). The tissues in which such increases in synthesis occur appear to be mainly splanchnic, from recent regional catheterization studies by Nair *et al.* (33). Likewise, these authors showed the *in vivo* effect of insulin to decrease protein turnover to be due to splanchnic tissues.

Glycine fluxes were significantly higher in "adequately treated" normoglycemic pregestational pregnant diabetic women, suggesting that plasma glucose levels do not necessarily reflect the static or dynamic parameters of other fuels affected by insulin, such as amino acids. Greater glycine fluxes were associated with delivery of fetuses with higher birthweights than those of control nondiabetic and gestational diabetic women (34).

In contrast to the considerable number of studies in type 1 diabetes, few previous studies have reported the kinetics of protein metabolism in type 2 diabetes. Those available led Bier in 1991 to conclude that "body protein metabolism is, by and large, essentially normal in" this type of diabetes, when studied in the fasted state (35). For example, Staten *et al.* (36), in studies of leucine turnover and oxidation, have found no difference between conventionally controlled, insulin-treated type 2 diabetic subjects, matched obese nondiabetic subjects, and normal weight subjects. Intensive insulin therapy sufficient to normalize blood glucose did not alter leucine flux and oxidation. This contrasts with the increased leucine flux and oxidation reported in hyperglycemic type 1 diabetic subjects, which could be normalized with insulin therapy. The authors concluded that despite similar levels of hyperglycemia, it is possible that in type 2 diabetes during conventional insulin therapy sufficient insulin action is present to control amino acid metabolism (36). In contrast to the other studies cited by Bier (35), Umpleby *et al.* showed increased leucine oxidation (although no other aspect of leucine kinetics was increased) when studied diurnally (37). Intensive insulin therapy was shown to decrease plasma glucose and glycerol levels, which, when taken together with the leucine data, was interpreted to suggest that the sensitivity of leucine metabolism to insufficient insulin action may differ from that of glucose and fat metabolism (36,38). Differential effects of insulin are known to occur at different plasma concentrations. Acute physiologic increases of insulin had no effect on nitrogen accretion in human skeletal muscle in healthy men during a protein meal. The major determinant of amino acid uptake across human forearm tissue appears to be the amino acid concentrations. However, more prolonged hyperinsulinemia (36–48 h) resulted in a significant increase in nitrogen accretion, indicating that a time-dependent induction of enzymes may be required for protein synthesis (39). Furthermore, Staten *et al.* (36) investigated a very specific obese diabetic population requiring insulin studied in the fasting state and during insulin therapy that maintained blood glucose at levels averaging 9.7 mmol/liter.

As noted above, one important limitation of the use of the ^{13}C-leucine kinetic methodology at present is that it can give useful data only in steady-state conditions. Thus, most studies in both type 1 and type 2 diabetes have reflected the fasted state and cannot be readily extrapolated to the fed-fasted, nonsteady-state that prevails in daily life. For this reason, we have chosen to use the longer and more tedious ^{15}N glycine method, because it gives data that are integrated over the fed and fasted states. For this (and other) reasons, we realize that the approach yields data that give rather imprecise inferences about the rates of protein synthesis and breakdown. It relies on end product ^{15}N enrichment in urine urea nitrogen, and on a number of assumptions relating to compartments of amino acids and to urea and its excretion. The calculations are based on the model of Picou and Taylor-Roberts [cited in (26)]. Of particular interest is the fact that this approach allows for repeated measurements in the same individual in different nutritional states and at different levels of diabetes control. It involves 3-hourly oral ^{15}N-glycine dosing, with corresponding timing of urine collections and meal consumption, over a total of 60 hours. We have chosen to include 3 days and 2 nights in the 60 hours, with nutrients in formula form divided into six equal meals during the day. The only other way of using the stable isotopic methodology with ^{13}C-leucine in the fed state would be to assure a continuously fed state during the tracer infusion, and this does not approximate to the physiological nonsteady-state related to meal consumption. Thus we have sacrificed the somewhat greater precision in estimating turnover parameters for the capacity to make "integrated feeding-fasting" estimations. We are not aware that anyone else has used this approach in persons with diabetes mellitus.

We first quantified protein turnover in this manner in obese nondiabetic persons in the isoenergetic weight-maintained state and then during the state of maximum endogenous fat mobilization with a protein-sparing modified fast (a very low energy, all protein diet, or VLED) (26). This approach was used because others have previously shown that such diets are capable of markedly reducing (and even normalizing) plasma glucose levels in people with type 2 diabetes (e.g., 40,41). Our strategy was thus to study such obese type 2 diabetic subjects first while markedly hyperglycemic and off all therapy, and then after 4 and 6 weeks of a VLED, to compare their nitrogen balance and ^{15}N-glycine results with those of the control obese subjects. The VLED contains a generous amount of protein. Having shown considerable differences, we then undertook to determine responses over one isoenergetic diet period in comparable subjects in whom intensive insulin therapy was employed, after which we allowed them to become hyperglycemic off insulin (again at isoenergetic intakes), and then again after 4 weeks of a VLED. This allowed us to compare the effects of rigorous short-term glycemic control with more moderate hyperglycemia, and then with near-euglycemia during the VLED.

In the first study, the isocaloric diet in the obese and type 2 diabetic subjects contained a fixed 80 g/day of good quality protein, and the VLED consisted entirely of 93 g/day of a collagen hydrolysate-based diet that provided 1.7 MJ/day (400 kcal/day). Collagen hydrolysate was used because of its palatability; it was methionine and tryptophan supplemented and provided sufficient essential amino acids to meet the current WHO recommendations. (We have since shown that such diets result in rather similar nitrogen balance and ^{15}N-glycine kinetic responses to those obtained during diets with the same protein content but with a higher proportion of essential amino acids, unpublished.) Since the subjects were comparable with respect to anthropometric variables and since the protocol was otherwise identical, the results of the seven nondiabetic subjects (26) can be directly compared with those of the seven type 2 diabetic subjects (42).

Figure 1 shows that off-treatment mean fasting and mean daily (premeal and bed-

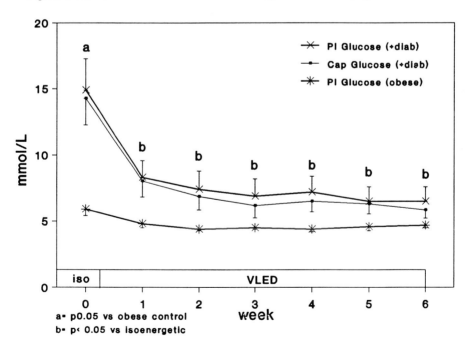

FIG. 1. Fasting plasma (PI) and mean daily capillary (Cap) glucose concentrations in obese subjects with type 2 diabetes and plasma glucose concentrations in obese control subjects during 1 week of isoenergetic feeding followed by a 1.7 MJ/day (400 kcal/day) collagen hydrolysate-based all-protein diet. Data are plotted as means ± SE.

time) glycemia in the diabetic subjects was markedly increased, at 15 ± 2 mmol/liter, compared with 5.9 ± 0.6 mmol/liter in the control subjects. Such hyperglycemia is not uncommonly encountered in certain treated patients. It was associated with polyuria and polydipsia (mean 24-h urine glucose 580 mmol/d) but with no undue discomfort in our subjects for the short duration of the study. Additional carbohydrate was given to approximate the measured urine glucose losses. Whereas fasting plasma free fatty acids were mildly raised (860 μmol/liter), blood, breath and urine ketone bodies were not increased in the diabetic subjects during the isoenergetic ^{15}N-glycine study.

With this protein intake, which was of the order of 0.85 g/kg/d, nitrogen balance was in equilibrium in both diabetic and nondiabetic subjects during the isoenergetic diet (Fig. 2). Had this been the only information available, the temptation would have been [as in the type 2 diabetic subjects previously studied, including the leucine kinetic data (35)] to infer a relative "resistance" of the untoward effects of type 2 diabetes on protein metabolism. However, as shown by the ^{15}N-glycine-derived data (Fig. 3), whole body N flux was increased by 13%, protein synthesis was increased by 16%, and protein breakdown was increased by 21%. This resulted in net synthesis (S-B) that was negative in the diabetic subjects and significantly different from that of the control subjects. Thus the maintenance of N balance in the diabetic subjects under the conditions of this study was at the cost of increased rates of protein turnover. We cannot extrapolate these results to what happens in a more chronic state

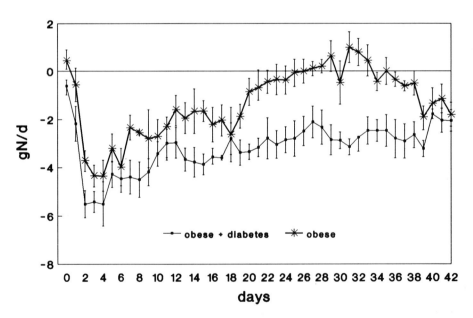

FIG. 2. Daily nitrogen (N) balance during the 1.7 MJ/day collagen hydrolysate-based protein diet in obese subjects with or without type 2 diabetes. Values at time 0 represent the last day of the isoenergetic diet. Data are plotted as means ± SE.

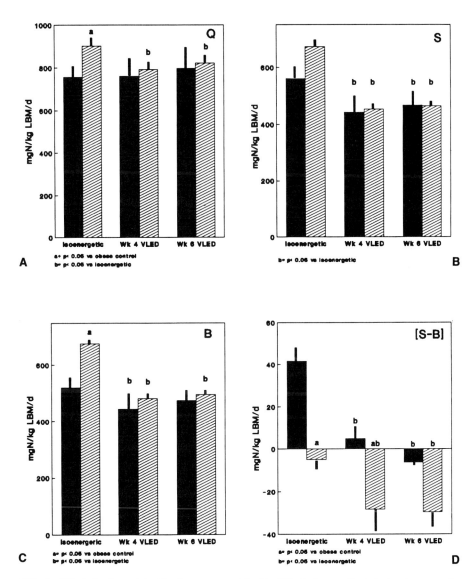

FIG. 3. Whole body protein kinetics measured by the ^{15}N-glycine method during isoenergetic feeding and at weeks 4 and 6 of 1.7 MJ/day collagen hydrolysate-based protein diet (VLED) in obese subjects without *(solid bars)* and with *(shaded bars)* type 2 diabetes. **(A)** N flux (Q); **(B)** rate of protein synthesis (S); **(C)** rate of protein breakdown (B); **(D)** net protein synthesis (S-B). Data are means ± SE.

of hyperglycemia, nor can we speculate upon whether the prior state of glycemic control was such that the subjects had already accommodated to a chronic challenge to maintain their protein metabolic status. Notably, within the group of seven diabetic subjects, there was no significant correlation between mean glycemia and the protein turnover variables. This is probably because their levels of hyperglycemia were rather comparable. However, significant correlations emerged when the data for the control and diabetic subjects were combined. Thus the possibility of there being such an association is raised, but clearly requires the study of a dose-response between graded levels of diabetic control and their effects on protein metabolism. This is presently being done in our laboratory. Having shown that comparing best (i.e., normal) with worst case glycemic conditions, we now address the responses of both groups to one approach to normalizing the hyperglycemia, the VLED.

There was a rapid decline in plasma glucose during the first week of the VLED to values similar to, but remaining slightly above, those of the control subjects (Fig. 1). Several of the subjects' values were superimposable upon those of the control subjects. The initial pattern of N balance response was similar to that of the control subjects, namely a shift toward greater negative balance, but it was sustained at a greater level in the diabetic subjects. Whereas a progressive improvement occurred in the control subjects, with N equilibrium being achieved at the third to fifth weeks, the mean values always remained negative in the diabetic subjects (Fig. 2). In both groups, the S and B declined, and total flux decreased in the diabetic subjects, such that at 4 and 6 weeks they no longer differed significantly (Fig. 3). However, S-B was more negative at week 4, and remained less than in controls at both 4 and 6 weeks.

The greater negative N balance for the first 2–3 weeks might have been due to the finite time required for the diet, and the weight loss it caused, to restore plasma glucose to near normal. The continued negative N balance, and the less favorable S-B at 4 weeks, was not due to the diabetic subjects with higher plasma glucose values at this phase. Nor was it directly attributable to plasma total immunoreactive insulin levels, since those were comparably high during the isoenergetic diet, falling rapidly during the first week of VLED and slightly thereafter in both groups (not shown). Clearly, the insulin resistance/insensitivity was markedly greater in the diabetic subjects while they were hyperglycemic, but we have no independent direct measure of this later in the VLED. It remains a tenable (and testable) hypothesis, however, that there is resistance to the effects of insulin on protein turnover (those components that are affected by insulin), and that this persists to a lesser degree during the VLED. Our insulin assay does cross-react with proinsulin, so the totals measured could also obscure the possibility of a greater proportion of proinsulin in plasma of the diabetic subjects. Whether or not this is a factor, hypoinsulinemia relative to that required for the maintenance of normal glucoregulation was also present. Insulin secretion was not assessed directly by other methods in this study. We cannot exclude the possibility that the diabetic subjects had been chronically adapted to the abnormal protein metabolism, and that their ability to respond to this protein conservation challenge had thereby been impaired. Although the protein intakes given were previously presumed to be in the range appropriate for both control and diabetic subjects, the present data further support the notion that a clinically inapparent abnormality is present, obscured by the fact that the amounts habitually ingested represent a surfeit (13). Finally, for analogous reasons, though 93 g/day (1.0 g/kg/day or 1.3 g/kg/day adjusted to a body mass index of 25 kg/m^2 per day) of the protein used was sufficient for control subjects to achieve a successful adaptation (at least until 5 weeks of VLED), it is conceivable that a higher quality protein might be required in the diabetic subjects. Nonetheless, these results add considerably to what has been reported previously with VLED (40,41).

In the next experiment, various changes were made to respond to these issues, and to test whether intensive insulin treatment aimed at rapid correction of the hyperglycemia would correct protein turnover in the isoenergetic state. In otherwise comparable type 2 diabetic subjects, high quality protein (45% versus 18% essential amino acids) was used at 93 g/day throughout. The energy intake was kept isocaloric for the first 14 days. Aggressive insulin therapy was used, with multiple daily injections of biosynthetic human regular and NPH, and a rapid increase in dose over the first week (mean 150 ± 13 U/day) aiming for normoglycemia during the last 3 days, during the ^{15}N-glycine study. This was followed by a period of equal duration off all therapy and remaining at isoenergetic intake, and finally a 4-week VLED, again off all other therapy. The glycemic responses were such that mean premeal capillary glucose values were about 6.0 mmol/liter with insulin, 13 mmol/liter off insulin, and again near normal with the VLED.

The N balance was positive with insulin therapy, suggesting that this group may have been in a state of previous protein depletion since such a response would not otherwise have been predicted at this level of protein intake (Fig. 4). N balance reverted to equilibrium off insulin, then showed negative values with failure to return to equilibrium during the VLED as was the case in the previous subjects. The ^{15}N-glycine results are shown in Fig. 5. A markedly greater total flux (Q) and B were observed off insulin, associated with a significant decline in net synthesis (S-B) despite an increase in mean S. All three parameters of turnover decreased with the VLED, but once again S-B remained negative as it had in the first study (Fig. 3).

The conclusions from these latter unpublished data are as follows: the more modest level of hyperglycemia that followed the insulin therapy is nonetheless still associated with an undesirable trend in N balance, and with the same abnormalities shown in the preceding study. Viewed in the reverse, correction of blood glucose with insulin, even in such insulin-resistant subjects, has marked beneficial effects on protein turnover. These effects occurred rapidly (within days), and at protein intakes well within the range likely to be consumed by a large proportion of type 2 diabetic persons. The VLED that followed the return to hyperglycemia was once again unable to normalize the ^{15}N-glycine responses completely, despite its effectiveness in normalizing glycemia and despite the administration of a high-quality protein. The latter again implies that the phenomenon under study is not one that can be demonstrated only under extreme conditions of hyperglycemia or during therapy with very large insulin doses.

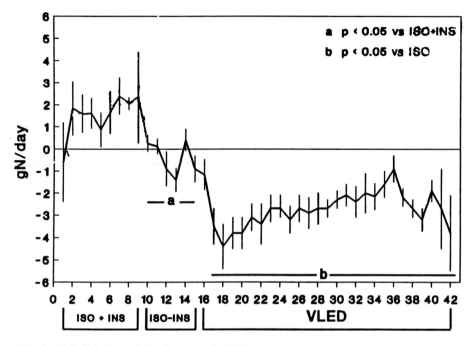

FIG. 4. Daily N balance during isoenergetic (ISO) feeding with and without insulin therapy and during the 1.7 MJ/day casein-soy protein diet (VLED) in obese subjects with type 2 diabetes. −INS signifies no insulin treatment; +INS signifies that insulin was given. Data are plotted as means ± SE.

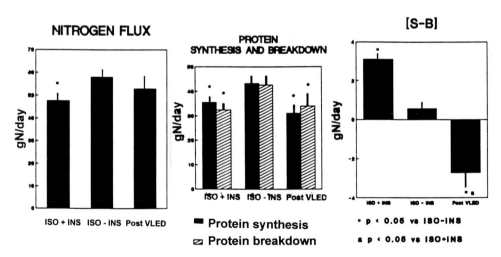

FIG. 5. Whole-body protein turnover measured by the ^{15}N-glycine method during isoenergetic (ISO) feeding with or without insulin therapy and at week 4 of the 1.7 MJ/day casein-soy protein diet (VLED) in obese subjects with type 2 diabetes. −INS signifies no insulin treatment; +INS signifies that insulin was given. Data are presented in g N/day as means ± SE.

CONCLUSION

In summary, the main thrust of this review has been to present current knowledge on whole-body protein metabolism in human diabetes mellitus. We propose that because protein metabolism can be shown to be abnormal in both type 1 and type 2 diabetes when moderate to marked hyperglycemia is present, this has potential clinical importance. The demonstration that improvement or correction of the protein metabolic abnormalities can be achieved by tight control of plasma glucose has implications for treatment. There are as yet insufficient data to allow us to correlate the magnitude of the abnormalities in protein metabolism with those of glucose (or fat) metabolism. However, data in type 1 diabetes (13,15,16), as well as that presented in this chapter, suggest that the previously held view that protein metabolism is less sensitive to the deficiency in insulin and/or to the actions of insulin than is the metabolism of glucose or fat must now be reassessed.

Hoffer has stated the case in relation to the possible impact on dietary protein requirements (13). The amounts required to optimize protein metabolism as well as the responses to experimental diets may be different in diabetic people and in normal individuals, even if the diabetes is rigorously controlled. The end points currently used in this type of clinical investigation have imprecisions, and none of the whole-body techniques is able to determine which of the multitude of body proteins are most susceptible to the abnormalities shown. What seems apparent to us, however, is that the previous failures to find abnormalities in type 2 diabetes were related to the methodologies used, which restricted the studies to the fasted state. The implication is that greater abnormalities occur in the markedly non-steady-state conditions that are related to ingestion and absorption of the exogenous protein. These are the times of the day when it is most difficult to achieve normalization of glucose metabolism as well, even during glycemic control using the "artificial pancreas" (43). Even with very precise glycemic control, the excursions of certain blood amino acids (including leucine) were actually overcorrected (*i.e.*, they did not rise as much as normal) (43). It is possible that the peripheral blood hyperinsulinemia that is required to normalize glucose excursions may have been responsible. More precise methods are needed to test fed-state amino acid metabolism in this setting. One of these might be the approach recently published by Hoffer's group (44), and others might be to study regional protein metabolism by the approach developed by Nair (33,45), or the synthesis of specific proteins as reported by De Feo *et al.* (25).

Even with a liberal protein intake, as used in our studies, the fact that hyperglycemia is associated with protein-kinetic and even N balance abnormalities provides yet another argument to support the conclusions of the DCCT in relation to the consequences of hyperglycemia and extrapolation of the results to type 2 diabetes. Future studies may define the amounts of dietary protein that seem to be required at different levels of glycemic control. We would argue that for both theoretical and practical reasons the management goals should include normalization of protein metabolism at the current usual intakes, by considering protein in addition to the glycemic, glycosylated protein, and lipid end points that are currently established.

This will require definition of the dose-response of level of glycemic control versus protein metabolism *in vivo* with the best tools available. As noted above, it could well be that an accelerated rate of protein turnover due to diabetes, even without ongoing net loss of body proteins, could place those proteins at greater risk of abnormal function through increased glycosylation resulting from the concurrent hyperglycemia. For the present, the chief therapeutic end point should still be to normalize glycemia, since this appears to have the greatest chance of normalizing protein metabolism at the usually taken and usually recommended intakes. The conundrum of incipient nephropathy remains; Brodsky *et al.* (16) have shown the risks of protein restriction, yet its benefits in slowing progression of nephropathy seem at this time to be reasonably well documented. Optimal diabetic control, with no more than 0.8 g/kg of reference body weight/day, would be the best compromise for the present, but this area, as well as the area in general, needs more research. This has been emphasized by the authors of the most recent review of the nutrition recommendations of the American Diabetes Association (46).

ACKNOWLEDGMENTS

The authors' studies have been supported by grants from the Canadian Diabetes Association (RG, EBM), and the Medical Research Council of Canada (MT-5466, PBP). We thank Madeleine Giroux, Anoma Gunasekara, and Marie Lamarche for expert technical assistance, Marla Myers PDt and Mary Shingler RN of the Royal Victoria Hospital Clinical Investigation Unit for support in the clinical studies, and Annie Oundjian for secretarial expertise.

REFERENCES

1. Atchley DW, Loeb RF, Richards DW, *et al.* On diabetic acidosis, a detailed study of electrolyte balances following the withdrawal and reestablishment of insulin therapy. *J Clin Invest* 1933; 12: 297–326.
2. Wood FC, Bierman EL. New concepts in diabetic dietetics. *Nutr Today* 1972; 7: 4–12.
3. Marsh PL, Newburgh LH, Holly LE. The nitrogen requirement for maintenance in diabetes mellitus. *Arch Int Med* 1922; 29: 97–130.
4. Anderson JW, Geil PB. Nutritional management of diabetes mellitus. In: Shils MS, Olson JA, Shike M, eds. *Modern nutrition in health and disease,* 8th ed. Philadelphia: Lea & Febiger, 1994: 1259–86.
5. Hollenberg CB, Carlston AM. Effects of dietary carbohydrate and fat intake on glucose and lipoprotein metabolism in individuals with diabetes mellitus. *Diabetes Care* 1991; 14: 774–85.
6. Mahaux J. Evolution du traitement diététique du diabète. *Hospitalia* 1946; 2: 41–54.
7. Zeller KR. Low-protein diets in renal disease. *Diabetes Care* 1991; 14: 856–66.
8. Brenner BM, Meyer TW, Hostetter TH. Dietary protein intake and the progressive nature of kidney disease. *N Eng J Med* 1982; 307: 652–9.
9. Walker JD, Dodds RA, Murrells TJ, *et al.* Restriction of dietary protein and progression of renal failure in diabetic nephropathy. *Lancet* 1989; ii: 1411–4.
10. Glasser JL, Smith M. Is dietary protein intake related to diabetic nephropathy? The Pittsburgh epidemiology of diabetes complications study. *Diabetes* 1990; 39 (suppl 1): 292A. (Abstract)
11. Kalk WJ, Osler C, Constable J, *et al.* Influence of dietary protein on glomerular filtration and urinary albumin excretion in insulin-dependent diabetes. *Am J Clin Nutr* 1992; 56: 169–73.

12. Forker LL, Chaikoff IL, Enterman C, *et al.* Formation of muscle protein in diabetic dogs. *J Biol Chem* 1951; 188: 37–48.
13. Hoffer LJ. Are dietary protein requirements altered in diabetes mellitus? *Can J Physiol Pharmacol* 1993; 71: 633–8.
14. Brodsky IG, Robbins DC. Safety of low-protein diets. Where's the beef? (Editorial) *Diabetes Care* 1989; 12: 435–7.
15. Larivière F, Kupranycz D, Chiasson JL, *et al.* Plasma leucine kinetics and urinary nitrogen excretion in intensively-treated diabetes mellitus. *Am J Physiol* 1992; 263: E173–9.
16. Brodsky IG, Robbins DC, Hiser E, *et al.* Effects of low-protein diets on protein metabolism in insulin-dependent diabetes mellitus patients with early nephropathy. *J Clin Endocrinol Metab* 1992; 75: 351–7.
17. Tessari P, Inchiostro S, Biolo G, *et al.* Differential effects of hyperinsulinemia and hyperaminoacidemia on leucine-carbon metabolism *in vivo. J Clin Invest* 1987; 79: 1062–9.
18. Pacy PJ, Garrow JS, Ford GC, *et al.* Influence of amino acid administration on whole-body leucine kinetics and resting metabolic rate in postabsorptive normal subjects. *Clin Sci* 1988; 75: 225–31.
19. Nissen S, Haymond MW. Changes in leucine kinetics during meal absorption: effects of dietary leucine availability. *Am J Physiol* 1986; 250: E695–701.
20. McMurlan MA, Garlick PJ. Influence of nutrient intake on protein turnover. *Diabetes Metab Rev* 1989; 5: 165–9.
21. Goodman MN, Del Pilar Gomez M. Decreased myofibrillar proteolysis after refeeding requires dietary protein or amino acids. *Am J Physiol* 1987; 253: E52–8.
22. Tischler ME, Desantels M, Goldberg AL. Does leucine, leucyl-tRNA or some metabolite of leucine regulate protein synthesis in skeletal or cardiac muscle? *J Biol Chem* 1982; 257: 1613–21.
23. Tessari P, Trevisan R, Inchiostro S, *et al.* Dose-response curves of effects of insulin on leucine kinetics in humans. *Am J Physiol* 1986; 251: E334–42.
24. Heslin MJ, Newman E, Wolf RF, Pisters PWT, Brenman MF. Effect of hyperinsulinemia on whole body and skeletal muscle leucine carbon kinetics in humans. *Am J Physiol* 1992; 262: E911–8.
25. De Feo P, Gaisano MG, Haymond MW. Differential effects of insulin deficiency on albumin and fibrinogen synthesis in humans. *J Clin Invest* 1991; 88: 833–40.
26. Gougeon R, Hoffer LJ, Pencharz PB, *et al.* Protein metabolism in obese subjects during a very low-energy diet. *Am J Clin Nutr* 1992; 56: 2495–545.
27. Nair KS, Garrow JS, Ford C, *et al.* Effect of poor diabetic control and obesity on whole body protein metabolism in man. *Diabetologia* 1983; 25: 400–3.
28. Robert JS, Beaufrère B, Koziet J, *et al.* Whole body de novo amino acid synthesis in Type 1 (insulin-dependent) diabetes studied with stable isotope-labelled leucine, alanine and glycine. *Diabetes* 1985; 34: 67–73.
29. Tessari P, Nosadini R, Trevisan R, *et al.* Defective suppression by insulin of leucine-carbon appearance and oxidation in Type 1, insulin-dependent diabetes mellitus. *J Clin Invest* 1986; 77: 1797–804.
30. Nair KS, Ford GC, Halliday D. Effect of intravenous insulin treatment on *in vivo* whole body leucine kinetics and oxygen consumption in insulin-deprived Type 1 diabetic patients. *Metabolism* 1987; 36: 491–5.
31. Luzi L, Castellino P, Simonson DC, *et al.* Leucine metabolism in IDDM: role of insulin and substrate availability. *Diabetes* 1990; 39: 38–48.
32. Umpleby AM, Boroujerdi MA, Brown PM, *et al.* The effect of metabolic control on leucine metabolism in Type 1 (insulin-dependent) diabetic patients. *Diabetologia* 1986; 29: 131–41.
33. Nair KS, Ford GC, Forbes E. Protein metabolism in the splanchnic and leg regions in Type-1 diabetic patients. *Diabetes* 1994; 43(suppl 1): 74A. (Abstract)
34. Hod M, Dorsman M, Friedman S, *et al.* Dynamic parameters of glycine metabolism in diabetic human pregnancy measured by [^{15}N] glycine and gas chromatography-mass spectrometry. *Isr J Med Sci* 1991; 27: 462–8.
35. Bier DM. Protein metabolism in type II diabetes mellitus. In: Nair SK, ed. *Protein metabolism in diabetes mellitus.* London: Smith-Gordon, 1992: 243–7.
36. Staten MA, Matthews DA, Bier DM. Leucine metabolism in Type II diabetes mellitus. *Diabetes* 1986; 35: 1249–53.
37. Umpleby AM, Scobie IN, Boroujerdi MA, *et al.* Diurnal variation in glucose and leucine metabolism in non-insulin-dependent diabetes. *Diabetes Res Clin Pract* 1990; 9: 89–96.
38. Groop LC, Bonadonna RC, Del Prato S, *et al.* Glucose and free fatty acid metabolism in non-insulin-dependent diabetes mellitus. *J Clin Invest* 1989; 84: 205–13.

39. Abumrad NN, Rabin D, Wise KL, *et al.* The disposal of an intravenously administered amino acid load across the human forearm. *Metabolism* 1982; 31: 463–70.
40. Henry RR, Wrest-Kent TA, Scheaffer L, *et al.* Metabolic consequences of very low calorie diet therapy in obese non-insulin-dependent diabetic and nondiabetic subjects. *Diabetes* 1986; 35: 155–64.
41. Bistrian BR, Blackburn GL, Flatt JP, *et al.* Nitrogen metabolism and insulin requirements in obese diabetic adults on a protein-sparing modified fast. *Diabetes* 1976; 25: 494–504.
42. Gougeon R, Pencharz PB, Marliss EB. Effect of NIDDM on the kinetics of whole-body protein metabolism. *Diabetes* 1994; 43: 318–28.
43. Hanna AK, Zinman B, Nadhooda AF, *et al.* Insulin, glucagon and amino acids during glycemic control by the artificial pancreas in diabetic man. *Metabolism* 1980; 29: 321–32.
44. Taveroff A, Lapin H, Hoffer LJ. Mechanism governing short-term fed-state adaptation to dietary protein restriction. *Metabolism* 1994; 43: 320–7.
45. Pacy PJ, Nair K, Ford C, *et al.* Failure of insulin infusion to stimulate fractional muscle protein synthesis in Type 1 diabetic patients. *Diabetes* 1989; 38: 618–24.
46. Franz MJ, Horton ES, Bantle JP, *et al.* Technical review: Nutrition principles for the management of diabetes and related complications. *Diabetes Care* 1994; 17: 490–518.

DISCUSSION

Dr. Jiang: What kind of natural food that is rich in fiber do you recommend?

Dr. Marliss: The source of fiber should be foods containing complex carbohydrates such as whole grain cereals and the like that are fairly typical dietary components in many parts of the world and have always been so. I do not at this stage recommend a supplement of fiber. I think Dr. J. Anderson who is a bit of an evangelist in relation to the use of fiber, probably recommends fiber more than other people do. One problem with very high intakes of the best kind of fiber in terms of plasma glucose control is that there is a substantial increase in flatulence.

Dr. Drash: Years ago, I had an interesting conversation with Ted Danowsky with regard to diet in diabetes. He said that diabetics ought to eat whatever a Chinese coolie eats. I think the point is a very good one. What he was saying was that diabetic people should eat a diet that makes them lean, mean, and fit. How does a long-term program of physical fitness change the diet?

Dr. Marliss: There are no really substantial differences in the diet required by an individual who engages in a fitness program as distinct from an intensive training program for competitive athletics, which is not I think what you were talking about. The kinds of recommendations that are made (such as in the US Recommended Dietary Allowances, or by various national diabetes organizations) are not meant to be what the mean of the population should be taking, but what the mean plus two standard deviations of the population might take in order to provide a margin of safety for the vast majority of individuals. The question becomes much more complicated when we are talking about diabetic individuals and trying to decide to what extent one should tailor intakes according to the level of diabetic control. The goal for most individuals is find a level that is very close to euglycemia, in which case the standard recommendations should apply. The activity issue is largely a calorie issue as much as anything, and how much more energy needs to be taken in to maintain homeostasis depends on the level of activity. That is pretty straightforward.

Dr. Karamanos: In the individuals in whom there is a defect in the balance of protein metabolism, can you change and improve this if you add a certain amount of exercise? And is there any difference between proteins of animal and vegetable origin?

Dr. Marliss: These are two very complicated questions. It would appear that acute bouts of exercise stimulate proteolysis in so far as this has been looked at. What then appears to happen is that between bouts of exercise, and most probably postprandially, repletion takes place, and the muscle will selectively take up the extra amino acids required to build up the necessary amount of protein. However, when you have a non-steady-state condition induced by exercise, it is a very complex problem to examine acute effects on protein balance. One of the points that I did not make about the leucine method is that it is really applicable only in the steady state, which would be either in the overnight fasted state or in a continuously fed state, which implies intravenous provision of amino acids up to the point at which blood levels are constant.

The problem with vegetarian diets is that the proportion of essential amino acids may be quite low and can in certain instances be limiting, particularly with respect to lysine and methionine. Therefore one would predict that individuals who have compromised protein metabolism to begin with, *i.e.*, persons with diabetes, and particularly those who are not in very good control, would be placing themselves at even greater risk if they chose a vegetarian diet. To my knowledge there are no data on this, but it would be prudent to look at the protein composition of those individuals' diets very carefully and make certain that, if they happen to be strict vegetarians, they are being supplemented with proteins that would complement any lack of particular amino acids in their diet.

Dr. Hoet: I should like to know whether you have any data on the specific patterns of plasma amino acids in vegetarians. The reason for asking this is that vegetarians have the lowest levels of taurine that one can see and in view of the new data accumulating that taurine may have a specific effect on glomerulonephropathy, at least in the rat, one has to be concerned.

Dr. Marliss: One has a tendency to defend fasting amino acid concentrations reasonably well in the face of fairly substantial changes in protein intake, and therefore it would not surprise me if there were no major changes in people on vegetarian diets. But I don't have data on taurine in particular.

Dr. Phenekos: We all know that apart from insulin there is another hormone with an anabolic action and that is growth hormone/IGF-1. I wonder if some of the abnormalities you have described may be mediated through the growth hormone IGF-1 axis.

Dr. Marliss: The answer is probably yes. It is clear that people with type 1 diabetes, particularly if it is in poor control, have significant abnormalities of growth hormone secretion. Corresponding abnormalities of IGF-1 and its binding proteins and the like have been identified, and it is entirely possible that these may be playing a role as well. To my knowledge, this has not been studied directly in such patients yet.

Dr. Christakopoulos: Would you please comment on protein intake and the progress of nephropathy?

Dr. Marliss: There is unfortunately no definitive evidence from a well-conducted multicenter controlled trial on protein restriction in diabetic nephropathy. In North America, nephrologists have moved *en masse* in the direction of protein restriction in individuals with early nephropathy. What we are talking about is the notion of protein restriction to prevent progression of nephropathy. Brodsky and Robbins (1) wrote an editorial raising this concern, shared by Hoffer (2), that we simply don't know enough about protein metabolism in people with diabetes to begin with, and we may be placing them at risk of protein malnutrition while trying to protect their kidneys. A study published in the *Journal of Clinical Endocrinology and Metabolism* by Brodsky *et al.* in 1992 (3) has been criticized because it was uncontrolled and because it was very difficult to obtain compliance with an extremely low protein diet of 0.6 g/kg per day. Although the study appeared to show benefit for incipient nephropathy, one cannot accept the evidence as definitive. It did show evidence of protein malnutrition.

It was the first study of its kind and one needs to be very careful about its interpretation. I think that if our incipient nephropathic patients are asked to restrict protein, they should probably not restrict it to as little as 0.6 g/kg, even if that 0.6 g is high quality protein with 45% essential amino acids.

Dr. Nattrass: One of the problems about metabolism is that it is very difficult to change one variable without altering a host of others, and very low energy intakes are quite ketogenic. I would like to ask you whether you have data on other gluconeogenic precursors in your studies and whether you think that what is responsible for the effect upon protein balance may be mediated through some of those other aspects of metabolism.

Dr. Marliss: Yes, of course we have considered the issue of the alternate sources of energy substrates in a hypoenergetic situation in some detail but we have no answers. As soon as one reduces the energy intake, the protein requirement for maintenance increases, so that in an obese individual on a hypocaloric diet the presumption is that the lower the energy intake the higher the protein requirement because of the well-known protein-energy interrelationship. The issue this raises is that if the protein-energy relationship in obese individuals who are not diabetic is such that there is a progressive increase in protein requirement as the energy intake falls, one would predict that, in a diabetic individual who is obese and receiving a low-energy intake, the slope of the curve of protein requirement with decreased energy intake would be steeper, so this puts another variable into the equation. The question of alternative energy substrates in relation to protein equilibrium is an extremely important one and what one would like to see happening is maximum fat mobilization to make up the energy deficit and minimum endogenous protein mobilization to maintain body protein homeostasis. What I have devoted 20 or more years of my career to trying to understand and still don't understand is what signals the body interprets to show that it is getting fewer calories than it needs. The other issue that arises is that we all adapt or accommodate to our particular level of protein intake and probably diabetics do this to a certain extent as well. If they then face a challenge such as a very low energy diet, this could be a factor in the sustained inability to maintain or reach a normal level of protein turnover and nitrogen balance, even later on. So what that suggests (which does not answer your question directly although it bears on it) is that individuals with conventionally controlled Type 2 diabetes may be in a state where, when challenged either by a low energy diet or by some other stress to their protein metabolism such as an activity program, they may be unable to mount a normal homeostatic response. This may relate to alternative substrates, or more likely to protein metabolism itself.

REFERENCES

1. Brodsky IG, Robbins DC. Safety of low-protein diets. Where's the beef? *Diabetes Care* 1989; 12: 435–7.
2. Hoffer LJ. Are dietary protein requirements altered in diabetes mellitus? *Can J Physiol Pharmacol* 1993; 71: 633–8.
3. Brodsky IG, Robbins DC, Hiser E, *et al.* Effects of low-protein diets on protein metabolism in insulin-dependent diabetes mellitus patients with early nephropathy. *J Clin Endocrinol Metab* 1992; 75: 351–7.

Diabetes, edited by Richard M. Cowett,
Nestlé Nutrition Workshop Series,
Vol. 35. Nestec Ltd.,
Vevey/Raven Press, Ltd., New York © 1995.

Pancreas and Islet Cell Transplantation

David Sutherland, Rainer Gruessner, and Paul Gores

*Department of Surgery, University of Minnesota, 420 Delaware Street SE,
Minneapolis, Minnesota 55455, USA*

Pancreatic and islet transplantation, either as an immediately vascularized organ graft or as a free graft of dispersed tissue, is the only treatment of type 1 diabetes that can establish an insulin-independent state (1). The success rate with pancreas organ transplantation is high relative to that with free islets (2). Of pancreas transplants done in the past several years, more than 70% of the recipients are insulin independent at 1 year after the procedure (3), while with islet allografts, even in the 1990s, long-term insulin independence has occurred in less than 10% (4). Many problems remain to be overcome before islet allotransplantation will be as successful as pancreas transplants (1).

PANCREAS TRANSPLANTS

After a successful pancreas transplant, euglycemia is constant and glycosylated hemoglobin levels are normalized as long as the graft is not rejected or afflicted by recurrence of disease (5,6). The penalty for achieving such a state is the need for immunosuppression (7). Thus most pancreas transplants are performed in diabetic patients with nephropathy in whom immunosuppression is obligatory because of a kidney transplant (8,9). Nonuremic patients whose problems of diabetes are (or predictably will be) more serious than the potential side effects of anti-rejection drugs (cyclosporin, azathioprine, corticosteroids) are also candidates for a pancreas transplant (10), but the proportion of pancreas transplant recipients in this category has been small to date (9).

In uremic diabetic patients, retinopathy and neuropathy are usually far advanced. Although eye function may stabilize over the long term (11) and nerve function may even improve (12), the main immediate value of adding a pancreas to a kidney transplant is the improved quality of life that comes with being insulin independent as well as dialysis free (13). A successful pancreas transplant also prevents recurrence of diabetic nephropathy in the new kidney, an additional benefit for the long-term survivor (14).

In nonuremic patients, the potential to influence the appearance or progression of secondary complications exists, but because the penalties associated with immuno-suppression or the specific side effects of the anti-rejection drugs may be greater in an individual patient than the complications of diabetes that were otherwise destined to appear, pancreas transplants are not usually done for this reason alone. This may change in the future as anti-rejection strategies with fewer side effects are developed; indeed, new drugs are currently being tested in clinical trials involving other organs. For now, however, pancreas transplants alone are primarily reserved for the nonure-mic patient whose diabetes is extremely labile, no matter what insulin regimen is tried, and whose day-to-day living is severely compromised for this reason alone.

The most extensive experience with pancreas transplantation in nonuremic diabetic patients is at the University of Minnesota (10). Even though extreme lability is the main indication, most patients have had diabetes for many years and have complica-tions. Autonomic neuropathy in this group is common and is usually associated with gastroenteropathy with erratic food absorption, defective glucose counterregulatory mechanisms, and hypoglycemic unawareness, making calculations of doses difficult and any method of exogenous insulin administration unsatisfactory or even haz-ardous.

The recipient of a pancreas transplant alone may or may not have other complica-tions, such as retinopathy or nephropathy. Cyclosporin is nephrotoxic, and this can be a problem in some patients. Patients with a creatinine clearance rate greater than 60 ml/min usually tolerate the dosage of cyclosporin necessary to prevent rejection of the pancreas (15). However, if the creatinine clearance rate is less, the functional deterioration already in progress from the underlying kidney disease may continue. At the University of Minnesota, approximately 80% of the recipients of pancreas transplants alone have had normal or nearly normal renal function, whereas, in approximately 20%, nephropathy was moderately advanced at the time of the trans-plant (16).

Graft Functional Survival Rates

Worldwide, more than 5000 transplants had been reported to the International Pancreas Transplant Registry (IPTR) by the end of 1993 (13), including more than 3000 in the United States (Fig. 1). Since October, 1987, it has been mandatory to report outcome on cases in the USA to the IPTR through the United Network for Organ Sharing (UNOS), the organization that operates the Organ Procurement and Transplant Network in the United States under the auspices of the Department of Health and Human Services (9).

Of approximately 2500 US pancreas transplants in the UNOS/IPTR database for analysis as of November, 1993, about 94% were in patients who also received a kidney transplant, either simultaneously (~2100) or prior to (~200) the pancreas transplant. With success defined as insulin independence, the best results have been with simultaneous pancreas and kidney (SPK) transplants with a 1-year pancreas

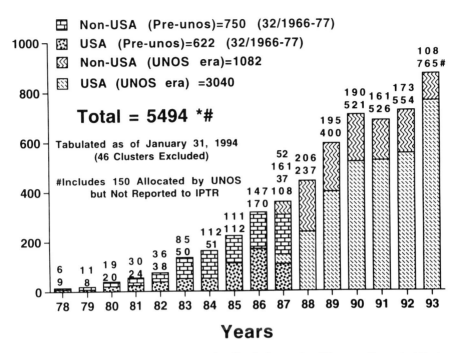

FIG. 1. Number of pancreas transplants tabulated by the International Pancreas Transplant Registry (IPTR) for 1966–1993 before and after the advent of the United Network of Organ Sharing (UNOS). The reporting for 1993 is incomplete. The total number of cases for the United States was 3662 (45 clusters) and for the non-United States was 1832 (one cluster). The world total with cluster cases included was 5540. From Sutherland DER, Moudry-Munns K, Gruessner A. Pancreas transplant results in United Network for Organ Sharing (UNOS) United States of America (USA) Registry with comparison to non-USA data in the International Registry. In: Terasaki P, ed. *Clinical transplants* 1993. Los Angeles: UCLA Tissue Typing Laboratory 1994: 47–69, with permission.

functional survival rate of over 75%, compared with approximately 50% in the pancreas after kidney (PAK) and pancreas transplant alone (PTA) categories (Fig. 2). The recipients can return to exogenous insulin therapy if the pancreas graft fails, and patient survival rates at 1 year have been greater than 90% in all categories (Fig. 3).

The higher pancreas graft functional survival rate in the SPK category appears to be related to the ability to use the kidney graft as a monitor for rejection episodes, the physiologic manifestations of rejection appearing earlier in the kidney (increase in creatinine) than in the pancreas. In addition, uremia itself may blunt the immune response.

The UNOS Registry as well as the US Renal Data System (USRDS) have calculated kidney- and patient-survival rates in recipients of SPK *versus* diabetic recipients of cadaveric kidney transplants alone (KTA) (9,17). In the slightly older USRDS database, the patient- and kidney-survival rates were similar in the two groups, whereas, in the UNOS analysis, kidney graft survival rates were significantly higher in the SPK group (82% at 1 year) than in the KTA group (78% at 1 year). This difference

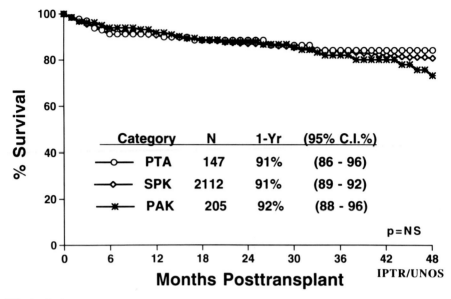

FIG. 2. Patient survival rates according to recipient category for bladder-drained (BD) cadaveric pancreas transplants reported to IPTR/UNOS 1987–93. SPK, simultaneous pancreas/kidney transplant; PAK, pancreas after kidney transplant; PTA, pancreas transplant alone.

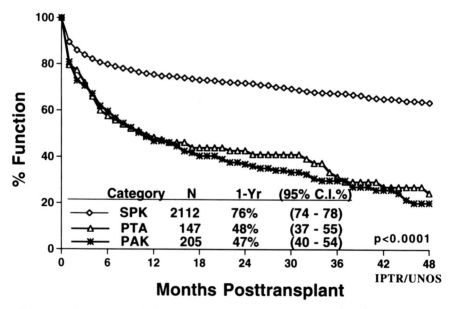

FIG. 3. Graft functional survival rates by recipient category for bladder-drained (BD) cadaveric pancreas transplants reported to IPTR/UNOS 1987–1993. SPK, simultaneous pancreas/kidney transplant; PAK, pancreas after kidney transplant; PTA, pancreas transplant alone.

may reflect the selection of uremic diabetic patients in better physiologic condition for the SPK than the KTA procedure, because analyses at individual centers have shown higher incidence of rejection episodes and surgical complications in SPK than in KTA recipients (1,18).

Most pancreas transplants are currently performed with the exocrine secretions drained into the bladder, allowing the level of urine amylase to be monitored. A decline in this level is a manifestation and a marker of rejection (19). In SPK recipients, an increase in the level of serum creatinine usually precedes a decrease in exocrine or endocrine function during rejection episodes, making monitoring of urine amylase largely superfluous for this group. In PTA recipients, however, serum creatinine cannot be used as a monitor for rejection. Fortuitously, a decline in exocrine function (decreased urine amylase) almost always precedes a decline in endocrine function (increased blood sugar) as a manifestation of rejection. Thus the possibility exists that the results of PTA procedures could be improved by treating rejection episodes on the basis of a decline in urine amylase before endocrine dysfunction occurs.

Such an approach (early treatment of solitary pancreas rejection episodes based on a decline in urine amylase) was taken at the University of Minnesota, beginning in 1988 (20). In addition, it was also noted that results of solitary pancreas transplants were better in recipients of grafts from donors who were well matched to recipients with respect to histocompatibility leukocyte antigens (HLA). Of 133 solitary, bladder-drained cadaver pancreas transplants performed at the University of Minnesota between November, 1984, and 1991 (21), the actuarial 1-year insulin-independent (graft function) rates were 80% for those mismatched for none or only one HLA, A, B, or DR antigen (n = 15) *versus* 56% for those mismatched for two to three antigens (n = 44) and 44% for those mismatched for four to six antigens (n = 74). Thus beginning in 1988 emphasis was also placed on doing the best matches possible for recipients of solitary pancreas transplants.

In the subgroup of PAK patients between 1988 to 1991 who received the kidney from a related donor followed by a primary bladder-drained pancreas from a cadaver donor (n = 17), the 1-year insulin-independent rate was 72% (22).

For uremic diabetic patients referred to the University of Minnesota Hospital, emphasis is placed on pursuing strategies that maximize the probability of long-term kidney function (23). Thus for patients who have a willing family member, we recommend a kidney transplant from a living, related donor with the option of subsequently receiving a pancreas transplant. Only if there is no living related donor for a kidney transplant do we recommend a simultaneous PAK transplant from a cadaver donor. Over a decade, the rejection rates are much lower for kidneys from living related donors than from cadaver donors. Thus by pursuing this strategy, the maximum number of patients can be rendered dialysis free for a lifetime. Furthermore, the insulin-independent rates with PAK transplants now approach those achieved with SPK transplants (17). The incentive to defer a pancreas transplant to achieve the advantage of a living donor kidney is therefore even greater than before.

Effect on Complications

Studies on the effect of pancreas transplantation on secondary diabetic complications have been mixed. Advanced retinopathy is present preoperatively in most patients, and progression has been observed in up to 30% of recipients during the first 3 years posttransplantation, whether the pancreas graft was successful or not. However, after 3 years, retinopathy in the patients with functioning pancreas grafts has been found to stabilize, whereas deterioration has continued to occur in those in whom grafts have failed (11).

With regard to neuropathy, improvement in nerve conduction velocities and stabilization of evoked muscle action potentials and of autonomic neuropathy have occurred in recipients of successful pancreas grafts, whereas deterioration has continued in those in whom grafts have failed (12,24). Indeed, in diabetic patients with severe neuropathy, those who undergo a successful pancreas transplant have a significantly higher probability of survival than those in whom transplantation is not done or is unsuccessful (25).

With regard to nephropathy, microscopic lesions of diabetes in the native kidneys of recipients with successful PTA procedures may stabilize or regress, but new lesions from cyclosporin can appear (26). Nevertheless, after an initial decline, renal function usually reaches a plateau. In recipients of kidney transplants, a successful pancreas transplant can definitely prevent recurrence of diabetic nephropathy (14).

Effect on Quality of Life

Many studies have been conducted on metabolism in patients following pancreas transplantation, and these are of great interest to endocrinologists (27). For patients and their physicians, however, the main question is what effect a successful pancreas transplant has on quality of life. Several studies have been published in this regard, and they are nearly unanimous in reporting that patients with successful transplants rate their quality of life to be better after the procedure than before (13,28–30). Pancreas transplants in patients with hyperlabile diabetes and extreme difficulty with metabolic control improve quality of life simply by inducing insulin independence (28,31). In uremic patients, kidney transplants alone can improve quality of life by obviating the need for dialysis (32). Some lability is not uncommon in uremic patents, and in such patients the effect of a double transplant can be dramatic; two difficult clinical problems are corrected for as long as rejection is prevented by immunosuppression (13,30).

For patients without nephropathy who undergo a PTA procedure, the price of ridding themselves of diabetes is the same, that is, chronic immunosuppression. The natural question to ask is whether the benefit is worth the price. Recipients of pancreas transplants have emphatically stated that it is (33,34). In the largest study to date (13,29), 131 patients were analyzed 1 to 10 years posttransplantation; half had functioning grafts (n = 65), and half had grafts that ultimately failed (n = 66). Overall,

92% felt that managing immunosuppression was easier than managing diabetes (13). When asked which was more demanding of their family's time and energy, 63% thought that the diabetes was more demanding, 29% thought that the two were equal, and 9% thought that the transplant was more demanding. Of the 65 patients with functioning grafts, 89% stated that they were more healthy than before the transplant. Indices of well-being, as quantified by standard tests, were significantly better in patients with functioning grafts than in those without. Virtually 10% of the patients with continuing graft function and 85% of those whose graft ultimately failed said they would encourage others with similar complications of diabetes to consider pancreas transplantation. In addition, most of the patients with failed grafts desired retransplantation, and those with functioning grafts said they would undergo a retransplant if their current graft failed.

Cost

Benefits must be weighed against the cost of the procedure (35). Many US Transplant Centers routinely offer pancreas transplants to uremic diabetic recipients of renal allografts. In many instances, the determining factor as to whether a pancreas transplant is added to the kidney transplant depends on whether financial coverage is available. Kidney transplants are routinely covered by Medicare or private insurance, but coverage of the pancreas transplant is highly variable. Approximately 50 insurance companies have covered pancreas transplants. The average hospital charges for cadaveric pancreas/kidney transplants is approximately $40,000 more than those associated with a kidney transplant alone, with $16,000 being for the organ procurement and $24,000 for the additional care required. For recipients of a pancreas transplant performed as a solitary procedure (nonuremic patients or nephropathic patients with a previous kidney transplant), the average cost of the hospital admission is $65,000. Following the transplant, there are also the ongoing costs of the immunosuppressive drugs. Patients who have also had a kidney transplant have this expense even without pancreas transplantation. However, for the nonuremic recipient, the costs of these drugs are assumed solely for maintenance of the pancreas, and this can amount to several thousand dollars per year.

Thus in uremic diabetic patients who receive a kidney, the only additional costs of adding a pancreas are those associated with the initial hospital admission. In nonuremic patients, all the costs associated with pancreas transplantation are directly related to treatment of diabetes.

It is more expensive to treat diabetes with a pancreas transplant than with insulin injections. If secondary complications are ameliorated, health care costs over a lifetime may be less than if the recipient remained diabetic, but individual variations are considerable. Although more expensive, the enhanced quality of life that ensues following a pancreas transplant in patients with hyperlabile diabetes makes the procedure worth the cost. Furthermore, in these patients, medical costs are high. Even though exogenous insulin itself is cheap, the need for hospital admissions and close monitoring by physicians and other health care personnel can approach the intensity of follow-up needed for posttransplant patients. This consideration is apart from the potential for amelioration of the secondary complications that may occur following a pancreas transplant. This benefit may translate into a financial one for individuals who were otherwise destined to develop such problems.

ISLET CELL TRANSPLANTS

Islet allografts, either purified or in the form of dispersed pancreatic tissue, are very successful in experimental rodent models, but are much less so in large animals and humans. Only 11 fully documented cases of insulin independence have occurred in the 139 attempts at clinical islet allotransplantation since 1974 (36). Slow progress is, however, being made (Fig. 4). When the achievement of a basal C-peptide level in excess of 1 ng/ml at 1 month is used in place of the more rigorous end point of insulin independence, steady improvement in clinical results has occurred. Analysis

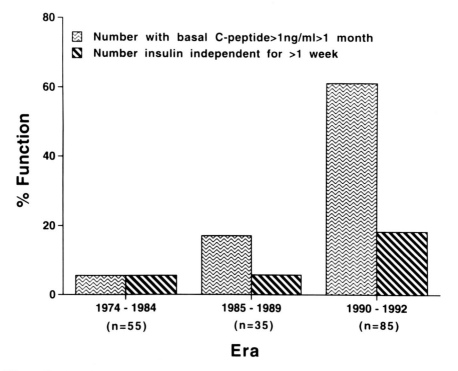

FIG. 4. Number of adult islet allograft cases worldwide and percent able to be insulin independent and with basal C-peptide after transplantation by era up to December 31, 1992 (adapted from Federlin KF, Bretzel RG, Hering BS. International islet transplant registry. *Newsletter* 1993: No 43. From Hering BJ, Browatzki CC, Schultz A, Bretzel RG, Federlin KF. Clinical islet transplantation—registry report, accomplishments in the past and future research needs. *Cell Transplant* 1993; 2: 269–82, with permission.

of International Islet Transplant Registry data shows that in the era of 1974–1984 only three of 55 cases (5%) achieved this end point in contrast to six of 35 (17%) in 1985–1989, and 52 of 85 (61%) in 1990–1992.

The problems preventing the stable engraftment of a sufficient number of islets to achieve a state of insulin independence may be broadly classified into four categories: 1. transplantation of an insufficient mass of viable islets; 2. immune-mediated destruction of transplanted islet tissue; 3. drug toxicity; and 4. metabolic exhaustion.

Transplantation of Insufficient Islet Mass

The precise number of transplanted islets required to render a type 1 diabetic patient insulin independent is not known. The relevant quantity is the amount of islet tissue effectively engrafted rather than the number of islets transplanted. The percentage of islets transplanted that are actually engrafted is likely to vary considerably according to the site chosen for transplantation. Most clinical islet transplants have used the portal circulation as the site of implantation.

Data from clinical studies of islet autotransplantation in patients undergoing total duodenopancreatectomy show that 3500 islets/kg are able to maintain fasting normoglycemia and normal glycosylated hemoglobin levels (37,38). In type 1 diabetic patients, islet engraftment may be adversely affected by the presence of longstanding microangiopathy, and insulin resistance may be present (39–41).

The normal human pancreas contains on average approximately one million islets of 150 mm equivalent diameter (I.E.) (42,43). However, the range varies by a factor of 5. The numbers of islets that are recovered after intraductal collagenase digestion of the gland and subsequent density gradient centrifugation are also extremely variable.

Currently islet yields are calculated by manually counting the number of islets (as identified by dithazone staining) in an aliquot of the preparation (44). This type of quantification is based on crude morphology and does not give an accurate determination of the number of the *viable* islets present. Islets may be irreversibly damaged during the period of collagenase digestion, or while undergoing centrifugation on hyperosmolar gradients.

The use of multiple donors poses certain logistic problems and is not desirable from an immunologic point of view. The survival of immediately vascularized pancreas allografts is enhanced by good HLA matching, and the use of multiple donors precludes good matching (45).

A practical alternative to the use of multiple donors is the use of unpurified dispersed pancreatic tissue prepared from one cadaver donor (46). This increases the islet yield approximately twofold, and since the tissue is not subjected to hyperosmolar density gradients, the yield of the viable islets is probably enhanced even more.

Little experimental work has addressed the question of the relative immunogenicity of exocrine and endocrine tissue. In a congenic mouse model, a hand-picked preparation consisting of 60% islets and 40% exocrine tissue survives just as well as a clean hand-picked preparation (47). However, if donor-strain splenocytes are added to either of the preparations, the islet allografts are in all cases readily rejected. Gotoh *et al.* conducted a similar experiment on an inbred rat model (48). They observed that purified, hand-picked islets survived significantly longer than a crude preparation consisting of islets, exocrine tissue, and contaminating lymphoid cells. They also showed that purified islets would be uniformly and rapidly rejected if donor-strain splenocytes were simultaneously injected intravenously. Taken together, these studies demonstrate that lymphoid and not acinar contamination significantly increases the immunogenicity of islet allografts.

However, it must be emphasized that the results above are relative. Purified islets are rejected and, when examined *in vitro* in a mixed lymphocyte/islet co-culture system, they elicit an immune response, albeit less than that evoked by crude islet preparations (49,50). Even rigorously purified β cells evoke an immune response *in vitro* unless responder (as well as simulator) antigen-presenting cells are removed from the system (49).

Since at the present time systemic immunosuppression of the recipient cannot be avoided in large animal models, a reasonable strategy is to use unpurified, dispersed pancreatic tissue, thereby dramatically increasing the yield of viable islets and enhancing the probability of the successful transplantation of islets from a single cadaver donor. Since pancreatic ductal cells function as the stem cell for islet neogenesis (51), this strategy also theoretically leaves open the possibility of expansion of the β-cell mass over time.

Immune Mediated Destruction

Allogeneic islet tissue may be destroyed by nonspecific inflammatory damage, antigen-specific T-cell-mediated cytolysis, or the recurrence of autoimmunity.

Nonspecific Inflammatory Damage

The cytokines interleukin 1 (IL-1), interleukin 6 (IL-6), and tumor necrosis factor alpha (TNFα) interact synergistically in their regulation of inflammation (52). IL-1 is a potent modulator of insulin secretion and at high concentrations is cytodestructive to pancreatic islet β and α cells (53,54).

Macrophages infiltrate freshly transplanted islet grafts and predominate in grafts showing poor initial function after transplantation (55). Most clinical attempts at islet transplantation use the portal circulation as the site of implantation. The islets become lodged in the presinusoidal space lined by Kupffer cells. When activated, these hepatic macrophages produce a variety of molecules toxic to β cells (56). Thus they may play an important role in the early destruction of transplanted islet tissue. In rodents, this early destruction is inhibited by the macrophage toxin silica (55), as well as by the novel immunosuppressive agent 15-deoxyspergualin (57), which has antimacrophage (58) as well as anti-T-cell effects. In addition, administration of a specific nitric oxide inhibitor (N-monomethyl-L-arginine) improves the early function of rodent isografts (59), as does injection of soluble TNF receptor (60).

Antigen-Specific T-Cell-Mediated Rejection

As is the case with all allogeneic tissue, islet grafts are susceptible to classic T-cell-mediated rejection. A major impediment to the successful application of islet transplantation in humans has been the lack of a suitable early means of detecting a rejection response. Currently, the only way to monitor islet allograft function is to determine serum glucose and C-peptide levels. By the time the serum glucose level is raised, the majority of the graft has been destroyed, and it is too late to initiate effective anti-rejection therapy. C-peptide levels are cumbersome since the assay is not widely available, and it requires several days before results are known. In addition, in the pre-bladder-drainage era of pancreas transplantation, C-peptides were not found to be useful as a means of early detection of rejection or disease recurrence in vascularized pancreatic allografts (61). Thus at the present time the best chance of success is when islets from only one donor are used and the kidney from the same cadaver donor is transplanted simultaneously so that serum creatinine can be used to monitor for the presence of a rejection response against donor tissue.

The successful application of islet transplantation in patients with previously transplanted functioning kidney allografts (IAK) or islet transplantation alone (ITA) in preuremic patients requires the development of a rejection-free protocol. Currently no such protocol exists for solid organ transplantation. However, 60% of patients receiving a renal allograft from a cadaver donor never experience rejection (62). Therefore, with current immunosuppressive protocols, one might expect that, if sufficient islets survive the initial generalized inflammatory reaction and stably engraft, 60% of the patients would experience long-term islet allograft function.

Various protocols using culture (63), antibody (64), or deoxyguanosine pretreatment (65), or irradiation (66), often in combination with a brief course of systemic immunosuppression, have been successful in rodent models. These protocols have been tried in large animal models, but there has been either no benefit or only slight prolongation of islet graft function (67,68).

A final approach, which is successful in rodent models, is intrathymic injection of donor antigen (islets or bone marrow) (69,70) in conjunction with a short course of immunosuppression prior to islet transplantation in the periphery. This appears to result in donor-specific transplantation tolerance; however, to date this approach has not been successful in large animal models.

Drug Toxicity

With human islet transplantation, the mass of viable islet cells is probably marginally adequate to maintain a normal metabolic state. The immunosuppressive therapy used after islet transplantation is based on the protocols that have been developed for solid organ transplantation. Many of these agents are diabetogenic, and when used in combination are even more so (71). For example, 19% of previously nondiabetic kidney transplant recipients develop altered glucose metabolism after being placed on the combination of cyclosporin, azathioprine, and prednisone (71).

Corticosteroids are known to induce insulin resistance in experimental animals and in humans (72,73). It is unlikely that islet transplantation will achieve significant levels of success as long as immunosuppressive regimens remain corticosteroid based. In order to maintain normoglycemia, nondiabetic kidney transplant recipients on triple immunotherapy must increase insulin secretion (as measured by C-peptide) 2.5-fold (74). When one considers that even with the use of unpurified islets, approximately half of the islet mass is lost during digestion, and invariably more is lost during the process of transplantation and engraftment, it is not surprising that single donor islet transplants rarely result in levels of insulin secretion sufficient to overcome the toxic effects of the drug used to prevent rejection.

Of the new agents currently being tested, FK506 is frankly diabetogenic (75); however, 15-deoxyspergualin does not impair glucose-induced insulin secretion from either normal human or rat islets and does not lead to insulin resistance in intact rats (76). Furthermore, in clinical studies to date, no evidence of a diabetogenic tendency has emerged. RS-61443 does not appear to disturb glucose metabolism *in vivo* (77), although it may reduce glucose-mediated insulin secretion *in vitro* (78). Rapamycin, when used in high doses, has been associated with the development of diabetes (79).

Metabolic Exhaustion

Sustained hyperglycemia renders β cells glucose unresponsive and, if hyperglycemia is severe and prolonged, it leads to direct β-cell destruction (80,81). The toxic effect is reversible if hyperglycemia is of short duration. However, prolonged exposure to hyperglycemia results in irreversible damage. Transplantation of insufficient islet numbers to maintain normoglycemia leads to a continuous decline in β-cell mass (82).

Furthermore, hyperglycemia itself has been shown, both *in vitro* (83) and *in vivo* (84), to lead to insulin resistance, which further exacerbates the hyperglycemia. Thus a vicious cycle occurs where the toxic effects of immunosuppressive drugs lead to hyperglycemia, which itself causes further insulin resistance and β-cell dysfunction. Fortunately, control of hyperglycemia by exogenous administration of insulin is able to reverse these effects (85,86), the hope being that insulin therapy may be withdrawn once the doses of immunosuppressive agents are lowered to baseline.

CONCLUSION

Pancreas transplantation is currently a routine form of treatment for diabetic renal allograft recipients. It is also used to treat selected nonuremic patients with extremely labile diabetes or other diabetic problems that are not well served by the alternative.

More widespread use of the procedure will depend upon advances in specific immuno-suppression and upon donor availability.

Transplantation of islets separately from the pancreas as free grafts has been successful in a few patients who also received kidney grafts (36), but there are many failures as well. Islet transplantation is clearly more difficult to apply clinically than pancreas transplants. From a recipient viewpoint, it is a much simpler procedure, but from the viewpoint of a transplanter, everything but the surgery is more difficult. Nevertheless, success has been achieved, and there is now a handful of patients with long-term insulin independence. In those who still need insulin, but who also have detectable C-peptide, diabetes management is easier, and it is possible to normalize glycohemoglobin, something rarely achieved by insulin alone. However, immunosuppression is still needed, and the indications for islet transplants at present are much fewer than for pancreas transplantation.

All of the problems with islet transplantation enumerated above are solvable. We would expect islet transplantation to replace pancreas transplantation in the future, first in association with cadaveric kidney transplantation and, later, as a solitary procedure.

For now the only treatment that can "cure" diabetes today with a high success rate is pancreas transplantation. It is applicable to virtually all diabetic recipients of kidney transplants and to selected nonuremic patients with difficult control problems.

REFERENCES

1. Sutherland DER. Pancreas and islet transplantation: an update. In: Auchincloss H, Bach F, eds. *Transplantation immunology*. New York: Wiley-Liss (in press).
2. Sutherland DER. Pancreatic transplantation: an update. *Diabetes Rev*. 1993; 1: 152–65.
3. Sutherland DER, Moudry-Munns K, Gruessner A. Pancreas transplant results in United Network for Organ Sharing (UNOS) United States of America (USA) Registry with comparison to non-USA data in the International Registry. In: Terasaki P, ed. *Clinical transplants 1993*. Los Angeles: UCLA Tissue Typing Laboratory 1994: 47–69.
4. Hering BJ, Browatzki CC, Schultz A, Bretzel RG, Federlin KF. Clinical islet transplantation—registry report, accomplishments in the past and future research needs. *Cell Transplant* 1993; 2: 269–82.
5. Morel P, Goetz FC, Moudry-Munns KC, Freier EF, Sutherland DER. Long term glucose control in patients with pancreatic transplants. *Ann Intern Med* 1991; 115: 694–9.
6. Sutherland DER, Goetz FC, Sibley RK. Recurrence of disease in pancreas transplants. *Diabetes* 1989; 38: 85–7.
7. Sutherland DER. Immunosuppression for clinical pancreas transplantation. *Clin Transplant* 1991; 5: 549–53.
8. Sollinger H, Stratta RJ, D'Alessandro AM, Kalayoglu M, Pirsch JD, Belzer FO. Experience with simultaneous pancreas-kidney transplantation. *Ann Surg* 1988; 208: 478–83.
9. Sutherland DER, Gruessner A, Moudry-Munns KC. Analysis of United Network for Organ Sharing (UNOS) United States of America (USA) Pancreas Transplant Registry data according to multiple variables. In: Terasaki PI, ed. *Clinical transplants—1992*. Los Angeles: UCLA Tissue Typing Laboratory, 1993: 45–59.
10. Sutherland DER, Kendall DM, Moudry KC, *et al*. Pancreas transplantation in nonuremic, type I diabetic recipients. *Surgery* 1988; 104: 453–64.
11. Ramsay RC, Goetz FC, Sutherland DER, *et al*. Progression of diabetic retinopathy after pancreas transplantation for insulin-dependent diabetes mellitus. *N Engl J Med* 1988; 318: 208–14.
12. Kennedy WR, Navarro X, Goetz FC, Sutherland DER, Najarian JS. Effects of pancreatic transplantation on diabetic neuropathy. *N Engl J Med* 1990; 322: 1031–7.

13. Gross CR, Zehrer CL. Impact of the addition of a pancreas to quality of life in uremic diabetic recipients of kidney transplants. *Transplant Proc* 1993; 25: 1293–5.
14. Bilous RW, Mauer SM, Sutherland DER, Najarian JS, Goetz FC, Steffes MW. The effects of pancreas transplantation on the glomerular structure of renal allografts in patients with insulin-dependent diabetes. *N Engl J Med* 1989; 321: 80–5.
15. Morel P, Sutherland DER, Almond PS, *et al*. Assessment of renal function in type I diabetic patients after kidney, pancreas or combined kidney-pancreas transplantation. *Transplantation* 1991; 51: 1184–9.
16. Wang TL, Stevens RB, Fioretto P, *et al*. Correlation of preoperative renal function and identification of risk factors for eventual native renal failure in cyclosporine-treated nonuremic diabetic recipient of pancreas transplants alone. *Transplant Proc* 1993; 25: 1291–2.
17. United States Renal Disease System. Simultaneous kidney-pancreas transplantation versus kidney transplantation alone: patient survival, kidney graft survival, and posttransplant hospitalization. *Am J Kidney Dis* 1992; 20: 61–7.
18. Cheung AHS, Sutherland DER, Gillingham KJ, *et al*. Simultaneous pancreas-kidney (SPK) transplant versus kidney transplant alone (KTA) in diabetic patients. *Kidney Int* 1992; 41: 924–9.
19. Prieto M, Sutherland DER, Fernandez-Cruz L, Heil JE, Najarian JS. Experimental and clinical experience with urine amylase monitoring for early diagnosis of rejection in pancreas transplantation. *Transplantation* 1987; 43: 71–9.
20. Sutherland DER, Dunn DL, Goetz FC, *et al*. A 10-year experience with 290 pancreas transplants at a single institution. *Ann Surg* 1989; 210: 274–85.
21. Sutherland DER, Gruessner RWG, Gillingham KJ, *et al*. *A single institution's experience with solitary pancreas transplantation*. Los Angeles:UCLA Tissue Typing Laboratory, 1992: 141–52.
22. Cheung AHS, Matas AJ, Gruessner RWG, *et al*. Should uremic diabetic patients who want a pancreas transplant receive a simultaneous cadaver kidney-pancreas transplant or a living related donor kidney first followed by cadaver pancreas transplant? *Transplant Proc* 1993; 25: 1184–5.
23. Sutherland DER, Gores PF, Farney AC, *et al*. Evolution of kidney, pancreas, and islet transplantation for patients with diabetes at the University of Minnesota. *Am J Surg* 1993; 166: 456–91.
24. Solders G, Tydén G, Persson A, Groth CG. Improvement of nerve conduction in diabetic neuropathy: a follow-up study 4 years after combined pancreatic and renal transplantation. *Diabetes* 1992; 41: 946–51.
25. Navarro X, Kennedy WR, Loewensen RB, Sutherland DER. Influence of pancreas transplantation on cardiorespiratory reflexes, nerve conduction, and mortality in diabetes mellitus. *Diabetes* 1990; 39: 802–6.
26. Fioretto P, Mauer SM, Bilous RW, Goetz FC, Sutherland DER, Steffes MW. Effects of pancreas transplantation on glomerular structure in insulin-dependent diabetic patients with their own kidneys. *Lancet* 1993; 342: 1193–6.
27. Diem P, Redmon JB, Abid M, *et al*. Glucagon, catecholamine and pancreatic polypeptide secretion in type 1 diabetic recipients of pancreas allografts. *J Clin Invest* 1992; 86: 2008–13.
28. Zehrer CL, Gross CR. Quality of life of pancreas transplant recipients. *Diabetologia* 1991; 34: S145–S149.
29. Gross CR, Zehrer CL. Health-related quality of life outcomes of pancreas transplant recipients. *Clin Transplant* 1992; 6: 165–71.
30. Nakache R, Tyden G, Groth CG. Quality of life in diabetic patients after kidney transplantation. *Diabetes* 1991; 39: 802–6.
31. Bolinder J, Wahrenberg H, Linde B, Tydén G, Groth CG, Ostman J. Improved glucose counter regulation after pancreas transplantation in diabetic patients with unawareness of hypoglycemia. *Transplant Proc* 1991; 23: 1667–9.
32. Jacobson SH, Fryd DS, Sutherland DER, Kjellstrand CM. Treatment of the diabetic patient with end-stage renal failure. *Diabetes Metab Rev* 1988: 4: 191–200.
33. Harmer N. Nonuremic pancreas transplantation (Letter). *Diabetes Care* 1990; 13: 452.
34. Loseke C. Quality of life after transplantation (Letter). *Diabetes Care* 1990; 13: 541.
35. Evans RW, Manninen DL, and Dong FB. An economic analysis of pancreas transplantation: costs, insurance coverage, and reimbursement. *Clin Transplant* 1993; 7: 166–74.
36. Federlin KF, Bretzel RG, Hering BJ. International islet transplant registry. *Newsletter* 1993: No 43.
37. Farney AC, Najarian JS, Nakhleh RE, *et al*. Autotransplantation of dispersed pancreatic islet tissue

combined with total or near-total pancreatectomy for treatment of chronic pancreatitis. *Surgery* 1991; 110: 427–39.

38. Pyzdrowski KL, Kendall DM, Halter JB, Nakhleh RE, Sutherland DER, Robertson RP. Preserved insulin secretion and insulin independence in recipients of islet autografts. *N Engl J Med* 1992; 327: 220–6.

39. Rayman G, Williams SA, Spencer PD, Smaje LH, Wise PH, Tooke JE. Impaired microvascular hyperaemic responses to minor skin trauma in type I diabetes. *BMJ* 1986; 292: 1295–8.

40. Cuthbertson RA, Koulmanda M, Mandel TE. Detrimental effect of chronic diabetes on growth and function of fetal islet isografts in mice. *Transplantation* 1988; 46: 650–4.

41. Moller DE, Flier JS. Insulin-resistance—mechanisms, syndromes, and implications. *N Engl J Med* 1991; 325: 938–48.

42. Hellman B. The frequency distribution of the number and volume of the islets of Langerhans in man. *Acta Soc Med Upsalien* 1959; 64: 432–60.

43. Saito K, Iwama N, Takahashi T. Morphometrical analysis on topographical difference in size distribution, number and volume of islets in the human pancreas. *Tohoku J Exp Med* 1978; 124: 177–86.

44. Ricordi C, Gray DWR, Hering BJ. Islet isolation assessment in man and large animals. *Acta Diabetol Lat* 1990; 27: 185–95.

45. Gores PF, Gillingham KJ, Dunn DL, Moudry-Munns KC, Najarian JS, Sutherland DER. Donor hyperglycemia as a minor risk factor and immunologic variables as major risk factors for pancreas allograft loss in a multivariate analysis of a single institutions's experience. *Ann Surg* 1992; 215: 217–30.

46. Gores PF, Najarian JS, Stephanian E, Lloveras JJ, Kelley SL, Sutherland DER. Insulin independence in type I diabetes after transplantation of unpurified islets from a single donor using 15-deoxyspergualin. *Lancet* 1993; 341: 19–21.

47. Gores PF, Mayoral JL, Field MJ, Sutherland DER. Comparison of the immunogenicity of purified and unpurified murine islet allografts. *Transplantation* 1986; 41: 529–31.

48. Gotoh M, Maki T, Satomi S, Porter J, Monaco AP. Immunological characteristics of purified pancreatic islet grafts. *Transplantation* 1986; 42: 387–90.

49. Stock PG, Ascher NL, Chen S, Field J, Bach FH, Sutherland DER. Evidence for direct and indirect pathways in the generation of the alloimmune response against pancreatic islets. *Transplant Proc* 1991; 23(1PT1): 819–20.

50. Ulrichs K, Muller-Ruchholtz W. Mixed lymphocyte islet culture (MLIC) and its use in manipulation of human islet alloimmunogenicity. *Horm Metab Res* 1990; 25: 123. (Abstract)

51. Bonner-Weir S, Baxter LA, Schuppin GT, Smith FE. A second pathway for regeneration of adult exocrine and endocrine pancreas: a possible recapitilation of embryonic development. *Diabetes* 1993; 42: 1715–20.

52. Arai KE, Lee F, Mijajima A, Myatake S, Arai N, Yokota T. Cytokines: coordinators of immune and inflammatory responses. *Annu Rev Biochem* 1990; 59: 783–836.

53. Bendtzen K, Mandrup-Poulsen T, Nerup J, Nielsen JH, Dinarello CA, Svenson M. Cytotoxicity of human pl 7 interleukin-1 for pancreatic islets of Langerhans. *Science* 1986; 232: 1545–7.

54. Ling Z, Veld PA, Pipeleers DG. Interaction of interleukin-1 with islet B-cells. Distinction between indirect, aspecific cytotoxicity and direct, specific functional suppression. *Diabetes* 1993; 42: 56–65.

55. Kaufman DB, Platt J, Rabe FL, Dunn DL, Bach FH, Sutherland DER. Differential roles of Mac-1 + cells, and CD4 + and CD8 + T lymphocytes in primary nonfunction and classic rejection of islet allografts. *J Exp Med* 1990; 172: 291–302.

56. Nathan CF. Secretory products of macrophages. *J Clin Invest* 1987; 79: 319–26.

57. Kaufman DB, Field MJ, Gruber SA, *et al*. Extended functional survival of murine islet allograft with 15-deoxyspergualin. *Transplant Proc* 1992; 24: 1045–7.

58. Walter PK, Dickneite G, Schorlemmer HU. Prolongation of graft survival in allogeneic islet transplantation by 15-deoxyspergualin in the rat. *Diabetologia* 1987; 30: 38. (Abstract)

59. Stevens RB, Lokeh A, Ansite JD *et al*. Role of nitric oxide in the pathogenesis of early pancreatic islet dysfunction during rat and human intraportal islet transplantation. *Transplant Proc* 1994; 26: 692.

60. Farney AC, Xenos ES, Sutherland DER. Inhibition of pancreatic islet beta cell function by tumor necrosis factor is blocked by a soluble tumor necrosis factor receptor. *Transplant Proc* 1993; 25: 865–6.

61. Sutherland DER, Sibley RK, Xu XZ, *et al*. Twin-to-twin pancreas transplantation: reversal and reenactment of the pathogenesis of type I diabetes. *Trans Assoc Am Physicians* 1984; 97: 80–7.

62. Frey DJ, Matas AJ, Gillingham KJ. Sequential therapy—a prospective randomized trial of MALG versus OKT3 for prophylactic immunosuppression in cadaver renal allograft recipients. *Transplantation* 1992; 54: 50–6.
63. Simeonovic CJ, Bowen KM, Kotlausk I, Lafferty KJ. Modulation of tissue immunogenicity by organ culture. Comparison of adult islets and fetal pancreas. *Transplantation* 1980; 30: 174–9.
64. Faustman D, Hauptfeld V, Lacy P, Davie J. Prolongation of murine allograft survival by pretreatment of islets with antibody directed to Ia determinants. *Proc Natl Acad Sci USA* 1981; 78: 51–6.
65. Al-Abdullah IH, Kumar AM, Al-Adnani MS, Abouna GM. Prolongation of allograft survival in diabetic rats treated with cyclosporine by deoxyguanosine pretreatment of pancreatic islets of Langerhans. *Transplantation* 1991; 51: 967–71.
66. Lau H, Reemtsma K, Hardy MA. Prolongation of rat islet allograft survival by direct ultraviolet irradiation of the graft. *Science* 1984; 223: 607–9.
67. Stegall MD, Chabot J, Weber C, Reemtsma K, Hardy MA. Pancreatic islet transplantation in cynomolgus monkeys. Initial studies and evidence that cyclosporine impairs glucose tolerance in normal monkeys. *Transplantation* 1989; 48: 944–50.
68. Kenyon NS, Strasser S, Alejandro R. Ultraviolet light immunomodulation of canine islets for prolongation of allograft survival. *Diabetes* 1990; 39: 305–s.
69. Posselt AM, Barker CF, Tomaszewski JE, Marmann JF, Choti MA, Naji H. Induction of donor-specific unresponsiveness by intrathymic islet transplantation. *Science* 1990; 249: 1293–5.
70. Posselt AM, Odorico JS, Barker CF, Naji A. Promotion of pancreatic islet allograft survival by intrathymic transplantation of bone marrow. *Diabetes* 1992; 41: 771–5.
71. Boudreaux JP, McHugh L, Canafax DM. The impact of cyclosporine and combination immunosuppression on the incidence of posttransplant diabetes in renal allograft recipients. *Transplantation* 1987; 44: 376–81.
72. Kahn CR, Goldfine ID, Neville DM, Demeyts P. Alteration in insulin binding induced by changes in vivo in the levels of glucocorticoids and growth hormone. *Endocrinology* 1978; 103: 1054–66.
73. Cigolini M, Smith U. Human adipose tissue in culture VIII. Studies on the insulin-antagonistic effect of glucocorticoids. *Metabolism* 1979; 28: 502–10.
74. Scharp DW, Lacy PE, Santiago JV. Results of our first nine intraportal islet allografts in type I, insulin-dependent diabetic patients. *Transplantation* 1991; 51: 76–85.
75. Mieles L, Gordon RD, Mintz D, Toussaint RM, Imventarza O, Starzl TE. Glycaemia and insulin need following FK506 rescue therapy in liver recipients. *Transplant Proc* 1991; 23: 949–53.
76. Xenos ES, Casanova D, Sutherland DER, Farney AC, Lloveras JJ, Gores PF. The in vivo and in vitro effect of 15-deoxyspergualin on pancreatic islet function. *Transplantation* 1993; 56: 144–7.
77. Platz KP, Sollinger HW, Mullett DA, Eckhoff DE, Eugu EM, Allison AC. RS-61443—A new potent immunosuppressive agent. *Transplantation* 1991; 51: 27–31.
78. Sandberg SS, Anderson A. Exposure of rat pancreatic islets to RS-61443 inhibits B-cell function. *International Congress on Pancreas and Islet Transplantation* Amsterdam, 1993. (Abstract)
79. Morris RE. Rapamycins: antifungal, antitumor, antiproliferative and immunosuppressive macrolides. *Transplant Proc* 1992; 6: 39–87.
80. Dohan FC, Lukens FEW. Lesions of the pancreatic islets produced in cats by administration of glucose. *Science* 1947; 105: 183.
81. Leahy JL, Bonner-Weir S, Weir GC. Beta-cell dysfunction induced by chronic hyperglycemia. Current ideas on mechanism of impaired glucose-induced insulin secretion. *Diabetes Care* 1992; 15: 442–55.
82. Montana E, Bonner-Weir S, Weir GC. Beta cell mass and growth after syngeneic islet cell transplantation in normal and streptozocin diabetic C57BL/6 mice. *J Clin Invest* 1993; 91: 780–7.
83. Garvey WT, Olefsky JM, Matthaei S, Marshall S. Glucose and insulin coregulate the glucose transport system in primary cultured adipocytes: a new mechanism of insulin resistance. *J Biol Chem* 1987; 262: 189–97.
84. Kahn BB, Shulman GI, Defronzo RA, Cushman SW, Rossetti L. Normalization of blood glucose in diabetic rats with phlorizin treatment reverses insulin-resistant glucose transport in adipose cells without restoring glucose transporter gene expression. *J Clin Invest* 1991; 87: 561–70.
85. Zeng Y, Ricordi C, Lendoire J. The effect of prednisone on pancreatic islet autografts in dogs. *Surgery* 1993; 113: 98–102.
86. Korsgren O, Jansson L, Andersson A. Effects of hyperglycemia on function of isolated mouse pancreatic islets transplanted under kidney capsule. *Diabetes* 1989; 38: 510–5.

DISCUSSION

Dr. Nattrass: You give the impression that if you can get kidneys from a cadaveric donor you can also get a pancreas. Is that correct?

Dr. Sutherland: From most, but not all. About 9000 kidneys are procured from 4500 donors annually in the United States. The other organs, heart, liver, pancreas, are procured in lower numbers. For example, we use kidneys from donors of 65 years but heart transplant surgeons may not want to use a heart from somebody of 65. However, there are also donors with nonfunctioning kidneys but with perfectly satisfactory heart or pancreas, so occasionally we take pancreas, liver, and heart from donors from whom we don't take kidneys. Last year in Minnesota, we had 130 donors for kidneys. The pancreas was suitable for transplantation in at least 100. In probably 80% of the donors, the pancreas is satisfactory. The management in the intensive care unit is important. The donors are frequently hyperglycemic because of being on steroids or being stressed, so it is not unusual to have a donor with blood glucose of 20 mM or more. Some of the donors have to be given large amounts of insulin to get their blood sugars down, so we know that there is a high degree of insulin resistance. Thus you don't know for certain how well the pancreas is working when there is insulin resistance. If you give 5 units of insulin and the blood sugar comes down straight away, I worry about that pancreas because it should have been able to achieve the same response on its own. The pancreas seems relatively resistant to ischemia. We can have up to 2 hours of ischemia in a dog pancreas and still be able to transplant it successfully, while with a kidney you have only half an hour.

Dr. Guesry: When you transplant kidney and pancreas simultaneously, is the rejection pattern comparable in the two organs?

Dr. Sutherland: Sometimes the rejection is discordant, which is a problem for the immunologists. We also see this in animal models, where you transplant two organs from the same donor at the same time, you would expect the rejections to be concordant. In 90% of the cases they are, but a 10% discordance has been shown for pancreas and kidneys as has also been the case for heart and lung transplants. There is a small percentage of patients who reject one organ and keep the other, that is, reject the kidney, keep the pancreas, or reject the pancreas and keep the kidney. However, if, when we have clinical evidence of renal allograft rejection, we do a biopsy of both kidney and pancreas, even if the pancreas is functioning well, in 90% of cases both pancreas and kidney have lymphocytic infiltration.

Dr. Drash: I feel that we ought to make a histological or immunological diagnosis at presentation of diabetes by pancreatic biopsy. How valuable do you think this might be?

Dr. Sutherland: I think it should be done. Biopsy techniques have improved so much in recent years that it is now feasible using computerized tomography (CT) guidance. We do pancreatic biopsies all the time for a variety of reasons, suspected cancer, for example. They can even be done transendoscopically.

Dr. Schwartz: What is the status of fetal islets, and are they as immunologically tolerant as the mature islets?

Dr. Sutherland: The outcome of fetal transplants has been extremely disappointing in animal models and in humans. First of all, it is a myth that fetal tissue is less immunogenic than adult tissue, and there are several experiments showing that fetal tissue is rejected just as readily as adult tissue. Fetal transplants do not work very well, and, in humans, the only reports of success are from China and Russia, but no one has been able to verify those cases and the ones that have been done in United States have met with no success. I am not sure what has to be done to make them successful.

Dr. Crofford: You equate being off insulin with a functioning graft. It may be possible to make this assumption reliably when these are your own patients and you have studied them and cared for them in other ways. But when you use this criterion in a worldwide registry, how confident are you that being off insulin does constitute a functioning graft, particularly if you don't know what the blood sugar is?

Dr. Sutherland: If you measure C-peptide in these patients and they have none, that is reasonably confirmatory. In the registry, 95% of the recipients are DR3 or DR4 or both, so they have got the genetic markers for type 1 diabetes. Many groups have reported data on metabolic studies, so I don't think there is much doubt that the vast majority of these are type 1 diabetic patients. Every group that has reported C-peptide in metabolic studies has shown that they are euglycemic if they have a functioning graft.

Dr. Crofford: You said that graft failure was random. I'd like a little more discussion on that.

Dr. Sutherland: One of the things we were criticised for was that we did not randomize our patients to pancreas transplants *versus* no transplant, especially when looking at secondary complications. If you do randomize patients, you can analyze by "intention to treat" in the pancreas transplant group, but you do have failures of the pancreas transplant. Early on when most of these studies were done, the success rate, instead of being 75%, was 50% or 40%, so even in your intention-to-treat group about half of the subjects would not have received the "intended treatment" of a functioning pancreas graft. So the patients weren't randomized, they were transplanted. However, the failures are random in that we cannot predict in advance who is going to reject or who is going to have a technical failure. Thus, 15% of the grafts would fail for surgical reasons early on and another 40% would fail from rejection fairly early, too, because most rejections occur in the first 3 months. And so the failures were random, but everyone got an operation and some had a "sham" operation and some had a successful operation.

Dr. Crofford: I don't think I would accept that the failures are random because I'm not sure that technical failures are truly random. However, it was probably the best control group that you could have under these circumstances, so I would certainly accept that.

Dr. Bergman: When you cut the pancreas in half and you give one person the head and one the tail, there are a lot more α cells in the head and very few in the tail. Does that make any difference?

Dr. Sutherland: The main difference in the islets of the head and the tail is probably the pancreatic polypeptide (PP) cells. There are many more PP cells in the islets in the head than in the tail. When we do islet autografts, we can hardly ever find a PP-positive cell, and we presume that this is because we do our autografts from the tail of the pancreas. The few patients in whom we have transplanted the head of the pancreas because the tail was damaged have generally remained euglycemic.

Dr. Bergman: Has anyone transplanted islets into the lymphatic system? Glucose levels in the lymphatic system are quite close to the levels in blood, and the site might be better protected.

Dr. Sutherland: From animal studies, islets can apparently work in the lymphatic system, but I don't think anybody has attempted this in the human.

Dr. Marliss: The concept of β-cell rest has been raised in another context here. A thought I have had is whether one might purposely keep insulin going after the graft, although that would of course create other kinds of problems in terms of assessing function early. Has any one been able to devise a way of doing this to see whether function might ultimately be improved and/or rejection made less?

Dr. Sutherland: Apparently β-cell rest is unnecessary with the whole pancreas graft. We do keep the patients on insulin initially to control the blood sugar if it goes above 7 mM, although other people working in this area don't give any. However, no one has systematically randomized patients to get insulin or no insulin after pancreas transplant. I think everybody can agree that the concept of insulin is good, but whether it has an immunological effect we don't know. We do know that insulin prevents diabetes in BB rats and NOD mice, and it may be valuable in humans in relation to the immune response, which is probably independent of β-cell rest. We also know from animal experiments that when the β-cell mass is marginal, as after a 90% pancreatectomy, eventually the animals become diabetic unless you give them insulin, and giving insulin under these circumstance definitely prevents diabetes' developing. So there is probably an effect of stress in a reduced β-cell mass independent of the immunological effect.

Diabetes, edited by Richard M. Cowett,
Nestlé Nutrition Workshop Series,
Vol. 35. Nestec Ltd.,
Vevey/Raven Press, Ltd., New York © 1995.

Education in Diabetes

Marian Benroubi

Athens Polyclinic, 3 Paraschou Street, Paleo Psychico, Gr. 154 52, Greece

Education is the process that will enable patients with diabetes to obtain the optimum metabolic control while continuing to maintain their chosen style of life. Education is not merely the process of informing and providing theoretical knowledge. Transmitting knowledge is part of the procedure, but it often covers only a very small segment. One must always keep in mind that *education is the means, not the end.* The end is the modification of patient behavior as well as the acquisition of a positive attitude toward diabetes.

Although there is increasing awareness of the need to educate people with diabetes, integration of patient education into health care programs is still unsatisfactory. Responsibility for this lack of integration has been attributed to all levels of the medical care system, from the doctor's office to the physicians' organizing national and international meetings on diabetes who do not recognize the importance of the subject when devising their programs (1). In our opinion, the belief among many diabetologists that patient education is unscientific and therefore irrelevant to the clinical management of diabetes is the main cause of this lack of integration.

Diabetes education, like insulin treatment, is not an easy task. Many educational programs for patients with diabetes concentrate too much on theory and on the acquisition of "knowledge," such as the genetics of diabetes and the biochemistry of ketoacidosis, and they pay insufficient attention to the practical aspects of day-to-day management.

The aim of education should be to improve knowledge, attitudes, and skills, thereby modifying behavioral attitudes and improving compliance with treatment. This will subsequently lead to better metabolic control.

There is increasing evidence that gain in knowledge by itself is not associated with metabolic improvement (2,3). Psychosocial and demographic factors contribute substantially to the variance in diabetic control (4).

PSYCHOSOCIAL VARIABLES INFLUENCING THE EDUCATIONAL PROCESS

Psychosocial factors affect the metabolic control of diabetes both directly and indirectly. Direct effects are those mediated by the psychophysiologic process implicated in the stress-coping-illness model (5). Factors that increase stress can increase glucose levels. Conversely, factors that attenuate the effect of stress, including social support and psychological coping responses, can enhance glucose control. (6–8).

Indirect effects of psychosocial factors on diabetic control are those implicated in the health-belief and illness-behavior model. Health knowledge, attitudes and beliefs (9,10), as well as social support and psychological traits, can influence the efficacy of self-care, as well as motivation for learning (11,12).

Health locus of control is another individual attribute affecting engagement in help-seeking and/or self-care behavior. By *health locus of control*, we understand whether the responsibility for health and health-related behavior is attributed to self or to others (13,14). Health locus can be internal, for example the patient believes that he or she is the person with the major responsibility for the outcome of the disease, or external, when the patient attributes responsibility to other key figures or to the physician.

Psychological arousability is another important factor affecting behavior. Some psychological arousal is required to motivate behavior, but, if arousal is too great, it may lead to denial and avoidance behavior as a means of anxiety management. The optimal level of arousability is one that leads to a state of arousal that is sufficient to cause motivation, for example to acquire knowledge, but not so great as to induce panic or denial.

The stages of a patient's acceptance of this disease should be seriously considered in the educational planning. Treatment can be successful only if the physician or nurse or dietician knows and takes into account the subjective experience of the patient. I have already mentioned above that psychological arousal can be a barrier to learning if it is too great. This is usually the case for newly diagnosed insulin-dependent diabetics. (Basic reaction: shock and denial of reality: "This cannot be happening to me. . . . I am not a diabetic.") At the stage of denial, it is an illusion to think that teaching will be effective when the disease is not real to the patient. The doctor or nurse should not force the issue at this stage but allow time for the patient to accept the new state (15).

A sequence of developmental stages leading toward acceptance of the disease has been observed. Five phases can arbitrarily be described in the process of accepting the disease after the diagnosis has been made. These five phases are as follows:

1. *Denial:* "Why me? I do not understand."
2. *Revolt:* "No, I do not have diabetes."
3. *Bargaining:* "OK, I've got the disease, but I refuse to do all this."
4. *Depression, inner questioning:* "Will I be able to cope with it?"
5. *Active acceptance:* "Even with the disease, I can lead an active life." (16).

Active acceptance of a disease is when the disease is integrated into daily life in the best possible way. The diabetic individual is then an active participant in the understanding and application of the treatment.

These stages are artificial in the sense that they describe in a simplistic way the dynamic process that normally occurs in the difficult period of disease acceptance

(17). One should remember that the developmental stages never occur in isolation, one at a time, but rather in relationship to the stages before and after.

Having accepted these characteristics of the newly diagnosed diabetic, a complete assessment of the patient's perception, knowledge, and skills is essential for the construction of an educational program. When making the assessment, it is possible to underestimate or overestimate the patient's capabilities; it may be difficult in the limited time available to evaluate the patient correctly.

The following must be identified:

the effect of diabetes and its treatment on lifestyle and mood, and a clear picture of the social context of the subject

the patients' attitudes to the need to learn about the disease

the patients' perceptions about standards of self-management, for example, whether their diets conform with the ideal

behaviors that have been "self-learned"; for example, aiming at higher than desirable blood sugar levels because they feel better at such levels

standards of knowledge

ability and performance of skills

the actual new learning needs (for example, potential pregnancy, driving etc.) and possible gains

the personal cost of the new targets, which may be unacceptable (18).

EDUCATIONAL OBJECTIVES

It is of the utmost importance to define our educational objectives, that is, what patients should be able to do at the end of the learning period that they could not do beforehand.

It is only by defining objectives that it is possible to plan a teaching program and to choose adequate means for instruction. The objective of a course should be defined in terms of the result sought; it should not be a description or summary of the program.

Types of Educational Objectives

General Objectives

These correspond to functional aims for the types of patients trained in a medical unit. Example: providing the best possible blood sugar control during day-to-day life.

Intermediate Objectives

These are arrived at by breaking down functions into activities. Example: organizing and carrying out a group discussion about planning a meal.

Specific (or Instructional) Objectives

These correspond to precise professional tasks, the results of which are observable and measurable against given criteria. Example: using the syringe to draw insulin from the vial and injecting it into the thigh.

Qualities of the Educational Objectives

- *Feasible:* It must be ensured that what the patients are asked to do can actually be done with the facilities at hand and be within their capabilities. Elderly people experience great difficulty in handling modern technological equipment for blood glucose monitoring, while this is very easy for younger people.
- *Relevant:* What we ask our patients to do should be relevant to their needs and not to our expectations. A male teenager, for example, is mainly interested in knowing how he can avoid a hypo during a football game with his team.
- *Measurable:* Even a rough assessment is better than none at all. If no assessment is made, instructors tend to assume that a goal has been achieved just because they have taught the subject.
- *Unequivocal:* Loaded words (words open to a range of interpretations) should not be used, to avoid any possibility of misunderstanding. What do we mean when we say we want the patient to "know" something? Do we want him to be able to recite, or to solve a problem (19)?

Once we have defined our educational objectives, having considered the above factors, we proceed by adopting the educational method that will facilitate learning and increase patient compliance.

Compliance is the term used to describe a patient's health behavior that follows medical advice. According to definition, compliance is the extent to which a person's health behavior coincides with medical or health advice.

In the conventional health transaction, it is thought that, if patients are not compliant, that is their responsibility. If problems arise, the patient is to blame. In recent years, there has been a change in the attitude of many physicians, and the concept has been put forward that the patient and the physician together should work out the procedures between them, and that they should solve, by mutual understanding, the difficulties of the therapeutic regimens.

It has been recommended that the phrase *levels of diabetes self-care behavior* should be used instead of the term *compliance*. Although cumbersome, this may remind us that there are many types of behavior, and furthermore that other variables, such as the frequency or the consistency of a certain type of behavior, may also have an impact on diabetes control. From recent research in the field, it seems that there is no single cause for noncompliant behavior. The noncomplier does not have a typical personality. Every patient is a potential noncomplier. The same patient may at some time of life comply, while at another time not comply. An awareness of factors that may influence compliance is important (20).

THE EDUCATIONAL PROGRAM: CONTENT AND METHODS

The course content will obviously differ for type 1 and type 2 cases. An outline program will include the following topics:

What is diabetes mellitus?
What is meant by *control*?
Why is control important?
How is control measured? Self-testing. What factors influence control?
Diet
Injections and syringes
Hypoglycemia
Sick days
Adjustment of insulin dosage
Exercise
Foot care
Complications

The program should be tailored to the specific characteristics of each patient, for example, age, occupation, family circumstances, and educational and cultural level.

An elderly patient will not need to learn how to adjust his insulin dose, since his pattern of activities is almost identical every day. Nevertheless, since he will most probably have peripheral neuropathy or angiopathy, he must be educated in foot care to prevent ulcer formation and eventually amputation.

Teaching sessions should not last more than half an hour. Because people have only a limited concentration span, not more than one or two messages should be delivered at each session. Patient education may be given either individually as an integral part of the one-to-one relationship between patient and health care provider, or else it may be given to a group. The number of participants in the group should not exceed eight to ten. The presence of the group promotes exchange of knowledge and experience, which are powerful educational tools. Belonging to a group of diabetic people facilitates the maturation of the patients and their families and helps them to come to terms with the disease. People within the group can teach one another, especially if they develop a commitment. The physician or any other health educator in the group should act as the catalyst for communication reactions, not the essential communicator or the initiator of every action. The group leader should allow the group freedom to determine its course of action and how it evolves, both in the choice of subjects and in the pace at which topics are dealt with in their discussion. The group leader should ensure that all the members of the group are given ample opportunity to express themselves. When questioned by an individual member, the leader should preferably not respond immediately but should look around the group, asking: "What do you think of this?" This enables as many participants as possible to formulate their ideas, thereby maximizing the stimulation of the group's activity.

Considerable time is saved when group education is given in selected topics such as diet or complications. On the other hand, education in skills and techniques, such as insulin injections or blood testing, can be done only in an individual setting (21).

Whether talking to groups or to individuals, it is always preferable to adopt a learner-centered approach, the principle of this approach being that education is most effective when people are encouraged to look at what they are doing, learn from it, and change if necessary. This requires those involved to reflect on their current practices, which generally has the effect of motivating them to want to know more about it. Once they understand what they are doing and why, they are likely to want to know what and how to change. In this way the educator does not pose as the expert who gives lectures and tells the learner what to do, but rather as the facilitator of the learning process.

MOTIVATION

Motivation is what makes people learn what they learn and behave in the way they do. Intrinsic motivation is related to the life and personality of the individual. It is to a large extent independent of his or her diabetes and is more powerful and persistently effective. Extrinsic motivation is constituted by reward or by threat or pressure on the individual from outside and can thus easily be offered by the diabetic clinic. Such motivation is short term and ultimately less effective.

How Can We Motivate Our Patients in Self-Care in Diabetes?

If we want our patients to follow an educational course, we must make sure that they clearly understand the aim of the course and what the results of their efforts will be. It is not sufficient to tell them: "You will learn the carbohydrate content of different foods." We have to be more specific and make our suggestions attractive for the patient; for example, "You will be taught how to choose your meals when eating out, without upsetting your blood sugar control." One cannot motivate in an abstract manner but must use real situations, giving attention to details that are sometimes considered boring. Motivation is strongly dependent on the relationship of the patient to the health care team.

EVALUATION

Evaluation is the process of determining whether certain previously defined objectives have been achieved. Evaluation must be an integral part of any educational process. The easiest but not necessarily the most significant part of evaluation is knowledge assessment. The methods used are 1. interviews, using open-ended questions that encourage patients to answer in words of their own choosing; 2. multiple-choice questionnaires, filled out by the patient or with the help of an intermediary.

The advantage of multiple-choice questionnaires is that they are easy to administer and score. The disadvantages are that the questionnaires cannot reveal the discrepancies between what patients say they would do and what they actually do. Only a small percentage of patients, knowing they should carry sugar, will actually do so. Patients with a low level of literacy find it difficult to fill out such questionnaires.

In comparison to knowledge assessment, attitude assessment represents a major challenge. Interviewing is the most commonly used approach. If the interviewer is not trained, this method is likely to be incomplete or inaccurate and the results not quantifiable. Patients' attitudes can be identified in the course of a structured consultation.

Practical skills, for example, giving an insulin injection, can be evaluated only by demonstration. The patient is asked to perform key procedures while being observed by a member of the health care team.

There has been much discussion on whether we should evaluate our teaching programs only by measuring the fall of glycated hemoglobin. A drop in HbA1c values is an index of one of our main goals, namely good metabolic control. It does not evaluate the general efficacy of the teaching program, that is, the overall changes in the patient's behavior that should lead to good metabolic control and better quality of life.

CONCLUSIONS

Knowledge of what has been written in this chapter is a necessary prerequisite for effective patient education, but it is by no means enough.

Patient education started as an informational process and evolved into a motivational one. Doctors assumed the role of educators only to discover that it is more difficult to change an attitude than to administer a pill. The enthusiasm of the first pioneers was often followed by frustration. They soon discovered that educating patients is a professional job and enthusiastic amateurs are very unlikely to produce constant and lasting results. Consequently they had to ask for help from the neighboring disciplines of pedagogy and psychology. They realized that before educating the patients, they had to educate the educators.

The results reported from the DCCT (Diabetes Control Complications Trial) obligate us, more than ever, to integrate education within the global concept of diabetes care. We might then invent new ways of approaching and motivating our patients for intensive care treatment.

REFERENCES

1. Assal JP, Aufsesser-Stein M. Patient education in diabetes therapy. In: Alberti KGMM, Kroll LP, eds. *The diabetes annual/2*. Amsterdam: Elsevier, 1986: 156–68.
2. Wise PH, Dowlatshahi DC, Farrant S, *et al*. Effect of computer based learning on diabetes knowledge and control. *Diabetes Care* 1986; 9: 504–9.

3. Meadows KA, Lockington TJ, Wise PH. Assessment of knowledge of diabetes by questionnaire. *Diabetic Med* 1987; 4: 343–7.
4. Wilson W, Ary DV, Biglan A, *et al*. Psychosocial predictors of self-care behaviors and glycemic control in non-insulin-dependent diabetes mellitus. *Diabetes Care* 1986; 9: 614–6.
5. Bradley C. Psychological aspects of diabetes. In: Alberti KGMM, Kroll LP, eds. *The diabetes annual/* 1. Amsterdam: Elsevier, 1985: 374–88.
6. Simonds J, Goldstein D, Wolker B, Rawlings P. The relationship between psychological factors and blood glucose regulation in insulin-dependent diabetic adolescents. *Diabetes Care* 1981; 4: 610–5.
7. Peyrot M, McMurry JF. Psychosocial factors in diabetes control: adjustment of insulin treated adults. *Psychosom Med* 1985; 47: 542–58.
8. Skyler JS. Psychological issues in diabetes. *Diabetes Care* 1981; 4: 656–7.
9. Alogna M. Perception of severity of disease and health locus of control in compliant and non-compliant diabetic patients. *Diabetes Care* 1980; 3: 533–4.
10. Sanders K, Mills F, Martin FIR, Del Horne DJ. Emotional attitudes in adult insulin-dependent diabetics. *J Psychosom Res* 1975; 19: 241–6.
11. Bloom Certoney KA, Hart LK. The relationship between the health belief model and compliance of persons with diabetes mellitus. *Diabetes Care* 1980; 3: 594–8.
12. Ruzicki DA. Relationship of participation preference and health locus of control in diabetes education. *Diabetes Care* 1984; 7: 372–7.
13. Bradley C, Brewin C, Gamsu DS, Moses JL. Development of scales to measure perceived control of diabetes mellitus and diabetes related health beliefs. *Diabetic Med* 1984; 1: 213–8.
14. Harris R, Linn MW. Health beliefs, compliance and control of diabetes mellitus. *South Med J* 1985; 78: 162–6.
15. Gfeller R, Assal JP. The diabetics' subjective experience. In: *Folia psychopractica*. Basel: Hoffman-La-Roche, 1980.
16. Gfeller R, Assal JP. Developmental stages of patient acceptance in diabetes. Diabetes Education. In: Assal JP, Berger M, Gay N, Canivet J, eds. *Diabetes education—how to improve patient education.* Amsterdam: Exerpta Medica, 1983: 207–19.
17. Hollender M, Hollender H. *The psychology of medical practice*. Philadelphia: WB Saunders, 1958.
18. Diabetes Education Study Group. Continuing and reinforcing patient education. *The Teaching Letter.* 1988: 81–5.
19. Guilbert J.J. *Educational handbook for health personnel.* Geneva: WHO Publications 1988; 35: 1.01–1.14.
20. Alivisatos JG, Benroubi M. Education: the most important form of treatment. In: Kroll LP, ed. *World book of diabetes in practice,* vol 2. Amsterdam: Elsevier, 1985: 92–7.
21. Dimou N. Individual, group and mass medical teaching: advantages and problems. In: *A better approach to a diabetic patient.* 6th EASD European Postgraduate Course on Diabetes. Geneva: Laboratoires Servier, 1980.

Subject Index

Subject Index